In Clinical Practice

Taking a practical approach to clinical medicine, this series of smaller reference books is designed for the trainee physician, primary care physician, nurse practitioner and other general medical professionals to understand each topic covered. The coverage is comprehensive but concise and is designed to act as a primary reference tool for subjects across the field of medicine.

Coziana Ciurtin • Janine Hackett
Editors

Adolescent and Young Adult Rheumatology In Clinical Practice

Second Edition

Springer

Editors
Coziana Ciurtin
Centre for Adolescent Rheumatology, Division of Medicine
University College London
London, UK

Janine Hackett
Division of Occupational Therapy
Queen Margaret University
Edinburgh, UK

ISSN 2199-6652 ISSN 2199-6660 (electronic)
In Clinical Practice
ISBN 978-3-031-82101-1 ISBN 978-3-031-82102-8 (eBook)
https://doi.org/10.1007/978-3-031-82102-8

This Springer imprint is published by the registered company Springer Nature Switzerland AG
The registered company address is: Gewerbestrasse 11, 6330 Cham, Switzerland

We would like to dedicate this book to the young people and their families who have been an inspiration in teaching us about what it is like to grow up in today's world with a long-term rheumatic condition. Given the space to have their voice heard, we have much to learn from adolescents and young adults (AYA) in relation to delivering and designing care, setting the research agenda, and policy design. We must therefore continue to ensure that their voices remain front and centre in all matters concerning them.

AYA regularly remind us to look beyond their diagnosis and consider them as AYA first and foremost, taking time to discover their strengths, interests, priorities, and future aspirations. This can only be done if we have the skills to communicate effectively to explore their lives at home, in school, at work, or in leisure.

We hope that by providing such a handbook, professionals in both paediatric and adult settings involved in delivering care for AYA in rheumatology will be inspired and commit to delivering developmentally appropriate, holistic, and person-centred interventions that support AYA to live a life not dominated by their condition and help them achieve their life goals and future potential despite their condition.

Foreword

It is great to see the arrival of a second edition of this vital resource for all members of the multidisciplinary rheumatology teams in both paediatric and adult settings involved in the developmentally appropriate care of young people with rheumatic conditions. Rheumatology professionals may be experts in their knowledge of the latest scientific advances in rheumatology, but without the knowledge and skills to communicate with and effectively engage young people, attempts to control the underlying inflammation or manage the condition are likely to be unsuccessful. Core to adolescent and young adult (AYA) rheumatology, as this book repeatedly reveals, is understanding young people and their lives, and how rheumatic conditions impact these lives. The editors and chapter authors of this book are all passionate advocates of both young people and of developmentally appropriate healthcare in rheumatology, ensuring clinically relevant content. This book will hopefully help ensure that young people feel listened to and understood by rheumatology professionals as they grow up and learn to manage their rheumatic condition themselves.

Janet E. McDonagh

Arthritis Research UK Centre
for Epidemiology,
Centre for Musculoskeletal Research
University of Manchester
Manchester UK
NIHR Manchester Biomedical Research Centre
Manchester University NHS Foundation Trust
Manchester UK
Manchester Academic Health Science Centre
Manchester UK
janet.mcdonagh@manchester.ac.uk

Preface

The Barbara Ansell National Network for Adolescent Rheumatology (BANNAR, Barbara Ansell National Network for Adolescent Rheumatology (versusarthritis.org)) is a UK-wide network that promotes research and clinical care in adolescent and young adult (AYA) rheumatology. BANNAR has initially facilitated and funded a youth advisory panel called YOUR RHEUM (Your Rheum | Versus Arthritis).

In 2020, a partnership between BANNAR, YOUR RHEUM, and Versus Arthritis, the largest UK charity supporting people living with arthritis and other rheumatic conditions, was created. The remit of BANNAR is focused on supporting education, research, and standards of clinical healthcare in AYA rheumatology, while YOUR RHEUM advises on research from priorities and inception through study design, recruitment, completion, and dissemination.

Many of the contributors to this book are members of BANNAR, including the previous two editors, Drs. Janet McDonagh and Rachel Tattersall, who are experts in adolescent health and transitional care in rheumatology. We also co-opted new members of the YOUR RHEUM youth panel, who lent their voices to provide us with their perspective on what's important when looking after them.

The second edition of the *Adolescent and Young Adult Rheumatology in Clinical Practice* brings the first edition of this unique book up to date, by incorporating new chapters focused on the management of pregnancy and that of childhood-onset Sjögren, addressing the need for neurodiversity awareness, as well as updating existent chapters and reference lists to reflect advances in clinical practice in AYA rheumatology.

We hope to make this second edition a valuable reference source as well as a practical guide for health professionals involved in the care of AYA with rheumatic conditions.

London, UK Coziana Ciurtin
Edinburgh, UK Janine Hackett

Introduction: Young People Have Their Say

Contributors

Amy Gallagher aged 17
Lydia Gahr aged 24
Caelan Batty aged 16
Angharad Bridges aged 17
Olivia Knight aged 16
Condoliza Tagedin aged 17
Isla Robbins aged 15
Rebecca Wibberley aged 17
Andrew Gordon aged 16
Evie Sandhu aged 14

Introduction

Childhood-onset RMD are often lifelong conditions, thus requiring developmentally appropriate care that is tailored and responsive to their developmental stage (see Chaps. 1, 2, 3, 22, and 23). Building effective and trusting relationships with AYA is key if we are to understand the wider context of living with an RMD, in addition to exploring individual aspirations to learn how best to support AYA. Opportunities for involvement and coproduction in matters affecting them and opportunities to participate in research were also seen as priorities, which is consistent with previous research, stressing the need for better alignment of AYA research priorities and the research agenda [1].

In this chapter, the editors have foregrounded the voice of AYA, who generously shared their time, experiences, thoughts, and ideas.

Young People Have Their Say

We are a group of ten young people, from England, Wales, and Scotland between the ages of 14 and 24, and all living with RMD.

We wanted to work together on this chapter to provide readers with an insight into our lives. Over a period of 4 months, we met online and in-person to develop a succinct overview of our experiences. In our first meeting, we produced a word cloud of initial ideas to help get discussion started (see Fig. 1).

In this chapter, we provide a summary of both our individual and shared experiences of RMD and how it has shaped our lives. Based on our experiences, this chapter details what we think is best practice for rheumatology professionals and how services might be improved. As AYA with a chronic condition, health care professionals (HCP) are a massive part of our lives for better or for worse. While we may only be 30 minutes of your day, you are a key part of our formative years. Your work has a lasting effect on

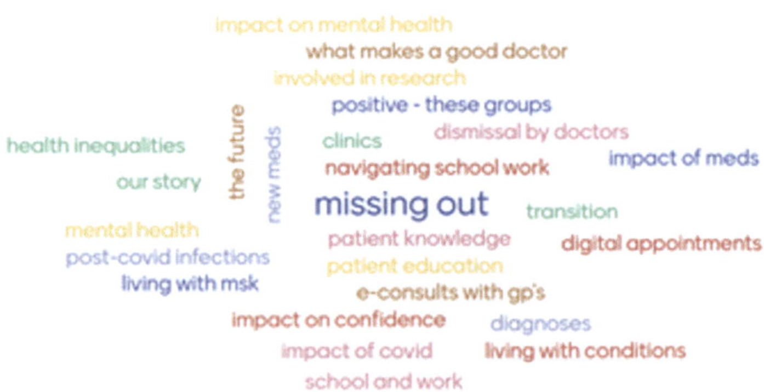

Fig. 1 Word cloud of our group key themes for this chapter

our lives, and we want everyone's experience of rheumatology care to be as positive as possible.

We have therefore created the following chapter, which focuses on key issues affecting our lives, and how you as a HCP can best help us. We start by focussing on how rheumatic illnesses can impact on our mental health, school, work, the unpredictability of our future, along with our experiences of medication and how communication between healthcare professionals could be improved. We then go on to outline the benefit of charities and finally finish with involvement in research and service development.

What It Is Like Living with RMD

This section aims to provide health professionals with a glimpse into what it is like to live with RMD and the impact this has on our health, well-being, participation, and quality of life.

Impact on Mental Health and Confidence

Having a disability or being diagnosed with a long-term medical condition is difficult for anyone, but particularly hard as a young person, and with this comes a 'mourning period'. RMD can take a huge toll on mental health and can affect all aspects of our life, including school, work, plans for the future, and ultimately how our life will turn out. As AYA living with this permanent, life-altering condition, we are at the stage of where we are figuring out our life, and we have this additional stress, pain, and feelings of isolation to deal with. The idea of the future can become overwhelming particularly when there is no certainty in our life or in our condition.

Receiving a diagnosis, which may not always be immediate, and the subsequent period in adjusting to the 'new normal' is stressful for us and can affect us in more ways than one. As young people with RMD, we feel we could be helped considerably if we are provided with access to psychological support. The importance of training, however, is key, and one young person in the group described the benefit of having a psychologist trained and experienced in RMD who was able to provide support for mental health issues specifically related to their RMD condition. For others, this was problematic as they felt they had to spend the majority of the session explaining the illness, rather than address the specific issue encountered. Whilst not all hospitals may be able to offer this service, it would be a significant help for psychologists to be part of the rheumatology team and be accessible during clinic appointments.

HCP need to recognise that in addition to physical symptoms, RMD conditions affect all aspects of our mental health (see Chaps. 2 and 3). A common experience within the group was a loss of confidence and loss of enjoyment in things we loved pre-diagnosis. Many members were previously part of sport clubs, enjoying activities such as karate, cricket, ice skating, and badminton; however, they had to give this up, either temporarily or permanently because of their condition and the physical pain of these sports. While we are advised there are lots of other, less active hobbies to join, it needs to be recognised that it is a struggle to give up our passion because of physical pain that is out of our control. We not only miss out on the activity but also seeing our friends and feeling a sense of belonging to that social group. Help is needed to suggest modifications to sustain our valued activities.

Impact on School Life

School life can also be hugely affected by the different aspects of our RMD condition. Importantly, there's a lack of understanding from teachers and peers alike, poor awareness that our condition is serious and that we shouldn't be made fun of or excluded from lessons, activities, or trips due to sickness and pain.

The important message here is that a high level of communication is required between our rheumatology teams and the schools we attend, so that support can be given for easier access around the school building, adaptations to lessons, and access to accommodations in exams. These might be permanent recommendations or only during times of flares, medication changes, or other procedures that require us to need extra support. Support might include breaks from lessons such as physical exercise (PE), drama, dance, etc., but it is important to ask us what our specific challenges are so that recommendations can be suggested. Contact between HCP and school staff could make a huge difference to our school lives and ensure we get the support we need and promote a more positive school experience. This is particularly important for those of us who are neurodivergent, who may find it difficult to communicate and advocate for ourselves, especially when already feeling overwhelmed. At times, it may also be hard for us to recognise if we are reluctant to go to school/college because of pain, or because we are feeling socially anxious. Getting the right level of support tailored to our individual needs will enable us to better cope physically and emotionally and enable us to participate in activities with friends and to improve our academic results and achievements.

Effective communication about school life during appointments would help us to feel listened to and believed. Prioritising conversations on topics such as asking us about our hopes for the future and possible careers plan could help guide us on which subjects to study. Similar conversations could also help some of us that are older students, with support to develop revision and exam strategies to help us cope with the effects of medications and flare ups. Whilst general exam advice we get from school would work for some people, those with RMD coping with medication side effects or dealing with certain pain need tailored support.

Impact on Work

It is important to recognise that AYA may be more negative about their condition compared to their rheumatologist. This is because it can feel like there's no light at the end of the tunnel. More encouragement about the future from HCP could make a huge difference on whether we choose to follow our dreams or not. We may not know what we can be physically capable of, which could lead us to limiting and excluding ourselves from potential career opportunities, or conversely, put us at risk of unnecessarily pain and deterioration of our condition by being too ambitious. Discussing our future plans and offering advice on different career paths could be very valuable when we're at a stage of considering our future.

Transitioning out of education and into the workforce should be an exciting part of any young person's life; however, for AYA with RMD, this often comes with heaps of worry and uncertainty. Finding jobs that are physically suitable for us is difficult, especially when we have to factor in the physical and mental requirements of the job, and whether the job is flexible enough to allow for hybrid working to accommodate fatigue or a flare. For those of us who are neurodivergent, these challenges can also be increased, and the combination of uncertainty of the work environment and the mental and physical fatigue can be highly overwhelming and can sometimes be a barrier to potential jobs and volunteering experiences.

During the clinic, having access to information about employment rights and legislation related to long-term health conditions, including how to make requests to employers for reasonable adjustments, becomes important and could make a big impact on the quality of our work life.

Unpredictability of the Future

In addition to education and work, the uncertainty and unpredictability that come with living with an RMD condition also affect other aspects of our lives. A standard part of our daily life involves figuring out alternatives and backup plans for every little thing we want to do in case things don't work out. This could be due to a flare of arthritis, fatigue, medication, or side effects. Anything we plan, whether it is a trip to the cinema, changing careers, or starting a family, all has to have a Plan B in case it doesn't work out.

Our social lives are heavily impacted by the unpredictability of our condition, which might mean missing out on social events due to flare and plans being ruined. Additionally, the side effects from medication, such as methotrexate, mean that there are days when we can't go out at all and don't have enough energy, and we often have to choose between having a social life or being able to study/work to the level required. Additionally, we can sometimes feel trapped due to the restrictions of our condition or feel we need to do lots of extra preparation. For example, before we travel, we must think about the practicality of bringing medication that may be temperature controlled, along with accessories such as sharps bins. The concern about unpredictability is prominent in our minds when travelling, because you need to plan for what happens if you get ill or have a flare when abroad and don't have access to the same health care, which could delay your progression and treatment.

The unpredictable nature of RMD can be terrifying for most people, let alone those with neurodiversity, who struggle with change and surprises. How our condition is going to improve or worsen over a single day, let alone a lifetime, is often foremost in our thoughts. We worry that as we get older, our condition could continue to get worse. This uncertainty extends to treatment plans, which may be unpredictable, with concerns about whether we'll be on or off certain medications and how this might affect other aspects of our lives and significant life milestones. When discussing treatment plans and other plans for the future, it is important that HCP explore our feelings and keep in mind how scared and worried we are about our futures and do their best to provide reassurance and support.

Impacts of Medication Regimes

From the AYA perspective, we feel there are lots of aspects to taking medications that are often left seemingly unconsidered by the rheumatology team. For many of us, the belief that medication will give us relief from pain and other effects of our conditions often means we take medication without a second thought, as the good typically outweighs the bad. However, there are many issues in relation to the impact of medication on our lives that we would like to highlight. Firstly, medications such as methotrexate are often the first to be prescribed due to their effectiveness; however, the side effects are often an annoyance to us as the sickness can cause us to miss out on school attendance and other social activities. Other side effects also mean taking additional medications to prevent our bodies from damage, which can often be scary.

Secondly, problems associated with storage of medication can also have a huge impact on us and those around us. Storage of medicines requiring refrigeration often means storing it in family fridges and other items such as sharps bins, and boxes of tablets can take up a lot of space within the home. This can sometimes feel like our homes are mini hospitals, which serves as a constant reminder of our RMD and a visible sign to our family and anyone who visits.

Another common experience is fear of needles, so helping us overcome this would be helpful. In addition, another issue we struggle with is the usability of some medicines, for example, injection devices are not designed to allow young people to use these independently. This can often cause increased levels of stress and anxiety for the whole day, due to the worry of taking medication later in the evening when someone else is available to help. Relying on a parent for help can sometimes make us feel like a burden to those around us and take away our sense of freedom and responsibility, which is the opposite of what we are trying to achieve.

The Modernisation of Medical Treatment

A positive take away from the recent pandemic was the capacity to adapt and modernise medical treatment. As face-to-face appointments became restricted, digital alternatives were offered, which were of benefit to both patient and HCP. We support the continued development of the use of technology for improved delivery of services as it offers a convenient alternative. For those of us with RMD, fatigue is a significant problem and may often be magnified for those of us who are also neurodiverse. Many of us find it difficult to attend appointments, especially if we are required to miss school or work and worry that this puts us at a further educational disadvantage.

HCP are asked to keep in mind that while their own appointment might be brief, it can take hours of our day to see you. Firstly, we need to arrange for time off for the appointment, travel to and from the hospital, and wait in the waiting room before even seeing the doctor, as well as wait for additional results or to see other health professionals post clinic. We then need to make up for lost time at school or work, possibly putting us behind and further disadvantaged.

The use of alternative methods of contact such as video calls, emails, or other online communication increases patient choice and access to medical support, which potentially could be more responsive to the condition we live with. Some of us have benefitted from video calls, which we feel work just as well as physical appointments and are ideal for check-ins. These are more useful than phone calls as they save time and allow for more face-to-face discussion. That said, more consideration may need to be given for neurodiverse AYA, who may find online and phone appointments more challenging due to finding it harder to read people's faces and understand tone of voice, underscoring the need for appointment type to be matched to individual need.

Often contact details are provided to a parent, but providing AYA with a small business card with rheumatology contact information was thought to be useful and potentially make a huge difference, as there was less likelihood of losing or misplacing vital contact information and would encourage independence and direct control over our own condition.

If virtual appointments are not possible, or when an AYA is required to be seen within a clinic, a quiet and uncrowded waiting area would be welcomed, as loud and crowded environments can be stressful and overwhelming particularly for those of us that are neurodiverse. Loud and busy waiting rooms can often cause anxiety and exhaust us before we have entered the clinic room. This can often affect the rest of the visit and influence how consultation will go. We may struggle to express what we originally wanted to, leading to an unsatisfactory experience for all. For all AYA, the uncertainty of who they might see in the clinic was also a source of stress, so ideally consistency or a named doctor can help.

One member of our group outlined another great service, which allowed her to call or email her queries to a general secretary account. This meant that she could contact the team at her own convenience, avoiding the need to wait on hold, and also allowing the doctors time to provide a more considered response via email rather than on the spot. This type of innovation is welcomed.

Investment in technology and the development of alternative methods of communication is key, as this allows us to get in contact with our rheumatology team quicker, allows us to access advice, but also helps us feel less isolated and less worried about our current medical state and treatment progression.

Importance of Good Communication and Effective Education

As we progress from children's clinics to adolescent ones and become more responsible for our health and treatment, we are aware we need to develop our understanding of RMD and our communication skills. This may also be a development need for health professionals. To aid effective communication and help us feel confident and included in our appointment, we suggest a few key strategies that would greatly benefit us.

These include:

Use of simple terminology Simple terminology will help us to better understand what's being said in relation to our condition and treatment plan and help us make better decisions. Care should be taken to ensure that simple language is not condescending or makes us feel stupid for asking questions.

Communication systems Self-rating assessment forms can sometimes be challenging, and we may need support to express our levels of pain or emotions in different ways beyond rating scales. For those of us who are neurodiverse, we can find that these scales don't always work. We may not know or be able to express our feelings as they are often fluid and seldom remain constant. When asked about our physical symptoms, we can struggle to remember or communicate how severe the pain has been since the last appointment. A more helpful way for us to express our symptoms may be to keep a record on a tracker style app or diary.

Be realistic without being blunt Aim to use language that is supportive and conveys empathy. Avoid minimising our experiences and take care to avoid paying unnecessary attention to areas that we might be self-conscious or feel awkward about. This will allow us to fully grasp the concepts being explained and allow us to make the best decisions without feeling anxious or under pressure from those around us.

Communicate key treatment goals Include us in goal setting and help us to understand why we are taking a particular medicine or doing something to achieve a goal, rather than just telling us to do it. Share the benefits of the treatment, setting short- and long-term goals and let us know how we're doing, as this can be motivating, and increase engagement with exercises and medication. Outline the side effects we might face, as this will help us to distinguish them from condition-related or other symptoms and also reduce stress and worry.

Speak to us not over us If we have the skills to lead our appointments, don't ignore us and speak to our parents. Speak directly to us, as we know our own bodies and can usually tell you a lot more than they can.

Listen when we say something isn't working If we suggest or ask for a change in our treatment plan, please listen and consider our point of view. Even if you disagree, work with us, and help us to understand why it may not be ideal and include us in creating a new plan that can work better. Look out for signs that we may be struggling with treatment and offer support, referring us to other services, which can help us overcome the issues that may affect us

Educate us in the early stages of our diagnosis and throughout our treatment Rather than throw leaflets and books at us, take time to sit and talk through what it means, what our options are, and what support systems are available. This can create a better prospect for us rather than us feeling fearful and anxious after the clinic appointment and wondering what might lie ahead in the coming weeks and months. Remember to revisit conversations as we get older to make sure we fully grasp important information about our condition, the treatment options, and what it means for us as we grow up and become more independent.

Engage us and listen to us It is important to include us in anything that affects us, so remember to give us opportunities to participate, so we can share our thoughts and you can hear our voice. This might be about how services can be improved, or you could include us in interview processes for new members of your team. It is also important to allow us to be involved in research, and we will go on to discuss this more in the next section.

Research

Being aware of, and being involved in, research is important, as it means that AYA know their condition is important, and that researchers are being proactive in working to improve our lives, which gives us hope and a much more positive outlook on life. The UK-based AYA research advisory group, 'Your Rheum', affords young people with an excellent opportunity to be part of an advisory group that offers thoughts, opinions, and advice to researchers. Not only does the group benefit researchers by providing them with unique insights, but it also benefits us as AYA and allows us to discover more about our condition, hot topics, and current research. Another benefit of the group is the opportunity to meet similar others and feel part of a small community sharing similar experiences, which can be empowering.

It's important when offering opportunities to be involved in group activities, however, to be mindful of the potential barriers to participation. For example, do we need to travel? Is it funded? Is it on the weekend (outside school time)? Is there a genuine benefit to the AYA and is there an opportunity to join remotely? Virtual participation through Zoom or Teams can reach a wider group of participants by being more accessible and time-saving, eliminating travel-associated barriers. Additionally, it would be ideal to ensure an inclusive and diverse representation within these groups and would be encouraging for underrepresented groups to see others like themselves included and participate in research studies that may lead to them being involved in more research, leading to better quality of research.

AYA are interested in participating in a range of activities that relate to their experience of RMD and are also keen to meet similar others. It is exciting for us to be able to see research about young people living with RMD. We just need assistance in finding out about research and other opportunities that we can join.

Access to Charity Support

Charities provide an indescribable amount of support to AYA and their families, and signposting to support groups charities, particularly at the early stages of diagnosis can be very reassuring and help us feel less alone. They also help our families better manage the effects of living with RMD and offer support, which reflects the changing nature of the condition throughout our life. From our experience, being signposted to charity and local support groups early is most useful around 6 months after diagnosis, as this allows some time to understand and come to terms with the diagnosis.

Some charities offer social activities that allow AYA to connect with similar others and encourage us to step outside our comfort zones and try new activities that we may not have previously had access to, due to the nature of our condition. This can feel daunting, and we may need encouragement and support to reach out to a charity and join activities. This may be especially challenging for some of us who are neurodiverse, as we can find it difficult to ask for help or have little confidence to make contact. Charity events and the connections we can make can have a positive effect on our mental health: we can feel included. The support from meeting other young people like us provides a huge confidence boost and allows us to push ourselves further than we thought possible, physically and mentally.

You can find information about charities working locally in your area by searching the following international website www.encanetwork.org/members.

Summary

We thank you for taking the time to read our chapter, which we hope highlights some of the key issues we face as AYA living with RMD. We hope this has helped you gain a greater understanding of our perspectives and experiences which will help you in your day-to-day work and allow you to consider where practice might be improved.

Table 1 provides a summary and quick reference point for how you can help improve healthcare for all young people in the future.

Table 1 Summary recommendations for the rheumatology multidisciplinary team

Areas to include in your assessments	Recommendations
Holistic assessment with review of mental health	Listen to us as AYA Encourage and support us Consider wider impacts on our life, including our social life Make psychological support accessible Signpost us to communities and charities
School life	Communicate our needs, outline our medical needs, and recommend adjustments to schools Advocate for us
Work and future work life	Help us plan for our future Help with progression to work Outline and signpost us to information about our work rights Work with occupational therapists, who can recommend reasonable adjustments and liaise with employers
Future focussed patient education	Be honest and open about the future and what might happen Encourage us about future possibilities as we will likely have a more pessimistic outlook Discuss future possibilities and be honest about any limitations Discuss family planning

(continued)

Table 1 (continued)

Areas to include in your assessments	Recommendations
Medication	Explain reasoning for choice of medication and offer alternative medication plans and/or allow negotiation Outline possible side effects Recognise the presence of side effects and acknowledge the wider impacts of medication (social life and mental health) Increase accessibility for making changes to medication Make travel support documents easily available and have a clear and timely process for provision
Young person friendly communication	Be patient and allow time for us to think and respond Present ideas/information to us in ways that are clear and understandable Be sensitive and be mindful of how young people could react to comments/information or communication style Review feedback/rating forms with us to check accuracy and consider our feelings
Involve us in research and other activities	Encourage and create opportunity for involvement as much as possible Involve us in research as this is positive and can help us be more active in our treatment Include us in any service development that involves us Use posters in clinic and social media to promote/signpost opportunities to get involved Support us and ensure there are no barriers that might prevent involvement
Signpost to charities	Be aware of charitable organisations that can provide support and signpost us to these Encourage us to get involved and meet others

Reference

1. Parsons S, Thomson W, Cresswell K, Starling B, McDonagh JE. What do young people with rheumatic disease believe to be important to research about their condition? A UK-wide study. Pediatr Rheumatol. 2017;15:53. https://doi.org/10.1186/s12969-017-0181-1

Scotland, UK — Lydia Gahr
Birmingham, UK — Amy Gallagher
Birmingham Women and Children's NHS Foundation Trust, Birmingham, UK — Claire Pidgeon
Pilkington Versus Arthritis, Birmingham, UK — Dawn Bovey-Pilkington

Contents

Part I

Implications of AYA Development to Clinical Practice

1 Impact of Rheumatic Musculoskeletal Conditions on Biological and Neurocognitive Development of Adolescents and Young Adults

Damien McKay and Katherine Steinbeck

Introduction

Puberty is the profound physical event during adolescence—the second decade of life. There are dramatic changes in height, weight and body composition, bone mass and reproductive capacity. Chronic physical illness may have an impact on puberty growth and development dependent on severity, inflammatory status, remission and exacerbation patterns, and medication prescribed for the chronic illness. RMD in adolescents and young

D. McKay
Department of Rheumatology, Liverpool Hospital,
Liverpool, NSW, Australia
e-mail: damien.mckay@health.nsw.gov.au

K. Steinbeck (✉)
Faculty of Medicine and Health, The University of Sydney,
Sydney, Australia
e-mail: katherine.steinbeck@sydney.edu.au

C. Ciurtin, J. Hackett (eds.), *Adolescent and Young Adult Rheumatology In Clinical Practice*, In Clinical Practice,
https://doi.org/10.1007/978-3-031-82102-8_1

adults (AYA) is no exception [1], but with the increasing use of biological disease modifying anti-rheumatic drugs (bDMARDS) the impact patterns are changing for the better.

Normal Growth at Puberty

Growth during puberty is characterised by significant linear growth, increased weight and changes in body composition under the influence of the gonadal hormones testosterone and oestradiol (see below), and growth hormone (GH) and insulin-like growth factor-1 (IGF-1) [2]. Body composition changes occur in lean mass (muscle, organs and bone) and fat mass proportions [3] with clear sex differences. Body fat distribution patterns also change. Females predominantly deposit fat at breast, hip and thigh locations. Males tend to deposit deep visceral fat that is more metabolically active and in excess predisposes to cardiovascular disease. The gonadal hormones enhance the stimulation of growth hormone from the anterior pituitary, which acts synergistically with these hormones to promote the pubertal height growth spurt. Growth hormone activity is expressed by the generation of growth factors, IGF-1 from the liver and a variety of growth factors produced at local tissue level. The growth spurt in females occurs in early puberty and in late puberty in males. For both sexes, height growth is halted by closure of the epiphyses or the growth plate of bone. Normal pubertal growth results in 15–20 cm and kilogram gains in females, and 25–30 cm and kilogram gains in males. Gonadal hormones have a major role in the acquisition of bone mass during adolescence and *into* the third decade where bone mass peaks (see Chap. 17).

Normal Secondary Sexual Development at Puberty

Pubertal onset is signaled by a rise above childhood testosterone and oestradiol levels, which are primarily responsible for secondary sexual development. This is clinically detected by an increase in testicular volume above 3mls in males, and the appearance of the breast bud in females. The hormone production pathways and organs necessary for puberty are present at birth. The neurons responsible for the production of gonadotropin releasing hormone (GnRH) migrate in utero to the hypothalamus, where their activity is kept in check by peptides from the arcuate nucleus, including MKRN3 and dynorphin [4]. This brake will ultimately be lifted with increasing production of kisspeptin and neurokinin B peptides allowing the initiation of puberty [4]. GnRH stimulates the pituitary in both sexes to produce luteinising hormone (LH) and follicle stimulating hormone (FSH). In males LH stimulates Leydig cell production of testosterone in the testes and FSH is responsible for the development of sperm forming tissue which makes up the main volume of the testes. In females FSH is responsible for the stimulation of oestradiol production from the ovarian follicles. LH is responsible for triggering ovulation under the positive feedback of rising oestradiol levels, and the production of progesterone and androgens, including testosterone, from the ovarian stroma.

Puberty typically commences between the ages of 8 and 13 in females and 9 and 14 in males and is considered delayed if there is no sign of physical puberty at 13 or 14 years in females and males respectively [5]. Menarche is considered delayed if not present by 15 years.

Growth and Pubertal Delay in Chronic RMD

Delayed onset and progress of puberty occurs in AYAs living with chronic rheumatic musculoskeletal disease (RMD), together with growth failure [6]. Delay in and progress through puberty are closely related to illness severity, and to therapy adherence. Despite newer therapies 10–20% of patients exhibit growth delay. In chronic RMD the aetiology of these states may be complex and multifactorial, with chronic inflammatory cytokines affecting both GH effect [7] and central appetite control through an anorectic effect, and inflammation may be exacerbated by failure to adhere to treatment regimens (see Chap. 21).

Low body weight may inhibit the onset of pubertal gonadotropin release in both sexes. Low body weight may be due to inadequate nutrition, especially protein, required to accommodate the major increase in height and weight during the pubertal spurt. Inadequate nutrition may be exacerbated by oral or gastrointestinal involvement that impairs intake, co-existent inflammatory bowel disease and malabsorption, and the development of disordered eating patterns or food aversions as part of a complex psychosocial response to chronic illness. In older adolescents or young adults, the positive response of others to lean and slight builds may promote unhealthy restrictive eating practices in females [8]. In males the use of supplements and non-prescribed anabolic steroids to enhance muscle mass may be a result of perceived or real inadequate muscle bulk [9].

The pattern of growth disturbance due to active disease in Juvenile Idiopathic Arthritis (JIA) can be localised or systemic and varies with disease subtype. Inflammatory cytokines act directly on growth cartilage causing premature fusion of the epiphyses. TNF–α inhibits *local* growth through its influence on growth plate chondrocyte dynamics/apoptosis [6], resulting in limb or digit length discrepancy, or micrognathia. Micrognathia may become apparent with rapid pubertal growth and affect self-image (see Chap. 2). Severe polyarticular or systemic JIA is associated with *generalized* growth impairment due to GH and IGF-1 resistance/insufficiency, together with IGF-1 binding protein abnormalities [10]. High levels of IL-1β result in general growth retardation through accelerated degradation of IGF-1 and development of phosphorylated IGF-binding protein (IGFBP1), which prevents IGF binding to its receptor, as well as alteration of growth hormone secretion. Effective control of inflammation with TNF-α antagonist therapy or IL-6 inhibition [11] together with adequate nutrition, especially protein, results in catch up growth and normalisation of IGF- 1 levels.

In the previous addition data on the efficacy of bDMARDs were promising [12, 13]. The data are considerably strengthened in later studies with clear improvements in catch-up growth, pain related disability and health related quality of life [6, 14, 15].

Endogenous and exogenous growth hormones remain relatively inactive, even if inflammation is controlled, if protein calorie malnutrition and/or supraphysiological glucocorticoid doses are present. These same scenarios reduce normal hypothalamic/pituitary production of GnRH/gonadotropins with a consequent reduction in oestradiol and testosterone production. This situation causes delay in or failure to progress in pubertal development in younger adolescents, together with a reduced peak height growth spurt. The induction or maintenance of puberty in these situations should be assessed and managed by an endocrinologist.

In adolescents and young adults this functional (reversible) hypogonadism also results in failure to optimize bone mass or loss of bone mass. A reduction in energy and wellbeing may occur with reduction in gonadal hormones and be falsely attributed to the disease process alone. In females, oligo- or amenorrhoea (infrequent or absent periods) and in males, loss of muscle strength and reduced libido are common effects of low gonadal hormones. Young males are unlikely to volunteer symptoms of erectile dysfunction. Replacement of gonadal hormones under the supervision of an endocrinologist may treat some of these issues but again will not improve bone mass unless accompanied by adequate nutritional intake and other supportive therapy for bone health [16].

Glucocorticoids still have a role as conventional therapeutic agents in RMD and have other profound effects than on health and wellbeing [17]. Gonadal hormone production is reduced through suppression of GnRH and LH and FSH production, and in young adults contributes to infertility. Glucocorticoids induce metabolic disturbances in glucose and fat metabolism with subsequent insulin resistance. It should be noted that normal growth hormone production during normal puberty produces transient insulin resistance which does not generally impair glucose metabolism [18]. Obesity, a family history of Type 2 diabetes and high dose GH therapy may all contribute to glucose dysmetabolism [19], and monitoring of both glucose and HbA1c levels should be considered. This importance of steroid sparing regimens using more targeted pharmacotherapies is clear progress, but in many countries access to more modern targeted approaches may be limited or absent, unlike low-cost glucocorticoids.

Non-rheumatic musculoskeletal conditions may be influenced by normal growth and maturation during adolescence. The increase in height velocity associated with early to mid-puberty appears to increase the risk of progression of spondylolisthesis [20]. Despite such specific examples of the influence of growth on non-rheumatic MSK disease the current evidence is at high risk of bias and impedes the ability to establish whether biological maturity and growth are independent risk factors for musculoskeletal conditions.

Sexual and Reproductive Health

AYAs living with RMD and their parents are keen to obtain specific sexual health information, but it may be hard for them to raise this, and clinicians may feel unprepared to discuss. Starting early with general questions is useful and this section provides information that can be a useful starting point. As with *all* young people, safe sex practices should be advocated such as condoms to avoid sexually transmitted infections and the importance of consent in sexual encounters. Especially consider where gender neutral language may be helpful as adolescent development includes the development of sexual identity. Such conversations indicate to the young person that the clinician is comfortable talking about sexuality and gender. A high percentage of unplanned pregnancies is present in the general AYA population and conversation around contraception and pregnancy planning should start early for all patients.

AYA Females with RMD

A regular, ovulatory menstrual cycle reflects overall wellness and adequate disease control. A high prevalence of menstrual disturbance is reported, varying from irregular menses and prolonged long cycle length to post-menarche amenorrhoea [13]. Periods may be present but not necessarily ovulatory if oestradiol levels fail to rise to the levels that trigger positive feedback to initiate the pre-ovulatory LH surge. This situation is often seen with falling or persistent low body weight. The use of NSAIDs impairs ovulation through inhibition of COX-2 which is the rate limiting step for prostaglandin formation. This inhibition is thought to cause luteinised unruptured follicle (LUF) syndrome, which may not be detected on routine endocrinology testing [21]. There is no published evidence of catamenial (peri-menstrual) exacerbation of disease effects in AYAs with RMD.

What is clear is that AYAs with RMD are keen to learn about sexual health and wellbeing while still in paediatric services but that this need is largely unmet [22, 23]. This means that their clinicians need knowledge and confidence to commence these conversations (see Chap. 19).

Contraception

Young women with chronic RMD need to understand their contraceptive options. The combined oral contraceptive pill (COCP) generally contains both synthetic oestrogen and progestogen compounds. COCPs increase the risk of venous thromboembolic phenomena (VTE) [24]. The COCP is absolutely contraindicated with a personal history of VTE or migraine with aura and/or paralysis and should not be used in AYAs with anti-phospholipid antibodies or other syndromes associated with chronic RMD that increase VTE risk. Long-acting reversible contraceptive agents (LARCs), either the subcutaneous rod or the intra-uterine system (IUS), contain progestogen. These are an important options where the COCP is contraindicated and more generally as no active therapy adherence is required [25]. Unlike the older intramuscular depot medroxyprogesterone acetate [26] the rod does not appear to impair bone formation. IUS acts locally and can be used in nulliparous females.

Fertility

Maximum ovarian follicle number is present at birth and follicles are primarily lost through apoptosis over the reproductive life span, rather than through ovulation. Anti-Mullerian hormone

(AMH) is secreted by the granulosa cells of the ovary and AMH levels in plasma are a marker of ovarian reserve and are relatively stable throughout the menstrual cycle [27] making it useful as a clinical indicator of reserve. A recent study has shown that ovarian reserves in AYAs on bDMARDs and/or methotrexate are similar to healthy controls [28], which is at odds with earlier literature in broader age groups. Low AMH levels require expert opinion around fertility preservation. Methotrexate is a known teratogen associated with an increased risk of major birth defects and spontaneous abortion at dosages used in treatment of RMD. As with any teratogenic drug, AYAs should be aware of this fact well before pregnancy is considered and discussed when reviewing contraception needs [29]. NSAIDs induced LUF should be considered in discussions around fertility, [21]. Data on safety in pregnancy for bDMARDs are limited with most sources calling for larger trials, but with initial data promising [30]. Prescribers should be aware of local advisory for their use. There is early evidence that these newer biological therapies may have a negative impact on decisions about pregnancy and breast- feeding for young women [31].

Sexual and Reproductive Health in AYA Males with RMD

Male sexual and reproductive health has received less attention than females, which may reflect the lower prevalence of chronic RMD and potentially lower ascertainment of partial hypogonadal states. These states, together with physical limitations of their condition may influence libido and sexual performance and directed history taking is important (See Chaps. 2 and 4). Methotrexate has received the most attention in the literature. With respect to male fertility, it is safe generally but may have a temporary impact on fertility with no impact on pregnancy outcomes [32]. The general instruction is to cease methotrexate for 3 months, considering the 90-day cycle of spermatogenesis, before attempting conception due to its general cytotoxic effect. At the time of writing there were no published data on the impact of bDMARDS on fertility. AYA males should be counselled about safe sex practices and offered specific consultation around fertility preservation where relevant.

Normal Brain Development in Adolescents and Young Adults

The dramatic brain development in AYA is second only to that in early childhood. This development parallels changes in brain structure and function which in turn are thought to underpin the characteristic behaviours of AYA (Fig. 1.1). The exact relationships and mediators between imaging data and the behaviours and the acquisition of skills that describe AYA neurocognitive maturation are still being elucidated [33]. These developmental changes begin in early adolescence and are not complete until after the second decade of life. In early adolescence there is a rapid increase in synapse formation. This is followed by synaptic pruning and increased long tract myelination in later adolescence and

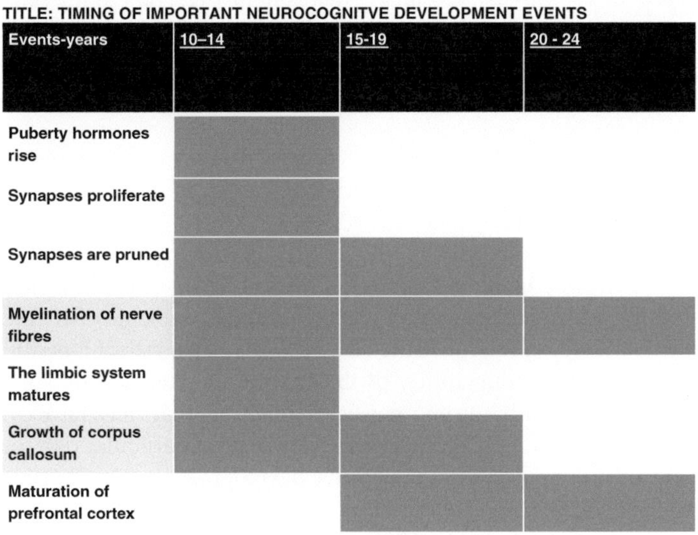

Fig. 1.1 Compiled from the literature by K Steinbeck

beyond. The overall result of this maturation is more efficient and effective neural pathways [34, 35]. The prefrontal cortex is the last area of the brain to develop, and by its functions modulates the emotional centres of the brain which mature earlier. The major prefrontal cortex function is an executive role, which includes abstract and long-term reasoning, decision making and assessment of risk. Risk taking and impulsivity are characteristic of mid to late adolescence. These should not always be perceived as negative, as taking some risks has positive influences on development of autonomy and independence. Risk taking is contributed to by adolescent hyper-emotionality and sensation seeking driven by other brain areas, including the amygdala and hippocampus [36]. There are other moderators of risk behaviours in adolescents, and these include performance based incentives and social context such as the presence or absence of peers, as well as inherent impulsivity [37]. Cortical maturation may also be affected by adverse childhood events, substance misuse and brain trauma [33]. Forward planning ability and an understanding of consequences relate to cognitive functions not fully developed until adulthood and are an aspect of cognitive development that is highly relevant to the self-management of chronic illness (see Chap. 20). The evidence base for the impact of puberty hormones on non-sexual behaviour is still being developed [33] and may be less than is assumed [38].

The Impact of RMD on Neurocognitive Development

The critical cognitive maturation period from late childhood through adolescence and into young adulthood coincides with the paediatric age spike for JSLE onset and may also reflect a period of exceptional vulnerability of the central nervous system. As a result, AYAs with chronic physical conditons that may have an impact on normal physiological functions are at particular risk for delays and impairments in cognitive development especially processing speed, response inhibition and working memory. The literature on neurocognition in AYAs with RMD is limited. There are potential temporary effects on neurocognitive function because of systemic inflammation in acute exacerbations of SLE [39], or with high dose glucocorticoid use. The possibility of sleep disturbance (see below) and its potential effects on behaviour and cognitive performance has been proposed, but to date has not been investigated further in AYAs with RMD.

Sleep in AYAs

Sleep deficit is a potentially modifiable risk factor in AYA health and wellbeing. Delayed sleep onset is a recognised normal developmental phenomenon of mid adolescence [40]. This delay is maximal in later pubertal stages and may reflect brain development, rather than a direct gonadal hormone effect. Adolescents want to go to sleep later and wake up later. This pattern does not fit with school or work hours, and adolescents tend to oversleep on weekends to make up their sleep deficit. In young adults, sleep deprivation is more likely due to exogenous factors including study and social activities. Sleep is essential to health and wellbeing as sleep deprivation lowers mood, increases impulsivity and unintentional injury, and has a negative impact on academic performance. In children with JIA causal relationships have been confirmed between reduced sleep and increased pain [41].

A sleep history should always be taken in AYAs with chronic inflammatory joint disease, as they will have additional risks for poor sleep hygiene: increased depression and anxiety (more common in chronic illness), inadequately treated pain, sleep disordered breathing due to malformation of upper airways, and glucocorticoid induced insomnia [42]. Also consider risk factors for poor sleep common to all AYAs, such as use of caffeine (including energy drinks) and small screen use.

Conclusion

RMD has different incidence, prevalence, and clinical phenotypes during adolescence. The influence of RMD and its treatment on physical, sexual, social, and neurocognitive development can be profound and should be considered and addressed. Developmental milestone assessment of AYAs over time is central to the initial assessment and ongoing management of young people presenting with RMD, given the number of potential interrupters detailed in this chapter.

The presence of any chronic condition may have an impact on the attainment of normal adolescent developmental milestones. Delayed pubertal development and growth can cause significant concern for both adolescents and their parents. Timely assessment and specialist referral where necessary is important to ensure windows of opportunity to treat pubertal delay and growth failure do not close, and that any psychosocial impact is minimised. Timing of normal adolescent neurocognitive development influences self-management of and attitudes to chronic illness. Parents must come to terms with their changing role, and support AYAs' transition to healthy and functional adulthood, including to adult health care, tertiary education, employment and romantic relationships.

Key Management Points

1. The dramatic biological and neurocognitive developments in AYAs have an impact on RMD management.
2. Age does not always reflect developmental stage.
3. Delayed pubertal development and partial hypogonadal states should be addressed. Close monitoring of growth and maturation is important in managing both the physical and psychosocial effects of chronic RMD.
4. There is limited knowledge on how chronic inflammatory processes impact on normal neurocognitive development. Further research is warranted in this area.

References

1. Simon D, Fernando C, Czernichow P, Prieur AM. Linear growth and final height in patients with systemic juvenile, idiopathic arthritis treated with long-term glucocorticoids. J Rheumatol. 2002;29:1296–300.

2. Bamba V, Kelly A. Assessment of growth. In: Kliegman RM, St Geme JW, Blum NJ, Shah SS, Tasker RC, Wilspn KM, Schor NF, editors. Nelson textbook of pediatrics E-book. Philedelphia: Elsevier; 2020. p. p151–7.
3. Biro FN, Kiess W. Contemporary trends in onset and completion of puberty, gain in height and adiposity. Endocr Dev. 2016;29:122–33.
4. Witchel SF, Plant TM. Neurobiology of puberty and its disorders. Handb Clin Neurobiol. 2021;181:463–96.
5. Faienza MF, Urbano F, Moscogiuri LA, Chiarito M, De Santis S, Giordano. Genetic, epigenetic and environmental influencing factors on the regulation of precocious and delayed puberty. Front Endocrinol. 2022;13:1019468.
6. D'Angelo DM, Di Donato G, Breda L, Chiarelli F. Growth and puberty in children with juvenile idiopathic arthritis. Pediatr Rheumatol Online J. 2021;19:28. https://doi.org/10.1186/s1296.
7. Dees WL, Hiney JK, Srivastava VK. IGF-1 influences gonadotropin-releasing hormone regulation of puberty. Neuroendocrinology. 2021;111:1151–63.
8. Hornberger LL, Lane MA. Identification and management of eating disorders in children and adolescents. Pediatrics. 2021;147(1):01. https://doi.org/10.1542/peds.
9. Ganson KT, Nguyen L, Ali ARH, Hallward L, Jackson DB, Testa A, Nagata JM. Associations between social media use, fitness and weight related content, and the use of legal appearance and performance enhancing drugs. Eat Behav. 2023;49:10173. https://doi.org/10.1016/j.eat.
10. Wong SC, Dobie R, Altowati MA, Werther GA, Farquharson C, Ahmed SF. Growth and the growth hormone-insulin like growth factor 1 axis in children with chronic inflammation: current evidence, gaps in knowledge and future directions. Endocr Rev. 2016;37:62–110.
11. De Benedetti F, Brunner H, Ruperto N, Schneider R, Xavier R, Allen R, et al for the Paediatric Rheumatology International Trials Organisation and the Pediatric Rheumatology Collaborative Study Group. Catch-up growth during Tocilizumab therapy for systemic juvenile idiopathic arthritis: results from a phase III trial. Arthrit Rheumatol. 2015;67:840–8.
12. Uettwiller F, Perlbarg J, Pinto G, Bader-Meunier B, Mouy R, Compeyrot-Lacassagne S, et al. Effect of biologic treatments on growth in children with juvenile idiopathic arthritis. J Rheumatol. 2014;41:128–35.
13. Rygg M, Pistorio A, Ravelli A, Maghnie M, Di Iorgi N, Bader-Meunier B, et al. A longitudinal PRINTO study on growth and puberty in juvenile systemic lupus erythematosus. Ann Rheum Dis. 2012;71:511–7.
14. Nguyen K, Barsalou J, Basodan J, Battish M, Benseler SM, Berard RA, et al. A decade of progress in juvenile idiopathic arthritis treatments and outcomes in Canada: results from ReACCh and the CAPRI registry. Rheumatology. 2023; https://doi.org/10.1093/rheum.

15. Brunner HI, Chen C, Bovis F, De Benedetti F, Espada G, Joos R, et al. Functional ability and health-related quality of life in randomized trials in patients with juvenile idiopathic arthritis. Arthritis Care Res. 2021;73:1264–74.
16. Zhang Y, Milojevic D. Protecting bone health in pediatric rheumatic disease: pharmacological considerations. Pediatr Drugs. 2017;19:193–211.
17. Ferraù F, Korbonits M. Metabolic comorbidities in Cushing's syndrome. Eur J Endocrinol. 2015;173:M133–57.
18. Kelsey MM, Zeitler PS. Insulin resistance of puberty. Curr Diab Rep. 2016; https://doi.org/10.1007/s1189.
19. Bismuth E, Chevenne D, Czernichow P, Simon D. Moderate deterioration in glucose tolerance during high-dose growth hormone therapy in glucocorticoid treated patients with juvenile idiopathic arthritis. Horm Res Pediatr. 2010;73:465–72.
20. Swain M, Kamper SJ, Maher CG, Broderick C, McKay D, Henschke N. Relationship between growth, maturation, and musculoskeletal conditions in adolescents: a systematic review. Br J Sports Med. 2018;52:1246–52.
21. Stone S, Khamashta MA, Nelson-Piercy C. Non-steroidal anti-inflammatory drugs and reversible female infertility; is there a link? Drug Saf. 2002;25:545–51.
22. Edens C. Early sexual health and reproductive implications in pediatric rheumatic diseases. Rheum Dis Clin North Am. 2022;48:91–112.
23. Savel C, Chausset A, Berland P, Guiguet-Auclair C, Cabane L, Fautrel B, et al. Survey of adolescents' needs and parents' views on sexual health in juvenile idiopathic arthritis. Pediatr Rheumatol Online J. 2023;21:95. https://doi.org/10.1186/s1296.
24. de Bastos M, Stegeman BH, Rosendaal FR, Hylckama V, Vlieg A, Helmerhorst FM, Stijnen T, et al. Combined oral contraceptives: venous thrombosis. Cochrane Database Syst Rev. 2014;3(3):CD010813. https://doi.org/10.1002/14651858.CD010813.pub2.
25. Margaritis K, Margioula-Siarkou G, Margioula-Siarkou C, Petousis S, Galli-Tsinopoulou A. Contraceptive methods in adolescence: a narrative review of guidelines. Eur J Contracept Reprod Health Care. 2023;28:51–5.
26. Bachrach LK. Hormonal contraception and bone health in adolescents. Front Endocrinol. 2020;11:603. https://doi.org/10.3389/fendo.2020.00603.
27. Cedars MI. Evaluation of female fertility- AMH and ovarian reserve testing. J Clin Endocrinol Metab. 2022;107:1510–9.
28. Ozer Y, Yildiz M, Turan H, Tarcin G, Bingol Aydin D, Gunalp A, et al. Ovarian reserve in children with juvenile idiopathic arthritis using biologic disease-modifying anti-rheumatic disease. Clin Rheumatol. 2024;43:399–406.

29. Nagafuchi H, Goto Y, Kiyokawa T, Ooka S, Kawahata K. Pregnancy outcomes in patients with rheumatoid arthritis who discontinue methotrexate to conceive. Clin Rheumatol. 2022;41:669–75.
30. Pham-Huy A, Sadarangani M, Huang V, Ostensen M, Castillo E, Troster SM, et al. From mother to baby: antenatal exposure to monoclonal antibody biologics. Expert Rev Clin Immunol. 2019;15:221–9.
31. Mills BS, Dao KH, Tecson KM, Beil EF, Tate R, Cush JJ. Perceptions of pregnancy and lactation from the Pregnancy and Lactation Autoimmune Network Registry. J Rheumatol. 2020;47:149–54.
32. Zaren P, Turesson C, Giwercman A. Methotrexate use among men—association with fertility and the perinatal health of their children: a Swedish Nationwide Register Study. Fertil Steril. 2023;120:661–9.
33. Dick AS, Lopez DA, Watts AL, Heeringa S, Reuter C, Bartsch H, et al. Meaningful associations in the adolescent brain cognitive study. NeuroImage. 2021;239:118262. https://doi.org/10.1016/j.neu.
34. Schilling KG, Archer D, Rheault F, Lyu I, Huo Y, Cai LY, et al. Superficial white matter across development, young adulthood and aging: volume, thickness and relationship with cortical features. Brain Struct Funct. 2023;228:1019–31.
35. Xia Y, Xia M, Liu J, Liao X, Lei T, Liang X, et al. Development of functional connectome gradients during childhood and adolescence. Sci Bull. 2022;67:1049–61.
36. Giedd JN. The amazing teen brain. Sci Am. 2015;312:32–7.
37. Towner E, Chierchia G, Blakemore SJ. Sensitivity and specificity in affective and social learning during adolescence. Trends Cogn Sci. 2023;27:642–55.
38. Hazell P, Balzer BWR, Garden F, Handelsman DH, Steinbeck PK. Association of urinary sex hormones with mood and behavior changes in a community adolescent cohort. PLoS One. 2023;18:e0293040. https://doi.org/10.1371/journ.
39. Nowling TK, Kral M, Wolf B, Gilkeson G, Ruth NM. Formal neurocogntive function and anti-N-methyl-D-aspartate antibodies in paediatric lupus. Lupus Sci Med. 2021;8(1) https://doi.org/10.1136/lupus-2020-000462.
40. Agostini A, Centofanti S. Normal sleep in children and adolescence. Psychiatr Clin N Am. 2024;47:1–14.
41. Clairman H, Dover S, Tomlinson G, et al. Lengthening sleep reduces pain in childhood arthritis: a crossover randomised controlled trial. RMD Open. 2023;9:e003352. https://doi.org/10.1136/rmdopen-2023-003352.
42. Saidi O, Rochette E, Bourdier P, Ratel S, Merlin E, Pereira B, Duche P. Sleep in children and adolescents with juvenile idiopathic arthritis: a systematic review and meta-analysis of case control studies. Sleep. 2022;45(2) https://doi.org/10.1093/sleep.

Impact of Rheumatic Musculoskeletal Conditions on Psychological Development in Adolescents and Young Adults

2

Ran Alice Cai and Hema Chaplin

AYA Psychological Development

Psychological development in AYA encompasses cognitive (see Chap. 1), emotional, and behavioural maturation [1]. A key process initiated by these psychological changes is the need to acquire a self-concept, which is how an individual perceives and thinks about the "self". It involves exploring and committing to identity-defining roles and values in a variety of life domains. Physical and hormonal changes during puberty also promote the development of body image and a sexual identity. As a result, social (see Chap.

R. A. Cai
Centre for Adolescent Rheumatology, Division of Medicine, University College London, London, UK

School of Human Sciences, University of Greenwich, London, UK
e-mail: r.a.cai@greenwich.ac.uk

H. Chaplin (✉)
Centre for Applied Health Research, University of Salford, Salford, UK
e-mail: h.chaplin@salford.ac.uk

C. Ciurtin, J. Hackett (eds.), *Adolescent and Young Adult Rheumatology In Clinical Practice*, In Clinical Practice,
https://doi.org/10.1007/978-3-031-82102-8_2

3) and physical components of the self-concept are of utmost importance during adolescence and have profound impacts on AYA psychological functioning [2].

Body image is based on a combination of one's own evaluation and the perception of others' attitudes towards one's physical characteristics [3]. A healthy body image means that the AYA accepts and appreciates their body and is generally satisfied with their appearance. Conversely, a negative body image occurs when there is a discourse between how the body is currently perceived and what the individual's preferences are.

Adolescence is also a time for discovering one's own sexual identity and for developing an interest in seeking intimate relationships. A sexual identity comprises cognitive and emotional understandings that individuals have about the meaning and significance of their sexual attractions, behaviours, and relationships, as well as how they value and adopt certain gender roles [4]. Social interaction with peers is essential for acquiring important milestones to developing a sexual identity and forming healthy romantic relationships in the future, such as increased dating competence, subjective awareness of sexual orientation, and exploratory sexual experiences.

AYA self-concepts are relatively fluid due to dramatic physical and psychosocial changes, and they may develop multiple, conflicting self-representations [2]. Not being able to integrate opposing identities into one consistent and resilient self-concept can decrease self-esteem, which is how we evaluate and value our self-worth. For example, body dissatisfaction can be high among adolescents as they are more influenced than adults by external feedback and tend to compare themselves to cultural and societal standards. This can contribute to feelings of inferiority and low self-esteem, which can render AYAs more vulnerable to psychological problems [5].

Mental health-related issues in AYA have been exacerbated even more by the COVID-19 pandemic, with clinically elevated levels of depression and anxiety potentially doubling compared to pre-pandemic estimates [6].

Factors Influencing Psychological Wellbeing in AYAs with RMDs

Whether or not AYA experience psychological issues depends on the balance of risk and protective factors [7, 8]. Negative life events that cause chronic, prolonged stress, such as the consequences of RMD, are significant risk factors for AYA wellbeing, which is why the prevalence of mental health issues are often higher in AYA with RMD compared to healthy counterparts [9]. One major issue is that the condition and its treatments can negatively impact physical appearance, including skin problems, delayed puberty, growth impairment, and increased risk of obesity compared to healthy peers [10–12]. The pain, fatigue, and mobility restrictions associated with RMD may also cause perceived physical weakness and poor fitness [13]. As a result, AYA with RMD might compare themselves negatively to their peers, feel ashamed for being "different", and may even be concerned about experiencing stigmatisation [14]. A negative body image can lead to low self-esteem and social withdrawal in adolescents of all genders and can be a precursor to developing anxiety and depression [15].

Managing RMD can also restrict educational, social, and leisure/sports participation, which can limit opportunities for psychosexual development that is often attained through interactions with peers [16, 17]. Moreover, physical limitations of RMD can interfere with an individual's ability to meet gender role demands. This may be particularly detrimental for boys, as small stature and thinness may be a significant source of sexual and gender-role anxiety due to embarrassment and fear of humiliation [18, 19]. Perceived challenges in forming long-term romantic relationships can decrease AYA abilities to establish this important source of social support and impact future wellbeing.

In addition, the unpredictable nature of physical symptoms related to RMD means that AYA need to accept the possibility of future flares or illness deterioration, and to continue a complicated treatment regimen (see Chap. 21). This can create uncertainties about whether or not they can achieve their full potential in personal and vocational endeavours despite the RMD. Worries about whether or not their illness will compromise employment opportunities exacerbates the primary source of stress among all adolescents, especially during the economic aftermath of the COVID-19 pandemic [17, 20]. Young adults with RMDs have reported lower rates of employment compared to pre-pandemic levels, as well as concerns regarding working conditions and occupational health and safety. Socioeconomic worries can also lead to guilt about potential dependency on intimate partners or on their parents, which further complicates the development of meaningful relationships. Economic stressors and disruptions from the pandemic can decrease AYA sense of control and security, which can have negative mental health implications.

An additional, often overlooked, issue is understanding the experience and support needed by neurodivergent AYA living with RMD. This is important given the health disparity between neurodivergent and neurotypical individuals due to co-occurring psychiatric and physical conditions [21, 22]. The term neurodivergence refers to differences in cognitive, emotional and social processes and functioning [23] and includes individuals with diagnoses such as autism spectrum condition (ASC), attention-deficit hyperactivity disorder (ADHD), and dyspraxia [24]. These individuals often have sensory perception and processing differences compared to neurotypical individuals, such as sensitivities to lights, sounds, smells and touch. However, the current medical model may not capture all types of diversities amongst the neurodivergent population and many individuals who experience the world differently compared to neurotypical people may not have received a formal diagnosis [25].

It is therefore necessary to recognise that communication with neurodivergent AYA, whether formally diagnosed or not, can be challenging, which reduces HCP ability to understand AYA needs and establish a positive relationship with AYA [26]. For example, neurodivergent AYA may find it difficult to be aware of and identify one's own emotions which then limits their ability to communicate how they feel to others verbally. This can increase feelings of distress, as well as displays of distressed behaviours, and their susceptibility to experiencing mental health issues [27].

This is unfortunate as neurodivergent AYA may experience greater levels of pain and fatigue compared to the neurotypical population [28]. These issues together can therefore exacerbate both physical and psychological symptoms in neurodivergent AYA, and worsened healthcare experiences due to mismanagement. As a result, AYA may feel misunderstood or disregarded, and these experiences can have negative long-term mental health consequences and reduces AYA ability to ask for help in later adulthood.

In order to prevent the escalation of chronic stress to psychological problems, AYA should be equipped with skills and resources to cope with these challenging situations. HCP can play an important role in providing AYA with important protective factors, such as identifying maladaptive thought processes, providing social support, and promoting self-efficacy and autonomy [29, 30].

Psychological Support in Routine Practice

Primary Prevention: Coping Strategies

One of the most important protective factors from experiencing mental health difficulties is developing resilience, which is the ability to employ adaptive coping strategies. Coping can be viewed as the effort to regulate psychological and physiological processes, such as emotions, behaviours, and cognition, in response to stressful situations [31]. In the realm of managing chronic illness in adolescence, three subtypes of coping have been identified (see Fig. 2.1) [32]:

- **Active:** efforts to directly influence the stressor
- **Accommodative:** efforts to adapt to the stressor
- **Disengagement:** efforts to deny/disengage with the stressor

Active and accommodative coping were found to increase resilience to stress, resulting in positive emotional and behavioural outcomes, whereas disengagement coping was associated with negative psychological adjustments [33].

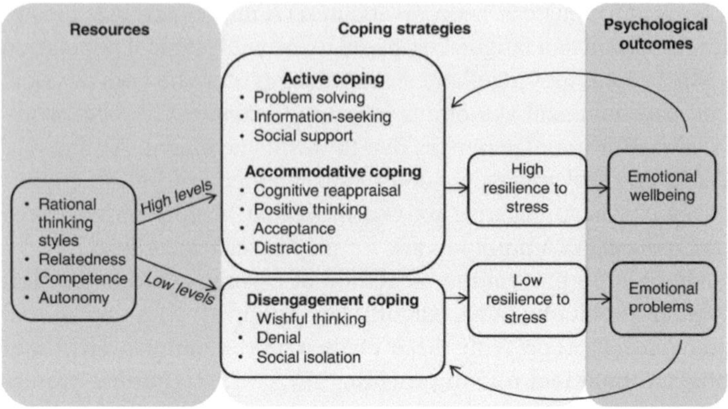

Fig. 2.1 Proposed relationships between cognitive processes, basic psychological needs, coping strategies, and mental health

Cognitive Distortions

The underlying principles of leading psychological therapies for AYA are identifying and modifying cognitive distortions in order to promote adaptive coping strategies [34, 35]. Two common distortions among AYA are:

- **Catastrophizing**: having an overly negative and pessimistic perception about how long symptoms will last and the consequences of illness.
- **Mental filters:** paying attention to and drawing conclusions from only one type of evidence, such as only focusing on personal failures and comparing these failures to other people's successes.

HCP can help AYA recognise and sensitively challenge these irrational thinking styles by encouraging alternative ways of thinking or reassessing the situation in a more flexible, optimistic and/or realistic way (see Chap. 4) [34, 35]. For example, AYA can be asked to consider all the evidence for and against their beliefs and assumptions, rather than evaluate a situation from only one perspective. It might also be helpful to reassure AYA that everyone has stress and worries and that they shouldn't be ashamed of how they feel. Normalising and validating negative feelings can encourage AYA to be more accepting of certain stressors. Instead of exerting energy on denying their feelings and problems, this attention can be refocused on learning to thrive despite limitations by developing personal values and interests [27]. Particularly for stressors that are outside of one's immediate control, such as managing unpredictable symptoms and outcomes of RMD, this type of accommodative coping was consistently found to lower levels of anxiety and depression [36, 37].

Psychological Needs

Resilience in AYA can also be promoted through satisfying three innate psychological needs [29, 30]:

1. **relatedness**; the need to feel connected to and cared for by others, satisfied through building relationships that are based on mutual trust and respect.
2. **competence**; the need to experience efficacy and mastery, such as having the skill to accomplish a goal.
3. **autonomy**; the need to make choices and take initiative for one's own decisions and behaviours.

Relatedness could be increased by developing an understanding and trusting relationship between AYA and HCP (see Chap. 4) and adopting a more person-centred care approach to consultations where HCP are sensitive to each AYA individual concerns, values, preferences and communication styles [38, 39]. It is important to be aware of the widespread impact of RMD on the young person's everyday life and avoid the application of adult values when assessing the impact of a potential stressor. For example, attributes affected by RMD, such as physical appearance, identity, and relationships, have greater impacts on AYA than adults' self-esteem [40, 41], and should be recognised and taken seriously. Especially in cases where an adolescent's pubertal development is affected by their RMD or treatment, HCP should ensure that the adolescent's sexual anxieties are addressed and not ignored. In addition, alternative, non-verbal ways for reporting symptoms should be offered by HCP to account for communication differences between neurodivergent and neurotypical AYA. This can help AYA feel understood and heard, and encourage young people to adopt active coping strategies by seeking help from HCP, and working together with the healthcare team to find a solution. Establishing a positive, supportive AYA-HCP relationship is important for all AYA, but especially for neurodivergent AYA as feelings of instability, disconnectedness and loss of control can lead to a disproportionately greater impact on their wellbeing.

Another essential predictor of psychological wellbeing in AYA is the feeling of competency or self-efficacy, which is how confident someone is in their abilities to achieve a goal [42]. Low self-efficacy creates feelings of helplessness and a tendency to avoid problems instead of adopting more positive coping techniques. One way to improve a sense of competency is to establish realistic goals for treatment and management. For example, if AYA expect to find a cure for their condition, they may develop low self-efficacy due to hopelessness. However, if the goal is more achievable, such as increasing adherence to treatments or adapting one's plans/goals according to disease activity, then this may enhance a sense of accomplishment and encourage better adjustment. High self-efficacy may also help AYA reappraise the situation by viewing the stressor as a challenge and opportunity to grow instead of a threat.

Self-efficacy in other life domains are extremely valuable as well, as participation in extracurricular activities increases AYAs' wellbeing, even after controlling for disease severity [43, 44]. This is especially true for activities that provide opportunities for developing new skills and relationships. Fostering internal qualities can reduce anxieties for some RMD-related issues by keeping their importance in perspective, such as decreasing the impact of physical appearance on self-esteem. Moreover, regular interactions with same-aged peers can help AYA acquire social skills necessary for psychosexual development. It is thus critical to help AYA identify, and encourage sustained participation in, hobbies such as sports and music. Therefore discussing and encouraging activity participation and signposting AYA to community services and patient organisations, such as peer support groups, can be beneficial. In addition to feeling competent in achieving a goal, AYA also need to have the autonomy to choose what goals to pursue and how they are achieved. HCP can increase autonomy by integrating AYA needs into treatment plans and allowing AYA to make informed decisions regarding their health. Being actively involved in the decision-making process can help AYA develop problem-solving strategies and empower them to take ownership of their wellbeing (see Chap. 4). HCP may also need to educate parents about the benefits of giving adolescents the freedom to participate in activities independently and of making lifestyle-related decisions. Control over treatment and lifestyle-related activities can help AYA acquire skills needed for active coping, such as how to seek relevant information, generate possible solutions, and weigh the pros and cons of an option, which are important skills for effectively managing RMD.

Secondary Prevention: Identifying Psychological Problems

Early Detection and Regular Screening

Even when efforts to prevent mental health problems in AYA are an integral part of care, guilt, rage, and hopelessness can arise at various stages due to the uncertain and chronic nature of RMD. Thus, early detection and management of emotional issues are vital in preventing further deterioration and encouraging rapid recovery. However, the difficulty of distinguishing normal emotional variabilities during adolescence and young adulthood from true psychological problems can often lead to late detection, and sometimes complete disregard, of mental health issues.

Normal AYA angst is transient, confined to a single setting such as home or school, and does not cause significant impairments. In contrast, mental health disorders persist over time, with symptoms presenting in various environments, negatively impacting important areas of life, and sometimes resulting in physical symptoms such as weight fluctuations, headaches, and sleep problems [45]. Additionally, AYA who are exposed to risk factors such as academic problems, abuse, issues with peers, bereavement, and family conflict, have higher psychological vulnerabilities [7, 8]. HCP should thus be vigilant in routine assessments for these stressful life events and for deteriorations in academic/work performance and relationship quality, as well as for physical symptoms not readily explained by RMD.

There is a growing interest in the use of patient-reported outcome measures (PROM) in daily practice to monitor psychological wellbeing. Regular screenings can also create a more accessible environment where AYA feel comfortable disclosing psychological problems, even when they are seeking treatment for a physical illness (see Chap. 4). PROMs such as the Centre for Epidemiological Studies Depression Scale and the Patient Health Questionnaire are brief (<10 min), free to use, and allow for longitudinal assessments in both adolescents and adults [46, 47]. However, PROMs are not all-encompassing and AYA may underreport negative feelings due to fear of mental health stigmatisation or by using denial as a coping strategy [38]. PROMs should therefore not substitute for thoughtful face-to-face assessments (see Chap. 4).

Management and Referrals to Psychological Therapies

Decisions for psychological referrals depend on the type of problem, duration, and severity. Emotional disorders, such as mild depression, can often remit spontaneously in AYA and a period of "watchful waiting" whilst providing general support for adaptive coping skills can be sufficient [48]. It is essential to approach the situation sensitively by speaking with AYA on their own before involving others, such as parents, friends, or teachers. Although help from others can be beneficial, it is important to respect adolescents' wishes and explore with them various ways in which they can receive support. In addition, AYA should be signposted to youth-friendly web-based resources around issues of mental health and organisations they can contact for confidential support. Information about how and where to obtain these resources should be readily available on the rheumatology centre's website or advertised in waiting areas.

If emotional problems persist and severely impair functioning, then HCP should consider referring AYA to psychological services. In these situations, it is important to ensure that psychological support is introduced as part of the multidisciplinary approach for managing the RMD, and that it will only supplement, not replace, medical support. Even if a psychological referral has been made, it is essential to continue reviewing AYA emotional state at each RMD appointment, since engagement with mental health referrals may be low or inadequate. It is therefore beneficial to adopt an integrated, holistic healthcare approach to reduce mental health stigma and increase awareness.

The bidirectional relationship between AYA emotional wellbeing and those of their parents and other family members should also be acknowledged [49, 50, 51]. Parental distress can have a profound impact on adolescents' own resilience and functioning, as well as predict treatment outcomes for mental health issues. It can therefore be beneficial to include close family members in the discussion and treatment of emotional issues in addition to providing one-to-one support for AYA.

Conclusion

Adolescence and young adulthood is an exciting and challenging phase of life, but it is also a period of heightened vulnerability. Being aware of the interplay between RMD and multifactorial sources of risks for psychological problems is central to the complete management of AYA. Although psychological issues can be complex and difficult to manage, disregarding them can have profound, negative impacts on AYA current and future quality of life [5]. Acknowledgement of the importance of good psychological health should thus be the responsibility of the healthcare team as a whole. This chapter has hopefully provided practical tools to help HCP improve psychological resilience and address AYA emotional needs during routine practice.

Key Management Points

1. Encourage active and accommodative coping by recognising and modifying cognitive distortions and by increasing levels of relatedness, competence, and autonomy.
2. Acknowledge AYA concerns. Stressors that may seem trivial to adults could be challenging for AYA as they value different attributes and are still developing cognitive and regulatory abilities.
3. Provide information for, and signpost AYA as well as close family members to web-based resources and support for managing RMD and psychosocial challenges. These resources should be AYA-appropriate, reliable, regularly reviewed/updated, and displayed in places where AYA can easily see and access.
4. Support participation in extra-curricular activities, patient organisations, community-led activities and/or peer support groups that won't aggravate RMDs but are still enjoyable, to help AYA develop new skills, social relationships, and a more positive outlook.
5. Adopt a person-centred approach by asking AYA about their individual opinions and preferences and help them make informed decisions about their treatments/management in order to promote autonomy and problem-solving skills.
6. Be aware of physical and behavioural changes, as well as of negative life events that AYA are experiencing, and encourage conversations around issues of mental health to help with early detection of psychological distress. This is especially important during, and in the aftermaths of, public health issues (e.g., the COVID-19 pandemic) due to their potential impact on AYA access to treatment and healthcare, physical health and safety, and socioeconomical wellbeing.

References

1. Somerville LH, Jones RM, Casey BJ. A time of change: behavioral and neural correlates of adolescent sensitivity to appetitive and aversive environmental cues. Brain Cogn. 2010;72(1):124–33. https://doi.org/10.1016/j.bandc.2009.07.003.
2. Harter S, Bresnick S, Bouchey HA, Whitesell NR. The development of multiple role-related selves during adolescence. Dev Psychopathol. 1997;9(4):835–53. https://doi.org/10.1017/S0954579497001466.
3. Cash TF, Smolak L. Body image: a handbook of science, practice, and prevention. 2nd ed. New York: The Guilford Press; 2011.
4. Dillon FR, Worthington RL, Moradi B. Sexual identity as a universal process. In: Handbook of identity theory and research. New York: Springer; 2011. p. 649–70. https://doi.org/10.1007/978-1-4419-7988-9_27.
5. Marques SC, Pais-Ribeiro JL, Lopez SJ. The role of positive psychology constructs in predicting mental health and academic achievement in children and adolescents: a two-year longitudinal study. J Happiness Stud. 2011;12(6):1049–62. https://doi.org/10.1007/s10902-010-9244-4.
6. Racine N, McArthur BA, Cooke JE, Patton GC, Coffey C, Cappa C, et al. Global prevalence of depressive and anxiety symptoms in children and adolescents during COVID-19. JAMA Pediatr. 2021;175(11):1–10. https://doi.org/10.1001/jamapediatrics.2021.2482.
7. Magson NR, Freeman JYA, Rapee RM, et al. Risk and protective factors for prospective changes in adolescent mental health during the COVID-19 pandemic. J Youth Adolescence. 2021;50:44–57. https://doi.org/10.1007/s10964-020-01332-9.
8. Cairns KE, Yap MBH, Pilkington PD, et al. Risk and protective factors for depression that adolescents can modify: a systematic review and meta-analysis of longitudinal studies. J Affect Disord. 2014;169:61–75. https://doi.org/10.1016/j.jad.2014.08.006.
9. Ferro MA. Major depressive disorder, suicidal behaviour, bipolar disorder, and generalised anxiety disorder among emerging adults with and without chronic health conditions. Epidemiol Psychiatr Sci. 2016;25:462–74.
10. Chua-Aguilera CJ, Moller B, Yawalkar N. Skin manifestations of rheumatoid arthritis, juvenile idiopathic arthritis, and spondyloarthritides. Clinic Rev Allerg Immunol. 2017;53:371–93. https://doi.org/10.1007/s12016-017-8632-5.
11. de Gruijter NM, Naja M, Peckham H, et al. A systematic review exploring the bidirectional relationship between puberty and autoimmune rheumatic diseases. Pediatr Rheumatol. 2021;19(47) https://doi.org/10.1186/s12969-021-00528-y.
12. Guzman J, Kerr T, Ward LM, et al. Growth and weight gain in children with juvenile idiopathic arthritis: results from the ReACCh-out cohort. Pediatr Rheumatol. 2017;15(68) https://doi.org/10.1186/s12969-017-0196-7.

13. Erkolahti RK, Ilonen T, Saarijärvi S. Self-image of adolescents with diabetes mellitus type-I and rheumatoid arthritis. Nord J Psychiatry. 2003;57(4):309–12. https://doi.org/10.1080/08039480310002101.
14. Pinquart M. Body image of children and adolescents with chronic illness: a meta-analytic comparison with healthy peers. Body Image. 2013;10(2):141–8. https://doi.org/10.1016/j.bodyim.2012.10.008.
15. Taal E, Rasker JJ, Timmers CJ. Measures of physical function and emotional well being for young adults with arthritis. J Rheumatol. 1997;24(5):994–7.
16. Packham JC, Hall MA. Long-term follow-up of 246 adults with juvenile idiopathic arthritis: social function, relationships and sexual activity. Rheumatology (Oxford). 2002;41(12):1440–3. https://doi.org/10.1093/rheumatology/41.12.1428.
17. Kaushansky D, Cox J, Dodson C, McNeeley M, Kumar S, Iverson E. Living a secret: disclosure among adolescents and young adults with chronic illnesses. Chronic Illn. 2017;13(1):49–61. https://doi.org/10.1177/1742395316655855.
18. Neufeld JA, Klingbeil F, Bryen DN, Silverman B, Thomas A. Adolescent sexuality and disability. Phys Med Rehabil Clin N Am. 2002;13(4):857–73. https://doi.org/10.1016/S1047-9651(02)00045-1.
19. Jordan A, Carter B, Fogeron P, et al. Romantic relationships in young people with long-term health conditions: a scoping review. J Pediatr Psychol. 2021;46(3):264–79. https://doi.org/10.1093/jpepsy/jsaa106.
20. Arif J, Tucker LB, Cynthia C, Gignac MAM. Impact of the COVID-19 pandemic on the employment of Canadian young adults with rheumatic disease: findings from a longitudinal survey. Arthritis Care Res. 2021;73(8):1146–52. https://doi.org/10.1002/acr.24617.
21. Buck TR, Joseph V, Megan F, Hilary C, McMahon WM, Jubel M, Bilder DA. Psychiatric comorbidity and medication use in adults with autism spectrum disorder. J Autism Dev Disord. 2014;44(12):3063–71. https://doi.org/10.1007/s10803-014-2170-2.
22. McLeod JD, Emily M, Amelia H. The experiences of college students on the autism Spectrum: a comparison to their neurotypical peers. J Autism Dev Disord. 2019;49(6):2320–36. https://doi.org/10.1007/s10803-019-03910-8.
23. Robert C. Neurodiversity and the social ecology of mental functions. Perspect Psychol Sci. 2019;16(6):1360–72. https://doi.org/10.1177/1745691620959833.
24. Polaris K. Genetics on the neurodiversity spectrum: genetic phenotypic and endophenotypic continua in autism and ADHD. Stud Hist Philos Sci Part A. 2021;89:52–62. https://doi.org/10.1016/j.shpsa.2021.07.006.
25. Susan Y, Jack H, Michael A, Patrick B, Polly B, William C, Emily C, Mayuri D, Quinton D, Emad F, Gisli G, Peter H, Ho-lan L, Clodagh M, Peri M, Marianna M, Fintan O'R, Dennis O, Patricia R, Nancy S, Eric T, Emma W. Guidance for identification and treatment of individuals with

attention deficit/hyperactivity disorder and autism spectrum disorder based upon expert consensus. BMC Med. 2021;18(1):146. https://doi.org/10.1186/s12916-020-01585-y.
26. Sala R, Amet L, Blagojevic-Stokic N, et al. Bridging the gap between physical health and autism spectrum disorder. Neuropsychiatr Dis Treat. 2020;16:1605–18. https://doi.org/10.2147/NDT.S251394.
27. Denise DB, Ameis SH, Meng-Chuan L, Casanova MF, Pushpal D. Interoception in autism Spectrum disorder: a review. Int J Dev Neurosci. 2016;52(1):104–11. https://doi.org/10.1016/j.ijdevneu.2016.05.001.
28. Failla MD, Gerdes MB, Williams ZJ, Moore DJ, Cascio CJ. Increased pain sensitivity and pain-related anxiety in individuals with autism. Pain Rep. 2020;5(6):e861. https://doi.org/10.1097/PR9.0000000000000861.
29. Tay L, Diener E. Needs and subjective well-being around the world. J Pers Soc Psychol. 2011;101(2):354–65. https://doi.org/10.1037/a0023779.
30. Lee CC, Enzler CJ, Garland BH, Zimmerman CJ, Raphael JL, Hergenroeder AC, Wiemann CM. The development of health self-management among adolescents with chronic conditions: an application of self-determination theory. J Adolesc Health. 2021;68(2):394–402. https://doi.org/10.1016/j.jadohealth.2020.05.053.
31. Compas BE, Connor-Smith JK, Heidi S, Harding TA, Wadsworth ME. Coping with stress during childhood and adolescence: problems progress and potential in theory and research. Psychol Bull. 2001;127(1):87–127. https://doi.org/10.1037/0033-2909.127.1.87.
32. Compas BE, Jaser SS, Dunn MJ, Rodriguez EM. Coping with chronic illness in childhood and adolescence. Annu Rev Clin Psychol. 2011;8(1):455–80. https://doi.org/10.1146/annurev-clinpsy-032511-143108.
33. Sarah N, Monica A, Iris K-G, Natoshia C. A scoping review and proposed framework for coping in youth with a history of psychological trauma and chronic pain. J Pediatr Psychol. 2021;47(4):469–82. https://doi.org/10.1093/jpepsy/jsab127.
34. Beck JS. Cognitive behavior therapy: basics and beyond. 3rd ed. New York: The Guilford Press; 2021. https://doi.org/10.1017/CBO9781107415324.004.
35. Rowan B, Vijaya M, Batterham PJ, Dusan H-P, Fiona S. Acceptance and commitment therapy universal prevention program for adolescents: a feasibility study. Child Adolesc Psychiatry Mental Health. 2017;11(1):11–27. https://doi.org/10.1186/s13034-017-0164-5.
36. Leona MG, Carolyn W, Leyla DA, Shannon C, Nuno F. Psychological mediators in the relationship between paediatric chronic pain and adjustment: an investigation of acceptance catastrophising and kinesiophobia. J Contextual Behav Sci. 2020;18:294–305. https://doi.org/10.1016/j.jcbs.2020.10.009.

37. Dufton LM, Dunn MJ, Slosky LS, Compas BE. Self-reported and laboratory-based responses to stress in children with recurrent pain and anxiety. J Pediatr Psychol. 2010;36(1):95–105. https://doi.org/10.1093/jpepsy/jsq070.
38. World Health Organization. WHO global strategy on people centred and integrated health services. 2015. http://apps.who.int/iris/bitstream/10665/155002/1/WHO_HIS_SDS_2015.6_eng.pdf. Accessed April 26, 2024.
39. The Health Foundation. Person-centred care made simple; What everyone should know about person-centred care, 2016.
40. McDonagh JE. Young people first juvenile idiopathic arthritis second: transitional care in rheumatology. Arthritis Care Res. 2008;59(8):1162–70. https://doi.org/10.1002/art.23928.
41. Hair EC, Jager J, Garrett SB. Helping teens develop healthy social skills and relationships: what research shows about navigating adolescence. Child Trends Res Br. 2002.
42. Albert B. Recycling misconceptions of perceived self-efficacy. Cogn Ther Res. 1984;8(3):231–55. https://doi.org/10.1007/BF01172995.
43. Ennett ST, DeVellis BM, Earp JA, Kredich D, Warren RW, Wilhelm CL. Disease experience and psychosocial adjustment in children with juvenile rheumatoid arthritis: children's versus mothers' reports. J Pediatr Psychol. 1991;16(5):557–68. http://www.ncbi.nlm.nih.gov/pubmed/1744805
44. Ingrid L, Danielsen AG, Birkeland MS, Oddrun S. Basic psychological need satisfaction in leisure activities and adolescents' life satisfaction. J Youth Adolesc. 2012;41(12):1588–99. https://doi.org/10.1007/s10964-012-9776-5.
45. Bailen NH, Green LM, Thompson RJ, et al. Understanding emotion in adolescents: a review of emotional frequency, intensity, instability, and clarity. Emot Rev. 2018;11(1) https://doi.org/10.1177/175407391876887.
46. Gemma V, Forero CG, Gabriela B, Jordi A, van der Feltz-Cornelis Christina. Screening for depression in the general population with the Center for Epidemiologic Studies Depression (CES-D): a systematic review with meta-analysis. PLoS One. 2016;11(5):e015543. https://doi.org/10.1371/journal.pone.0155431.
47. Luigi C, Cesira P, Anna O, Eugenia CM, Alessandra C, Gianluca S, Andrea A, Martino BM, Vlasios B, Mario A, Nassir GS, Andrea A. Screening for depression in primary care with Patient Health Questionnaire-9 (PHQ-9): a systematic review. J Affect Disord. 2020;279:473–83. https://doi.org/10.1016/j.jad.2020.09.131.
48. Phipps S, Srivastava DK. Repressive adaptation in children with cancer. Health Psychol. 1997;16(6):521–8. https://doi.org/10.1037/0278-6133.16.6.521.
49. Kaveh A, Oluwatosin A, Wahezi DM, Caliendo AE, Curran ML, Jessica N, Susan K, Correll CK, Brunner EJ, Knight AM. Parent perspectives on

addressing emotional health for children and young adults with juvenile myositis. Arthritis Care Res. 2021;73(1):18–29. https://doi.org/10.1002/acr.24466.

50. D'Angelo CM, Sylvie M, Daniel G, Schwebel DC, Nina R, Kimberly GR. Coping attributions and health functioning among adolescents with chronic illness and their parents: reciprocal relations over time. J Clin Psychol Med Settings. 2019;26(4):495–506. https://doi.org/10.1007/s10880-018-9597-0.
51. Dikla E, Krumholz ML, Jessica S, Weisz JR. Parental depressive symptoms as a predictor of outcome in the treatment of child depression. J Abnorm Child Psychol. 2018;46(4):825–37. https://doi.org/10.1007/s10802-017-0323-4.

3 Impact of Rheumatic Conditions on Social Development in Adolescents and Young Adults

Hema Chaplin and Ran Alice Cai

Social Development of AYA and the Influence of RMD

As discussed, (see Chaps. 1 and 2) biological changes during adolescence interact with psychosocial development to set up a range of new behaviours not seen in childhood or often dealt with in paediatric care [1]. These biopsychosocial interactions include puberty, neurological maturation, abstract thought, self-identity, peer identification and autonomy. The main factors of typical adolescent social development can be broadly categorised as 'independence', 'emotional adjustment' and 'identity formation' [2]. By late adolescence and early adulthood, several developmental

H. Chaplin (✉)
Centre for Applied Health Research, University of Salford, Salford, UK
e-mail: h.chaplin@salford.ac.uk

R. A. Cai
Centre for Adolescent Rheumatology, Division of Medicine, University College London, London, UK

School of Human Sciences, University of Greenwich, London, UK
e-mail: r.a.cai@greenwich.ac.uk

C. Ciurtin, J. Hackett (eds.), *Adolescent and Young Adult Rheumatology In Clinical Practice*, In Clinical Practice,
https://doi.org/10.1007/978-3-031-82102-8_3

tasks should be in progress or achieved during this period of profound psychosocial transformation [2–4]:

- Emergence of autonomous behaviour and social independence;
- Intimate relationships and secure friendships;
- Experimentation with personal and sexual identity,
- Self-development;
- Emotional skills development;
- Development of the social brain – the network of brain areas involved in social perception and cognition developed through the social environment; and
- Vocational capability, including financial independence

AYA are at a critical point in their social and communication development which may mean that they face difficulties in understanding their internal experiences and symptoms, and the importance of articulating these for diagnostic pathways for physical health conditions [5]. Chronic childhood-onset conditions often disrupt young peoples' sense of normality and impair their capacity for social participation [6]. This results in delayed social maturation leading to knock-on effects into adolescence and young adulthood, as AYA with RMD can feel misunderstood and stigmatized from an early age. The physical and psychosocial challenges experienced with RMD are particularly salient and difficult for AYA compared to either children or adults, because of peer pressure to "fit in", cultural associations between youth and health, exposure to social stigmas around disability and limited experience in adjusting to adversity [7]. Some AYA with RMD can be at risk of experiencing social difficulties, due to physical and psychological effects of disease and its treatment, including disruptions and restrictions to daily life and functional outcomes [8].

Social functioning has been ranked as a top area impacted by RMD in those aged 16–25, with this effect on their lives more important than pain/stiffness and functional impairments [9]. Table 3.1 shows the range of social impacts due to RMD, meaning opportunities available for healthy peers can be missed in AYA. These negative social consequences occur during any point of the fluctuating disease course, even during disease inactivity, as

Table 3.1 Effects of RMD, including disability and/or medications on typical social development in AYA [4, 13–19]

Hindered development of independence, including delayed independent living;
Reduced self-esteem;
Affected self-confidence and heightened self-consciousness, resulting from side effects of medications impacting body image (e.g. weight gain and hair loss);
Forced locus of control to be external, rather than internal, i.e. AYA believe that external elements have more control over the outcome of events in their lives than they do;
Less opportunities for participation in social activities and consolidation of social skills, due to impact of pain, fatigue and reduced mobility;
Medication impeding daily activities, such as side-effects, medication times, administration, storage or restrictions due to interactions (e.g. alcohol intake and methotrexate);
Transport issues, e.g. relying on parents for transport when friends can use public transport self-sufficiently;
Feeling isolated and potentially bullied causing social anxiety, especially if experiencing long or multiple absences from school/university/work caused by ill health or healthcare utilisation;
Overprotective family and/or peers imposing restrictions;
Problematic relationships with friends, family and professionals;
Difficulties with intimate relationships, potentially due to additional pressure or guilt of having someone be concerned and caring for you;
Educational difficulties and subsequent greater problems with vocation, either in finding employment or experiencing discrimination;
Struggles with identity, as misrepresented self being defined by disease;
Restricted major life decisions, such as narrowed career options, threat to parenthood and/or travelling considerations;
Unable to be as spontaneous or experimental as peers, with disease-related anxiety caused by unpredictability of disease and side effects of treatment

a result of affected quality of life from symptomatology not directly driven by inflammation [10, 11]. AYA with RMD are often unable to achieve the same level of autonomy as healthy peers, as the shift in balance of independence and identity development is affected [8]. There can be a reliance on parents for involvement in their treatment that is either driven by the young person not feeling confident in self-management or due to parents not letting go. A balance between family involvement to be supportive but not too overprotective needs to be achieved [12] to not limit the AYA own autonomy.

Childhood illness may influence a typical child–parent interaction (see Chap. 5) and parenting styles particularly in regard to fostering independence, especially in terms of managing the AYA own health and relationships with HCP [12, 16]. Parents' and close others' concerns can restrict activities and overprotect AYA [20]. This overprotection can have detrimental effects on achieving autonomy and hindering experimentation that results in completion of social development tasks. The main challenge for AYA with RMD is achieving an identity not defined by their illness. This involves developing their ability to accomplish desired activities, experience positive relationships [7], manage pain, use social support and live one day at a time [14, 18]. Otherwise AYA can resent the restrictive impact of disease on limiting physical and social capacities, career opportunities and parenthood goals [15]. Adapting, planning and pacing activities are required to maintain social involvement and prevent additional pain and fatigue from exerting excessive energy when attempting to keep up with peers [18]. Positive emotions and self-esteem can be maintained through acceptance of their abilities and limitations. HCP should encourage a discussion on realistic goal setting, e.g. SMART goals (Specific, Measurable, Attainable, Relevant, Time-bound). Despite the numerous barriers mentioned in this section, most AYA with RMD are socially competent and comparable to healthy counterparts on social functioning, acceptance and behaviour [16, 18], adjusting and coping quite well with the psychological and social sequelae of their RMD over time.

RMDs, Neurodivergence and Learning Disabilities in AYAs

Neurodivergence influences an individual's behaviour in social situations and is associated with atypical emotional responses. Co-morbid physical and health conditions occur in neurodivergent AYA, with RMD accounting for a significant proportion of these [5, 21], in particular hyper-mobility, connective tissue disease and chronic pain. Difficulties in interactions occur because of different ways of experiencing the world and processing information creates mismatch in communication styles with both peers and health professionals [22]. Communication challenges, misattributing physical health symptoms as a part of neurodivergence, sensory processing differences, masking and a history of not being believed, can limit reporting of symptoms or problems affecting diagnosis and management of RMD [5, 21]. The interaction between neurodivergence and fatigue associated with physical health conditions as well as school absences, may make socialising increasingly difficult and force some neurodivergent AYA to socially withdraw completely [5].

A learning or intellectual disability affects the way a person learns new things throughout their life, which is problematic when diagnosed with a RMD. Understanding complicated health and medication information, learning self-management skills and looking after themselves or autonomy can be difficult to achieve. Children with Down syndrome are at increased risk of developing associated arthritis [23], and therefore may be the most common learning disability seen in AYA Rheumatology clinics. However, as hypermobility, loss of range of movement and muscle tone, and differences in pain expression are features of Down Syndrome, coupled with poor verbal skills, may make clinical consultation and examination more challenging. AYA with specific learning disabilities experience significant social, emotional, and/or behavioural concerns in addition to achievement deficits, whereas others seem to possess adequate psychosocial functioning [24]. No one size fits all and management strategies need to be appropriately tailored for AYA with RMD and neurodivergence or learning disability.

Social Aspects of Health Behaviours, Disease Course and HCP Management Strategies for AYA with RMD

During the AYA developmental stage, independent health behaviours begin and can be established as lifelong habits [25]. Adolescent social development can lead to egocentric behaviour and a disregard for the consequences of their behaviour on others.

This change in attitude and hindered forward planning, due to delayed neurological development (see Chap. 1), can increase risk-taking health behaviour [4]. The extent to which typical adolescent issues affect illness management and control will depend on how AYA balances competing priorities. For example, the need for social support and acceptance can tempt AYA to give into peer pressure by undertaking exploratory behaviours [26] that can put RMD management at risk. These risky health behaviours can include chaotic, nutritionally poor eating habits, smoking, alcohol, drug use and sexual risk-taking. Conversely, some AYA report being able to use their condition or medications as a convenient excuse not to participate in behaviours they don't want to [26], with peer pressure lessened when the adverse effects were explained to peers. Treatment can be seen as both an opportunity for living a 'normal' life and also a threat to achieving this [27]. Another unique issue in this population is transitioning from paediatric to adult services (see Chap. 23) and it has been found that those who have better social support and family functioning are associated with greater transfer readiness [28].

Rheumatology HCP have the unique, ongoing opportunity to assess social, psychological and emotional functioning, in addition to physical outcomes, and intervene early in a nonpsychiatric environment to improve clinical outcomes [16, 28, 29]. This should start once RMD diagnosis is confirmed with an initial comprehensive psychosocial assessment (see Chap. 2 for other areas to monitor). During routine clinic visits, some patients may benefit from a more unstructured opportunity to express their illness experience, but following a structured psychosocial screening assessment such as HEEADSSS (see Chap. 4) is useful for AYA and HCP alike.

Differences in communication styles may also not be understood, especially those without appropriate neurodivergent or learning disability training. For example, a neurodivergent AYA may be non-verbal, or AYA with a learning disability may have reduced/altered communication and, therefore, struggle to verbally communicate symptoms in a manner that Rheumatology professionals expect [5]. Their ability to describe their feelings may differ significantly from those who are neurotypical and they might struggle to verbalise their symptoms in a logical or consistent manner. Additionally, they may find it hard to deal with persistent questions that occur during consultations that try to disentangle what may sometimes seem like a jumble of symptoms without a firm timeline [21]. Therefore, is it important to allocate longer time for appointment and work with Social Workers and Special Educational Needs Co-ordinators as appropriate.

The Importance of Peer Support and Social Media for AYA with RMD

Due to symptomatic and illness-related absences, AYA with RMD miss out on social aspects of their education [5] that may typically provide peer support. Peer support through strong peer relations is vital during adolescence to promote typical social development [2, 14, 30], since friendships nurture self-development separate from familial identity. Peers offer practical, emotional and social support [17], and can facilitate adjustment to chronic disease through normalisation (if peers themselves are also living with a chronic condition), coping with pain/illness and adherence by reducing general and illness-related stress [12, 26].

Supportive peers can provide understanding, reassurance, shared learning and increase self-efficacy in terms of their confidence in one's ability to manage their RMD and acting as role models [31]. They can increase optimism and alleviate feelings of social isolation, especially for AYA with RMD which are uncommon chronic illnesses [12]. This can assist the adoption of healthy behaviours, disease management skills [29], and acceptance of help with disease management [32]. Conversely problematic unsupportive relationships lead to increased distress and disease activity [30, 33], by being oppressive, underestimating the disease and not providing useful advice [34]. However, even without an RMD, socialising may pose difficult for many AYA who have learning disabilities or are neurodivergent and may struggle with peer relationships [5]. Regardless of social network size, AYA primarily disclose their illness to family members and only to a few peers, although some feel more comfortable expressing issues and concerns online through social media [19].

Peer support from other AYA with similar RMD can provide meaningful emotional and social support due to a shared understanding of living with a chronic unpredictable disease, reducing isolation and negating the problems in support from friends without a RMD diagnosis [35]. However, no one size fits all and it is important to provide varied access to peer support [31]. This support can involve discussions around acknowledging and overcoming concerns for the future (education, occupation or relationships), strategies around taking medication, and developing positive lifestyles in terms of physical activity and psychological wellbeing through goal setting and action-planning [36]. This can be disease specific or regarding areas indirectly impacted such as school/work and social life.

Good support from peers is key to adjustment, whereas support from the wider network (e.g. teachers, employers AHP's and nurses) becomes more important when family functioning is less positive [32]. Reasons for withholding and not seeking support can include fear of rejection, pity, perceptions of being seen as vulnerable or different, dismissal of their problems/concerns as unimportant or alternatively overreactions and limiting of social activities/involvement. Sometimes others do not perceive these AYA as chronically ill, in part due to the fluctuating and invisible nature of disease or not understanding the emotional impact of coping with daily pain and taking medications [29]. Disclosure can be influenced by [30, 37]:

- Perceived trust and familiarity;
- Possibility of experiencing stigma or negative consequences;
- Shared experience with illness/disability;
- Visibility of the condition and practical needs;
- Recipient's anticipated response; and
- Decision that disclosure is justified.

It is important that appropriate information regarding RMD, and the specific impact it has on that young person including pain and mood, is shared with peers, school, and work to enable appropriate support [29, 38]. Greater support beyond educational attainment is needed [13, 39], such as focusing on finding and keeping employment. AYA and parents can be supported to disclose information in an appropriate and stepwise manner depending on their preferences and needs. For example, with the AYA consent, the school nurse or university doctor should be fully notified, whereas teachers or employers could be given information on supporting the AYA during absences or coping with critical events [29]. The healthcare team are in a position of authority and can facilitate this disclosure by examining how the organisation (school, university, or work) and the content of the treatment can be modified according to the AYA lifestyle, suggesting dialogue for the young person to say or providing supporting clinical letters of recommendation to schools or local authorities.

Support groups, peer mentorship, residential weekends and virtual forums provide opportunities for peer networking, sharing inner thoughts to strengthen self-development and self-management confidence [14, 17, 35]. Moreover, many AYA are more open to recommendations from near-peer mentors versus adult mentors or professionals and may see other young adults coping successfully with a similar diagnosis as a sign of hope, which increases motivation and confidence that they too can manage their illness [35]. Social media and/or online resources can provide peer support and information electronically which can promote self-management skills [18, 19, 31, 40], although there can be issues in terms of safeguarding, misinformation, and digital exclusion. For more instrumental support, e.g. healthcare advice, it is important to make sure the accounts are somewhat monitored or aligned with patient organisations, although social media is a good medium for general/emotional support. Use of digital media is also particularly useful for those with physical restrictions or during unique health situations, such as hospitalisations or shielding/lockdowns as experienced during the COVID-19 pandemic, when physical interactions with peers are not possible [3].

Impact of COVID-19 on Social Development of Those AYA with RMD

Although it is still too early to tell the longer-term impacts of the COVID-19 pandemic for AYA with RMDs, there is some evidence for the substantial effects on mental and physical health from the social deprivation caused by consecutive lockdowns, disruptions to education, changes to peer interaction, being labelled as 'vulnerable' due to being immunocompromised, shielding and reduced healthcare access/interactions [3, 41–44]. As highlighted throughout this chapter, peer interaction and support is a vital aspect of typical development that was negatively impacted in an unprecedented and extreme manner for all AYA (with and without RMD) that clinicians should remain aware of and sensitive to during their consultations [3].

Summary

It is extremely positive that many AYA are doing well with regard to psychosocial adjustment and are comparable to peers in several areas. However, those at risk need to be identified and intervention measures introduced as early as possible [16], as impact on behaviour and management of disease can still be profound. Therefore, regular screening/discussions to assess the psychosocial burden impacting quality of life are important to personalise treatment [33]. It is imperative to match the needs and preferences of the AYA with the support provided [30], with HCPs providing a flexible and youth-friendly approach (see Chap. 22).

Key Management Points

1. Explore social functioning and support, screen for social issues and identify areas needing support and appropriate referral, e.g. nurse or psychologist:
   - Follow HEEADSSS psychosocial interview [45] to assess social issues and changes to a patient's social situations that might impact wellbeing.
   - Use brief screening questionnaires in clinic to quickly assess impact of illness on functioning by assessing work, home management, leisure activities and family/relationships, to highlight areas needing discussion and support.

(continued)

- Allow time for unstructured discussion, and encourage questions to gain further understanding of their perceptions of impact and distress, especially if the AYA is neurodivergent or has a learning disability.
- Decide whether to escalate beyond patient education and whether to refer to mental health services or psychologist, particularly if disease is active or symptoms are severe.

2. Ensure the AYA has routine access to a key worker (such as a clinical nurse specialist, AHP, special educational need co-ordinator or social worker), to develop appropriate education, health and care plans to support continued engagement with activities and/or return to school or work.
3. Signpost AYA to further information and support from charities, trusted up-to-date social media accounts, and other organisations for general information about living with RMD and further resources and support.
4. Enable peer-to-peer support with other AYA with RMD, and help the young person make connections through charities and organisations.
5. Encourage parents, family members and/or partners to be supportive in helping the young person gain independence and social contacts in line with typical AYA social development.
6. Engage AYA in shared decision-making regarding treatment options, including seeing the young person alone for a portion of the consultation, to encourage independence from parents and promote self-management.

References

1. Viner R. Life stage: adolescence. In: Chief Medical Officer annual report 2012: children and young people's health. London: Department of Health; 2012. p. 1–11.

2. Eccleston C, Wastell S, Crombez G, Jordan A. Adolescent social development and chronic pain. Eur J Pain. 2016;12(6):765–74. https://doi.org/10.1016/j.ejpain.2007.11.002.
3. Orben A, Tomova L, Blakemore S-J. The effects of social deprivation on adolescent development and mental health. Lancet Child Adolesc Health. 2020;4(8):634–40. https://doi.org/10.1016/S2352-4642(20)30186-3.
4. Eleftheriou D, Isenberg DA, Wedderburn LR, Ioannou Y. The coming of age of adolescent rheumatology. Nat Rev Rheumatol. 2014;10(3):187–93. https://doi.org/10.1038/nrrheum.2013.202.
5. Donaghy B, Moore D, Green J. Co-occurring physical health challenges in neurodivergent children and young people: a topical review and recommendation. Child Care Pract. 2023;29(1):3–21. https://doi.org/10.1080/13575279.2022.2149471.
6. Armon K. Outcomes for Juvenile idiopathic arthritis. Paediatr Child Health. 2014;24(2):64–71. https://doi.org/10.1016/j.paed.2013.07.008.
7. Snelgrove R. Living with a chronic illness in adolescence and emerging adulthood. Doctoral thesis 2012.
8. Jones A, Caes L, McMurtry MC, Eccleston C, Jordan A. Sociodevelopmental challenges faced by young people with chronic pain: a scoping review. J Pediatr Psychol. 2020;46(2):219–30. https://doi.org/10.1093/jpepsy/jsaa101.
9. Hema C, Rosemarie B, Yiannis I, Debajit S, Heidi L, Alice CR, Sam N. 299 The impact of juvenile idiopathic arthritis on adolescents and young adults: a qualitative study. Rheumatology. 2018;57(suppl_3) https://doi.org/10.1093/rheumatology/key075.523.
10. Bromberg MH, Connelly M, Anthony KK, Gil KM, Schanberg LE. Self-reported pain and disease symptoms persist in juvenile idiopathic arthritis despite treatment advances: an electronic diary study. Arthrit Rheumatol. 2014;66(2):462–9. https://doi.org/10.1002/art.38223.
11. Consolaro A, Ravelli A. Paediatric rheumatology: juvenile idiopathic arthritis—are biologic agents effective for pain? Nat Rev Rheumatol. 2013;9(8):447–8.
12. Bitencourt N, Kramer J, Bermas BL, Solow BE, Wright T, Makris UE. Clinical team perspectives on the psychosocial aspects of transition to adult care for patients with childhood-onset systemic lupus erythematosus. Arthritis Care Res. 2021;73(1):39–47. https://doi.org/10.1002/acr.24463.
13. Díaz-Mendoza AC, Modesto Caballero C, Navarro-Cendejas J. Analysis of employment rate and social status in young adults with childhood-onset rheumatic disease in Catalonia. Pediatr Rheumatol. 2015;13(1) https://doi.org/10.1186/s12969-015-0026-8.
14. Sällfors C, Hallberg LR-M. Fitting into the prevailing teenage culture: a grounded theory on female adolescents with chronic arthritis. Int J Qual Stud Health Well Being. 2009;4(2):106–14. https://doi.org/10.1080/17482620802431862.

15. Tunnicliffe DJ, Singh-Grewal D, Chaitow J, Mackie F, Manolios N, Lin M-W, O'neill SG, Ralph AF, Craig JC, Tong A. Lupus means sacrifices: perspectives of adolescents and young adults with systemic lupus erythematosus. Arthritis Care Res. 2016;68(6):828–37. https://doi.org/10.1002/acr.22749.
16. Kietz D. Psychosocial aspects in pediatric rheumatology. Curr Opin Rheumatol. 2004;16(5):555–9.
17. Hackett J, Johnson B, Shaw KL, McDonagh JE. Friends united: an evaluation of an innovative residential self-management programme in adolescent rheumatology. Br J Occup Ther. 2005;68(12):567–73. https://doi.org/10.1177/030802260506801206.
18. Beneitez I, Nieto R, Hernández E, Boixadós M. Adolescents' social needs living with juvenile idiopathic arthritis and their views about digital resources. Adv Rheumatol. 2020;60(1) https://doi.org/10.1186/s42358-020-00138-4.
19. Modica R, Lomax KG, Batzel P, Cassanas A. Impact of systemic juvenile idiopathic arthritis/Still's disease on adolescents as evidenced through social media posts. Open Access Rheumatol Res Rev. 2018;1073-81 https://doi.org/10.2147/OARRR.S165010.
20. Jetha A, Badley E, Beaton D, Fortin PR, Shiff NJ, Rosenberg AM, Tucker LB, Mosher DP, Gignac MAM. Transitioning to employment with a rheumatic disease: the role of independence overprotection and social support. J Rheumatol. 2014;41(12):2386–94. https://doi.org/10.3899/jrheum.140419.
21. Martin R, Taylor R, Kelly C. Recognising the rheumatological needs of neurodivergent females: commentary. Rheumatology. 2023;3(4):221–7. https://doi.org/10.3390/rheumato3040017.
22. Davis R, Crompton CJ. What do new findings about social interaction in autistic adults mean for neurodevelopmental research? Perspect Psychol Sci. 2021;16(3):649–53. https://doi.org/10.1177/1745691620958010.
23. Foley Charlene M, Deely Derek A, Jane MDE, Killeen Orla G. Arthropathy of down syndrome: an under-diagnosed inflammatory joint disease that warrants a name change. RMD Open. 2019;5(1):e000890-10.1136/rmdopen-2018-000890.
24. Backenson EM, Holland SC, Kubas HA, Fitzer KR, Wilcox G, Carmichael JA, Fraccaro RL, Smith AD, Macoun SJ, Harrison GL, Hale JB. Psychosocial and adaptive deficits associated with learning disability subtypes. J Learn Disabil. 2015;48(5):511–22. https://doi.org/10.1177/0022219413511861.
25. AYPH. Ten reasons to invest in young people's health. London: Association for Young People's Health; 2017.
26. Stinson JN, Toomey PC, Stevens BJ, Kagan S, Duffy CM, Huber A, Malleson P, McGrath PJ, Yeung RSM, Feldman BM. Asking the experts: exploring the self-management needs of adolescents with arthritis. Arthritis Care Res. 2008;59(1):65–72. https://doi.org/10.1002/art.23244.

27. Hart RI, McDonagh JE, Thompson B, Foster HE, Kay L, Myers A, Rapley T. Being as normal as possible: how young people ages 16–25 years evaluate the risks and benefits of treatment for inflammatory arthritis. Arthritis Care Res. 2016;68(9):1288–94. https://doi.org/10.1002/acr.22832.
28. Howsley P, Dunkley L, Calvert R, Hawley S, Tattersall R, McMahon A-M, Hawley D. Psychological/social factors associated with transfer readiness in young people with juvenile idiopathic arthritis. Clin Rheumatol. 2022;41(12):3777–82. https://doi.org/10.1007/s10067-022-06237-5.
29. Nabors L, Ige Teminijesu J, Fevrier B. Peer support and psychosocial pain management strategies for children with systemic lupus erythematosus. J Immunol Res. 2015;1-5 https://doi.org/10.1155/2015/238263.
30. Camara M, Bacigalupe G, Padilla P. Int J Adolesc Youth. 2016;22(2):123–36. https://doi.org/10.1080/02673843.2013.875480.
31. Waite-Jones JM, Swallow V. Peer-based social support for young-people with juvenile arthritis: views of young people parents/carers and healthcare professionals within the UK. J Pediatr Nurs. 2018;43e85-e91 https://doi.org/10.1016/j.pedn.2018.07.012.
32. Nabors LA, Iobst EA, Weisman J, Precht B, Chiu P, Brunner H. School support and functioning for children with juvenile rheumatic diseases. J Dev Phys Disabil. 2007;19(2):81–9. https://doi.org/10.1007/s10882-007-9038-8.
33. van Middendorp H, Evers AWM. The role of psychological factors in inflammatory rheumatic diseases: from burden to tailored treatment. Best Pract Res Clin Rheumatol. 2016;30(5):932–45. https://doi.org/10.1016/j.berh.2016.10.012.
34. Mazzoni D, Cicognani E. Problematic social support from patients' perspective: the case of systemic lupus erythematosus. Soc Work Health Care. 2014;53(5):435–45. https://doi.org/10.1080/00981389.2014.888124.
35. Sara AK, Jennifer S, Paula F, Stephanie L, Lauren H. Been there done that: the experience of acting as a young adult mentor to adolescents living with chronic illness. J Pediatr Psychol. 2017;42(9):962–9. https://doi.org/10.1093/jpepsy/jsx062.
36. Stinson J, Ahola Kohut S, Forgeron P, Amaria K, Bell M, Kaufman M, Luca N, Luca S, Harris L, Victor C, Spiegel L. The iPeer2Peer Program: a pilot randomized controlled trial in adolescents with juvenile idiopathic arthritis. Pediatr Rheumatol. 2016;14(1) https://doi.org/10.1186/s12969-016-0108-2.
37. Kaushansky D, Cox J, Dodson C, McNeeley M, Kumar S, Iverson E. Living a secret: disclosure among adolescents and young adults with chronic illnesses. Chronic Illn. 2017;13(1):49–61. https://doi.org/10.1177/1742395316655855.

38. Alessia A, Paul S, Elena N, Petra B, van Linda N, Sofia R, Francesco C, Christophe R, Nele C, Laure G, Marios K. Person-focused care for young people with rheumatic and musculoskeletal diseases: young rheumatologists' and EULAR Young PARE perspectives. RMD Open. 2017;3(2):e000514. https://doi.org/10.1136/rmdopen-2017-000514.
39. Packham JC, Hall MA. Long-term follow-up of 246 adults with juvenile idiopathic arthritis: education and employment. Rheumatology. 2002;41(12):1436–9. https://doi.org/10.1093/rheumatology/41.12.1436.
40. Hausmann JS, Weitzman ER. The promises and perils of social media for pediatric rheumatology. Rheum Dis Clin North Am. 2021;48(1):233–43. https://doi.org/10.1016/j.rdc.2021.09.005.
41. Hider S, Muller S, Gray L, Manning F, Brooks M, Heining D, Menon A, Packham J, Roddy E, Ryan S, Scott IC, Paskins Z. Exploring the longer-term impact of the COVID-19 pandemic on physical and mental health of people with inflammatory rheumatic diseases: a cross-sectional survey. Clin Rheumatol. 2023;42(7):1903–9. https://doi.org/10.1007/s10067-023-06565-0.
42. Caton E, Chaplin H, Carpenter L, Sweeney M, Tung HY, de Souza S, Galloway J, Nikiphorou E, Norton S. The impact of consecutive COVID-19 lockdowns in England on mental wellbeing in people with inflammatory arthritis. BMC Rheumatology. 2022;6(1) https://doi.org/10.1186/s41927-022-00266-y.
43. Sloan M, Harwood R, Gordon C, Bosley M, Lever E, Modi R, Blane M, Brimicombe J, Barrere C, Holloway L, Sutton S, D'Cruz D. Will 'the feeling of abandonment' remain? Persisting impacts of the COVID-19 pandemic on rheumatology patients and clinicians. Rheumatology. 2022;61(9):3723–36. https://doi.org/10.1093/rheumatology/keab937.
44. Shukla M, Crew A, Wu A, Riddleston L, Hutchinson T, Kumari V, Hughes LD, Lau JYF. Self-reported worries in young people during the COVID-19 pandemic. Cogn Ther Res. 2023;47(4):531–42. https://doi.org/10.1007/s10608-023-10396-3.
45. Doukrou M, Segal TY. Fifteen-minute consultation: Communicating with young people—how to use HEEADSSS a psychosocial interview for adolescents. Arch Dis Child Educ Pract Ed. 2018;103(1):15–9. https://doi.org/10.1136/archdischild-2016-311553.

4 Engaging Young People: Consultation Skills

Rachel S. Tattersall

Factors Affecting Successful Engagement with Adolescents and Young Adults

What Are the Issues for AYA in Communicating with Their Healthcare Professionals?

Adolescence and young adulthood is a time of great challenge and change for young people (see Chaps. 1, 2 and 3) as neurocognitive development proceeds and AYA identity and autonomy evolve. Advances in neuroscience (see Chap. 1) show that the challenges in communicating with young people may, at least in part, result from changes in the AYA brain related to social communication [1, 2], decision-making and threat perception [3]. HCPs need to know that young people may have difficulty in reading facial expressions and some find it difficult to express emotion. Language is also a key issue for HCPs; within peer groups, specific youth language may evolve as a marker of unity and identity.

R. S. Tattersall (✉)
Department of Rheumatology, Royal Hallamshire Hospital, Sheffield, UK

Sheffield Teaching Hospitals and Sheffield Children's Hospital, Sheffield, UK
e-mail: rachel.tattersall@nhs.net

C. Ciurtin, J. Hackett (eds.), *Adolescent and Young Adult Rheumatology In Clinical Practice*, In Clinical Practice,
https://doi.org/10.1007/978-3-031-82102-8_4

Healthcare professionals should not try and use such language but to take an open, inquisitive and non-judgemental approach, actively asking about the meaning of language or terms that AYA use.

Hallmarks of the adolescent trajectory such as risky behaviours and developing resilience are normal and necessary to adolescent development (see Chap. 3). A recognised barrier, both for AYA and their health care professionals can be the exploration of personal and intimate information and experiences that can impact on health and healthcare interventions [4]. Setting up consultations with upfront assurances of confidentiality and routine, expected assessment of psychosocial history to explore risky behaviours helps reduce barriers to communication. Resilience has become an increasingly important concept in adolescent medicine (see Chap. 2) and has neurobiological and psychosocial determinants. Fostering resilience is an important part of interactions with, and interventions offered to, adolescents [5]. Identifying resilience factors in particular can inform strategies and interventions to support management such as medicines adherence (see Chap. 21).

Framing healthcare communication, and especially active listening to AYA, in a psychosocial framework acknowledges the multifaceted nature of adolescent development. The lives of young people are complex, and health care is just one aspect. A psychosocial framework can help guide successful communication with young people and screening tools such as HEEADSSS [6] are freely available and well validated. They can be used in different ways depending on the context of the consultation [7]. All domains can be explored fully when there are concerns or known risky behaviours affecting health domains for example. Equally the screen can be used in an abbreviated form to give an important message that you are there to talk about those things should someone wish to discuss them at a later date. Either way, starting from a position that a clinical encounter has a psychosocial context, and you are interested in the young person's whole world and not just their illness is likely to ensure the best possible consultation outcome. Evidence shows that effective communication with AYA can be learned and sustained [8] and results in improved attendance, treatment adherence (see Chap. 21) and overall health. As with people of all ages, it is important to remember AYA have a right not to answer your questions!

What Do YP Want/Need from Consultations?

AYA with long-term conditions want to be active participants in their own health care but the evidence suggests they are often 'bystanders' in clinical consultations. Triadic consultations—where parents, young people and healthcare professionals engage together—can lead to young people's voices being unheard [9]. These consultations can generate tensions and differences of opinions and often health professionals control the turn taking and agenda, while parents control their child's participation. Dyadic consultations where young people engage on a one-to-one basis with healthcare professionals enable young people to have a voice but need to be introduced and managed carefully. There can be mixed perspectives on the parent/carer role in the communication that happens in consultations. Where it is useful to the young person, that involvement should be fostered but always with the young person front and centre [10]. This is particularly important where young people may have learning disability or cognitive impairment, where strategies to ensure maximal engagement are key (see Chap. 3).

Young people are more likely to engage with, and return for, care when they trust their health care professionals [11]. They need to feel that HCPs are honest, respectful and empathetic and particularly that they are assured of confidentiality [12]. Structuring consultations on the split model where young people are seen alone for some of their consultation with assured confidentiality, but which their parents/carers are also part of, enables conversations that address key psychosocial and medical concerns [13, 14]. Health care professionals often worry about the impact and practicalities of their duty of confidentiality. A concept of conditional confidentiality can be helpful to reduce blocks to addressing this in consultations. Here the conversation with young people centres on the concept that an HCP will respect

Table 4.1 Key points on confidentiality in consultations with young people

AYA have a right to confidentiality, even if they lack capacity
Confidentiality is conditional: information will always be kept confidential unless the YP wants to share it or when not sharing would cause them or someone else harm
YP should be informed if information is to be shared, with whom and the justification for the decision to share
Confidentiality should not be kept if YP disclose significant issues that threaten their safety or that of others: examples of such disclosures include suicidal or homicidal ideation or significant self-harm
Questions to use in discussing confidentiality 'During our discussion I am going to ask you some personal questions…' 'What do you understand by confidentiality?' 'Whatever you say will be kept private between us; I won't tell anyone else unless you give me permission but there are three occasions I would have to tell someone else—if you were seriously harming yourself, if someone was harming you or if you said you were going to harm someone else'

their confidentiality *unless* young people want disclosure to their parents or there is a risk that what is disclosed could harm the patient or another person. Sometimes young people want clinicians to help them tell their parents important information and a consultation with a clinician that is based on trust and good communication can facilitate this. The key issue is to explore with the young person, while they are alone, what information they wish to be shared and with whom (see Table 4.1).

Practical Approaches to Improve Communication and Engagement with Young People in Clinical Consultations

A practical approach to developing both youth-friendly communication skills and strategies for clinical consultations that promote young people's participation include:

- 'Ice-breaking' or 'problem-free talk' openers to consultations in the context of the young person's cognitive context and attending to issues such as neurodiversity

- establishing how young people like to be addressed and what they can call you
- explanations about confidentiality and seeing young people routinely alone later in the consultation (dyadic or split consultations)
- motivational interviewing
- using aids to encourage YP to set the agenda in consultations

It can be particularly helpful to set up consultations to recognise the 'critical first two minutes' of a young person-centred consultation:

- Arrange seating so that the young person is in the prime position to enable communication
- Introduce yourself first to the young person (my name is X, you can call me Y—Preferred pronouns can be addressed here)
- Ask the YP what they prefer to be called, how they like to be addressed and who they have brought with them
- Open the consultation with some 'ice-breaking' 'problem-free talk'—talk to the YP first and then their parents/carer. e.g. other than your arthritis, how have you been? This enables you to begin to establish the developmental level at which the YP is operating and to frame your approach accordingly. It also begins the process of establishing trust and rapport and illuminates the skills and resilience a YP possesses
- Explain what will happen in the consultation and that it is routine for you to split the clinic time to spend some time alone with the YP later in the consultation. At this point you can discuss confidentiality.
- If a parent is present: Agenda setting—first I will let you (the young person) tell me your story, then I will ask you (the care giver) to add anything else……

Specific communication techniques that may help in a young person-centred consultation include motivational interviewing, agenda setting tools such as question prompt lists, psychosocial screening tools, engaging with parents and wrapping up a consultation; a practical approach to these is given next.

Motivational interviewing (MI) is a patient-centred communication skills approach. It works on engaging the patient's' intrinsic motivation and readiness to change, helping YP to recognise and do something about their current or potential problems [15]. Clinicians using MI are actively pursuing a strategy in consultations working towards change whilst recognising that there are different stages of motivation and readiness to change (e.g. pre-contemplation, contemplation, preparation, action and maintenance). MI is collaborative, evocative, empathic and explicitly recognises patient autonomy. Critical principles include clinicians expressing early empathy and using open ended questions and agenda setting techniques (see below). Questions and discussion are aimed at recognising and developing discrepancies that YP raise, rolling with resistance and supporting self-efficacy. Rather than a didactic approach of giving advice and directing treatment, an MI approach involves asking permission to offer advice while actively discussing and raising change on the assumption that YP are autonomous and self-efficacious. MI can improve adherence, symptom severity and quality of life in adolescents [16].

Examples of questions include

- **Looking for resources and resilience rather than problems**: ask about times when YP have taken positive steps to address and control their health. Find out how they did this, what resources they used and how they might do it again. Positive reinforcement of their skills is likely to promote similar engagement in the future
- **Discussing expert advice in a collaborative rather than didactic way:** here the HCP is a conduit for good information rather than telling a patient what to do. Giving YP choices in their health care improves their engagement. An open discussion is more likely to enable YP to ask questions that are important to them

Question prompt lists (QPL) are lists of topics either generated by healthcare teams or patients or both used just before a consultation to enable patients to select priority areas they wish to discuss. There is evidence that such aids may increase patients question asking and lead HCPs to offer more information [17]. There is emerging evidence that QPLs in conjunction with web-based video educational information are particularly effective in helping engage YP [18].

Psychosocial screening; this addresses all aspects of YPs lives and helps to understand what factors might put them at risk and which characteristics they possess which make them resilient, able to withstand challenge and change and ultimately protect themselves (see Chap. 3). HEEADSSS is a validated screen which is easy to use in clinical consultations [6, 7]. Questions are asked with the YP alone and in the positive, open, empathic, respectful and resilience-seeking approaches described above. HEEADSSS covers the following domains:

Home	'Who lives with you at home?'
Education	'Are you at school, college or at work?'
Eating	'How is your appetite?' 'Is your weight stable' 'do you ever struggle with food?'
Activity	'What kinds of things do you like to do outside school/work?' 'Who do you do those things with?' 'How much physical activity do you do?'
Drugs (including alcohol and tobacco)	'Do your friends drink alcohol—Do you drink alcohol? If so when and how much do you drink?' 'Do your friends smoke? Do you? Just tobacco or anything else?'
Sexuality, sexual and reproductive health	'Do you have a partner?' 'Are you sexually active/having sex?' 'Do you know about safe sex?' 'What does safe sex mean to you?' 'Can we talk about using condoms?'
Suicide/low mood	'How are you in yourself?' 'Do you ever feel stressed or distressed? Have those feelings been so bad you worried you might not cope?' 'Have you ever harmed yourself—anything from pinching or punching yourself to cutting?' 'Have you thought about taking your own life?'

(continued)

Safety (including social media)	'Which social media platforms do you use?' 'Have you ever been uncomfortable with what others, have posted about you or been bullied online?' 'What did you do about that? How would you ask for help if you felt you were in a dangerous situation?'
Training app	https://app.appinstitute.com/heeadsss

For some HCP a barrier to psychosocial screening is the worry that YP answers to some questions may be challenging and that the HCP won't know the answer or be able to help. A key approach in young-person friendly services is the 'no wrong door approach' meaning that HCPs are able to signpost YP correctly. For example, if a young person discloses they are sexually active, then signposting to local sexual health services for contraceptive and safe sex advice is crucial. Having readily available, locally applicable signposting information gives several important messages to YP that are likely to improve their engagement; that your service is knowledgeable, you care, can be trusted and that you are interested in all aspects of their life.

It is also important to remember that you are unlikely to be able, in a single consultation, to cover all psychosocial aspects in detail. Flexibility of approach and the ability to uncover and adapt to the YP priorities on the day are best in ensuring the necessary work is done and the scene set for future consultations. Once the standard is set that psychosocial screening is a routine part of clinical care this helps YP trust and understand healthcare services and empowers them to access and use such services effectively.

There are increasing reports of the potential of digital technology in this area including tools which enable psychosocial screening based on HEADSSS to be collected before the clinical consultation [19]. In our experience, this helps with agenda setting and pitching the consultation at the right level to match the young person on a particular day.

Engaging with parents; once you have seen YP alone you may then bring parents back into the room. Parents and carers have often had to coordinate and navigate care for their young people and need help to detach from them and help their YP become empowered to manage their own healthcare. This process, and the parents'/carers' trust in you and your service, will be helped if you actively listen to and support parents whilst being clear that the YP is your primary focus. A useful strategy with parents anxious that their young person will forget to tell you something is to suggest they prepare a list of questions together the night before their appointment and decide who will ask what. If the young person is seen alone, prepare them to tell the parent the management plan when they join the consultation at the end. That way you can assess their understanding of what you have discussed and also demonstrate to the parent their developing competency in negotiating consultations independently.

Wrapping up the consultation; having completed the consultation and with the AYA alone it is important to sum up the information you have discussed and reflect this back. Firstly, this ensures you have understood them correctly and secondly it enables a focus on both the positive factors and resilience factors you have discussed as well as the difficulties and medical issues. Then confirm what information you will share and with whom, especially if you are going to see the YP again with their parents as part of the consultation. Check that the AYA has someone they can confide in, and they have the contact details for your team in case they have further questions. Confirm the date of the next appointment and if possible, offer the AYA some choice in timing. Remind YP that your clinical correspondence will be (preferably) addressed directly, or at least copied, to them and ensure that letters you write are comprehensible and as jargon-free as possible. Encourage them to keep them together in a file or folder so it becomes a "patient-held record".

Summary

Engaging with AYA requires health care professionals to recognise the kinds of understanding of the world that YP have, the pressures and priorities they experience and the different ways in which they think. Taking time to address communication skills and strategies and embracing a positive, respectful and open approach to consultations over time enables good communication with AYA. This communication is an essential part of good quality, young person-friendly care.

Key Management Points

1. Ensure consultations are young person centred (whilst listening to parents and carers and supporting their roles) and developmentally appropriate
2. Ensure the consultation is set up and tailored to the AYA needs and that the clinician has effective communication and listening skills to enable trust and rapport
3. Encourage AYA to speak and ensure clinicians listen and hear
4. Ensure neither the medical nor parental agenda is dominant
5. Ensure that young people are seen alone for some or all of the consultation (dyadic consultation)
6. Conditional confidentiality should be discussed and assured
7. Taking a psychosocial history is key in consultation with AYA and should address resilience factors as well as risk

References

1. Blakemore SJ. The social brain in adolescence. Nat Rev Neurosci. 2008;9(4):267–77. https://doi.org/10.1038/nrn2353.
2. Blakemore SJ. Inventing ourselves: the secret life of the teenage brain penguin. London: Black Swan; 2019. ISBN: 9781784161347
3. Colver A, Longwell S. New understanding of adolescent brain development: relevance to transitional healthcare for young people with long term conditions. Arch Dis Child. 2013;98(11):902–7. https://doi.org/10.1136/archdischild-2013-303945.
4. Bora K, White K. How can health professionals enhance interpersonal communication with adolescents and young adults to improve health care

outcomes?: systematic literature review. Int J Adolesc Youth. 2018;23(2):198–218. https://doi.org/10.1080/02673843.2017.1330696.
5. Malhi GS, Das P, Bell E, et al. Modelling resilience in adolescence and adversity: a novel framework to inform research and practice. Transl Psychiat. 2019;9:316. https://doi.org/10.1038/s41398-019-0651-y.
6. Klein DA, Goldenring JM, Adelman WP. HEEADSSS 3.0 the psychosocial interview for adolescents updated for a new century fueled by media. 2014 http://contemporarypediatrics.modernmedicine.com/contemporary-pediatrics/content/tags/adolescent-medicine/heeadsss-30-psychosocial-interview-adolesce?page=full
7. Doukrou M, Segal TY. Fifteen minute consultation: communicating with young people—how to use HEEADSSS, a psychosocial interview for adolescents. Arch Dis Child Educ Pract Ed. 2017;0:1–5. https://doi.org/10.1136/archdischild-2016-311553.
8. Sanci LA, Coffey CM, Veit FC, et al. Evaluation of the effectiveness of an educational intervention for general practitioners in adolescent health care: randomised controlled trial. BMJ. 2000;320:224–30.
9. Van Staa AL. Unraveling triadic communication in hospital consultations with adolescents with chronic conditions: the added value of mixed methods research. Patient Educ Couns. 2011;82:4555–464. https://doi.org/10.1016/j.pec.2010.12.001.
10. Lee RR, Mountain D, Connelly M, Palermo TM, Peters S, Cordingley L, McDonagh JE. 'That's what makes me better': investigating children and adolescents' experiences of pain communication with healthcare professionals in paediatric rheumatology. Eur J Pain. 2023;27:111–28. https://doi.org/10.1002/ejp.2043.
11. Hardin HK, Bender AE, Hermann CP, Speck BJ. An integrative review of adolescent trust in the healthcare provider relationship. J Adv Nurs. 2021;77:1645–55. https://doi.org/10.1111/jan.14674.
12. Ford CA, Millstein SG, Halpern-Felsher BL, Irwin CE Jr. Influence of physician confidentiality assurances on adolescents' willingness to disclose information and seek future health care. A randomized controlled trial. JAMA. 1997;278:1029–34. https://doi.org/10.1001/jama.1997.03550120089044.
13. Gilbert AL, Rickert VI, Aalsma MC. Clinical conversations about health: the impact of confidentiality in preventive adolescent care. J Adolesc Health. 2014;55:672–7. https://doi.org/10.1016/j.jadohealth.2014.05.016.
14. Agostino H, Toulany A. Considerations for privacy and confidentiality in adolescent health care service delivery. Paediatr Child Health. 2023;28(3):172–7. https://doi.org/10.1093/pch/pxac117.
15. Rubak S, Sandboaek A, Lauritzen T, et al. Motivational interviewing: a systematic review and meta-analysis. Br J Gen Pract. 2005;55:305–12.
16. Schaefer MR, Kavookjian J. The impact of motivational interviewing on adherence and symptom severity in adolescents and young adults with chronic illness: a systematic review. Patient Educ Couns. 2017;100:2190–9. https://doi.org/10.1016/j.pec2017.05.037.

17. Sanasoni J, Grootemaat P, Duncan C. Question prompt lists in health consultations: a review. Patient Educ Couns. 2015;98(12):1454–64. https://doi.org/10.1016/j.pec.2015.05.0150738-3991/.
18. Sleath B, Carpenter DM, Davis SA, et al. Acceptance of a pre-visit intervention to engage teens in pediatric asthma visits. Patient Educ Couns. 2017;100(11):2005–11. https://doi.org/10.1016/j.pec.2017.05.013.
19. Waller D, Bailey S, Zolfaghari E, et al. Psychosocial assessment of adolescents and young adults in paediatric hospital settings: patient and staff perspectives on implementation of the e-HEEADSSS. BMC Health Serv Res. 2023;23(1):683. https://doi.org/10.1186/s12913-023-09621-2.

5 Adolescents, Young Adults and Their Parents

Helena Fonseca and Filipa Oliveira Ramos

Introduction

Although the concept of family has evolved over time, there is evidence that parents remain their child's first role model. Parenting involves the care and guidance that enable young people to grow, develop and make appropriate choices. In recent years, there has been an increasing interest in promoting parental involvement in the lives of AYA within a resilience perspective. Tips for parents in the process of raising adolescents have been developed by several authors to address these resilience factors. When appropriate, some of them can be used in the clinical setting

H. Fonseca (✉)
Unidade de Medicina do Adolescente, Departamento de Pediatria, HSM-CHLN, Lisbon, Portugal

Unidade de Investigação em Reumatologia, Instituto de Medicina Molecular, Faculdade de Medicina, Universidade de Lisboa, Centro Académico de Medicina de Lisboa, Lisbon, Portugal

F. O. Ramos
Unidade de Investigação em Reumatologia, Instituto de Medicina Molecular, Faculdade de Medicina, Universidade de Lisboa, Centro Académico de Medicina de Lisboa, Lisbon, Portugal

Unidade de Reumatologia Pediátrica, Serviço de Reumatologia, HSM-CHLN, Lisbon, Portugal

C. Ciurtin, J. Hackett (eds.), *Adolescent and Young Adult Rheumatology In Clinical Practice*, In Clinical Practice,
https://doi.org/10.1007/978-3-031-82102-8_5

in order to facilitate parental adaptation to this life cycle stage and to their AYA living with a RMD (Table 5.1) [1].

Steinberg defined four main styles of parenting: authoritative (warm and firm); authoritarian (firm but not warm); indulgent (warm but not firm); and neglectful (neither warm nor firm). He found that AYA raised in authoritative households are more psychosocially competent, more successful in school, and less prone to internalizing or externalizing problems than their peers who have been raised in other styles [2]. AYA with RMD are no exception and their parents have to deal not only with the normal developmental challenges of adolescence (see Chaps. 1, 2 and 3) but also with their AYA's chronic condition.

Table 5.1 Ten golden rules for parents raising adolescents

Ten top tips for parents of adolescents
1. Listen to your adolescent. Always be available to talk and listen.
2. Be kind. Don't be inhibited when showing affection, provided that you do not embarrass your adolescent before friends.
3. Get involved in your adolescent's life and follow his/her academic performance. Your involvement is as important if not more so than during childhood.
4. Make an effort to get to know your adolescent's friends. That is the only way you can have to better understand his/her behavior.
5. Be firm. Set up limits and establish clear and adequate rules.
6. Avoid too much control and don't be too bossy. Autonomy is essential for an adolescent to grow up well. Provide him/her with enough room to learn how to be self-confident and to make decisions without looking for your constant advice.
7. Guide your adolescent on the most difficult decisions. He/she may not be ready or mature enough to plan, set up priorities, organize thoughts, manage impulses, and/or be thoughtful about every consequence of his/her own actions.
8. Have positive and realistic expectations about your adolescent. But be realistic: your expectations should be neither too high nor too low.
9. Help your adolescent to become a sensible and responsible citizen. Help him/her to improve his/her respect for everyone, regardless of race, gender, status, or religion.
10. Love your adolescent unconditionally.

Adapted from Fonseca [1]

RMD has a significant impact on families because the ongoing care and management rests primarily with the AYA and their family [3]. Many healthcare professionals and especially adult providers have not been sufficiently trained to assess the developmental and psychosocial challenges faced by AYA and their families with chronic conditions. The Family Adjustment and Adaptation Response Model developed by McCubbin and Patterson [4] is especially useful for examining the impact of the condition on the family as well as which resources and coping behaviors inside the family may facilitate a successful adaptation of the family unit to AYA with RMD. Throughout the life cycle of the family, the unit (like all social systems) attempts to maintain balanced functioning by using its capabilities (resources and coping behaviors) to meet its demands (stressors and strains). The seriousness and chronicity of the AYA's illness will influence the intensity of the demand and how much it interferes with the family's homeostatic state.

A variety of theoretical models dealing with a systems perspective on the family have been developed. Olson's circumplex model was developed as an attempt to bridge the gap between theory and practice. It is basically based in two dimensions (adaptability and cohesion) with a third dimension (communication) considered as a facilitating dimension [5].

- *Cohesion* is the emotional bonding that family members have toward one another. Four levels of cohesion have been defined, ranging from disengaged (very low) to enmeshed (very high) with both of these extreme levels potentially being problematic.
- Optimal functioning, comprising 'low to moderate' (separated) and 'moderate to high' (connected) levels of cohesion, means achieving a balance of togetherness and separateness. Family members are connected yet separate. The hypothesis is that too much or too little cohesion will lead to problems in the long term.
- *Adaptability/flexibility* is the ability of the family system to change in response to situational and developmental stresses. The rigid dominant pattern of family functioning is characterised by a very low level of adaptability, authoritarian

leadership, with roles seldom changing, strict discipline and too little change. In the other extreme, the chaotic dominant pattern is characterised by lack of leadership, dramatic role shifts, erratic discipline, too much change. Structured and flexible levels of adaptability are those at the centre, more conducive to healthy family functioning.

- Optimal family functioning involves a balance of stability and change. Both are necessary.
- *Communication* is the third dimension, which facilitates a family's ability to change its levels of cohesion or flexibility. The hypothesis is that communication skills make it possible for families to change in response to situational stressors and developmental transitions.

The model serves as a typology to distinguish different types of families, falling into three categories: (i) balanced; (ii) midrange; and (iii) extreme or unbalanced, as follows:

(i) Types of balanced families: flexibly connected, flexibly cohesive, structurally connected, and structurally cohesive.
(ii) Types of midrange families that are balanced on one dimension and extreme on the other. The types are chaotically connected, chaotically cohesive, flexibly enmeshed, structurally enmeshed, rigidly cohesive, rigidly connected, structurally disengaged, and flexibly disengaged.
(iii) Types of extreme or unbalanced families: chaotically disengaged, chaotically enmeshed, rigidly enmeshed, and rigidly disengaged.

A double balance of togetherness/separateness and of stability/change, portray the most protective scenario. Extreme levels of family functioning were associated with poor medication adherence, for example, in the treatment of juvenile arthritis [6], which is consistent with the findings concerning families with children who live with other conditions, such as diabetes.

Family dynamics highly influence the way AYA with RMD and their parents interact, with a significant impact on the AYA autonomy and identity construct.

There is a wide spectrum of family typologies (traditional, single, divorced, reconstructed, same-sex), coming from different cultures and backgrounds. The roles of their caregivers, however, do not differ much. A combination of a warm and firm (being able to set limits and define rules in a consistent way) style of parenting; a family functioning balanced between stability and change, togetherness and separateness, are key components of a successful parenting in all sorts of families and irrespective of having a AYA living with a chronic condition.

Case Report 1

DS, currently 21 years old, presented at age 15 with systemic lupus erythematosus (SLE) and lupus nephritis treated with corticosteroids, hydroxychloroquine, mycophenolate mofetil and enalapril with good effect. At age 17 DS became depressed, addicted to computer games and had progressive weight gain. He was in denial and began missing his treatment. He was an only child living alone with his mother (his father with alcohol dependence was living abroad). His mother was always very supportive and concerned, but felt she had no control over him. DS lost 1 year at school and had a relapse of his SLE with cerebral vasculitis. The depression worsened, and he had suicidal ideation. He was treated with cyclophosphamide and antidepressants with good adherence this time, as he became scared about the severity of his SLE.

The transition process to adult care had been initiated 2 years before but delayed until the disease was controlled. Currently, he is proceeding with his studies, never misses a clinical appointment, comes by himself and has good adherence to treatment.

The psychosocial impact of SLE on an adolescent like DS is significant (see Chaps. 1, 2, 3 and 8). His personal and family history deeply influenced his experience. When he first came to the Clinic his mother was feeling alone, despaired, concerned about DS lack of a male role model and clearly asking for external support. DS was at risk of dropping out from health care and he ultimately shared with us that he was fed up with having to come to the Clinic so often, as well as with his mum controlling him all the time. Although the tension between them was high and communication quite difficult, he readily identified his mother as the "trusted and significant other" in his life, feeling a strong sense of support from her and perceived she was someone with whom he could share his problems.

For the team managing DS, risk factors were seen to outweigh protective factors in his life, so they decided to reinforce the protective factors by providing support, relationships, experiences, and opportunities to promote positive outcomes.

The team acknowledged the mother's difficulty in allowing her son to take control of his own healthcare management, and in facilitating his autonomy to negotiate treatment plans. A family intervention was started based on:

- supporting DS and his mother in clarifying their respective demands
- modulation of empathy towards DS and his mum
- raising questions in a non-judgemental and open way
- enabling and empowering each of them to express themselves.

DS and his mother benefited from a patient and family centered care treatment plan, acknowledging that a progressive transition from parental management to self-management should happen throughout adolescence.

Because communication was difficult/damaged, some systemic therapy techniques were applied:

(i) Neutrality: health professional's neutrality has to be preserved at all cost, by challenging everyone and everything while siding with no one.
(ii) Turn-taking: involving each family member in turn, avoiding questions that invite yes/no responses, checking back with each participant and asking how they see something that others have commented on.
(iii) Circular questioning to see clearly what the definition of the problem is for each family member; for example *"What do you think X will say the problem is? … Who agrees with him?*

... Who disagrees? ... How would you put it? ... In what way is this problem a problem? ... What makes the problem a problem? ... How is it a problem for you? ... Who is it most a problem for?"

(iv) Problem solving: by asking each member *"If you could change one thing ... what would it be?"*, negotiation can be facilitated. Ideally, the adolescent/family create the solution, but if not, the health professional can make a proposal for discussion.

Case Report 2

JG, a 12 year old girl was diagnosed with polyarticular Juvenile Idiopathic Arthritis (JIA), and treated with methotrexate with a very good response. She experienced nausea on the day of her methotrexate injection and started refusing treatment at 13 years of age. The arthritis got worse and her life at school became quite difficult. Her teachers were asked to give her extra time for work, but her classmates did not understand this allowance and started bullying her. She lived with her parents and with her younger brother and sister. Her parents were very engaged in helping her cope with treatment. They invited friends over on the day of the injection and this positive distraction worked well with no more resistance to treatment and complete remission 1 year later. At school JG was asked to tell a story to the class and her parents encouraged her to present the story of an adolescent with JIA. Her classmates were very understanding, and the bullying stopped. She is now 15 years old, doing very well at school and in complete remission with a very good knowledge about her condition and management.

JG's family style of parenting could be defined as authoritative and her parents were quite involved and warm, but simultaneously able to set rules and define limits. The family was characterised by moderate to high levels of cohesion, and positive communication skills, including empathy, reflective listening, supportive interaction, maximizing the ability of family members to share their feelings with high levels of adaptability. They were able to facilitate the process of adherence to treatment such as inviting friends over and helping JG develop coping strategies. Family interaction with the school was crucial for a better understanding of the impact of JIA on her ability to partake in education and involvement with peers.

Parents often lack support in the difficult and complex task of supporting their AYA living with RMD as well as going through their own transition of relative detachment. Unmet parental needs include lack of tools to deal with difficulties related to autonomy and issues around relative attribution to disease versus normal adolescent development (e.g. parents of AYA with RMD suffering from psychosocial difficulties may be more inclined to relate these problems to their RMD) [7].

The struggle for autonomy can be stressful both for AYA and their parents and may be exacerbated by the limits implied by their RMD, and the specific medical care while longing for normality comparable to that of their peers [8].

Parents experiencing high levels of anxiety concerning 'letting go', tend to overprotect their AYA, making the road to autonomy more difficult to travel. This should be identified and supported by healthcare professionals. Peer-to-peer support should be considered for parents and in more severe cases referral to psychology services should take place [9].

In summary, there is increased evidence of the benefits of shared patient/family-centered management in chronic conditions in general [10–12]. AYA living with RMD should be viewed as any other AYA as regards the relationship they establish with their parents, acknowledging not only that this interaction changes throughout adolescence/young adulthood but also the potential impact of RMD on the development of the interaction.

Key Management Points

1. There is evidence that being raised in authoritative (warm and firm) households, leads to more psychosocially competent AYA, less prone to internalizing or externalizing problems.
2. Optimal family functioning involves a balance of stability and change, as well as a balance of togetherness and separateness. Both are necessary.
3. Parenting interventions are an unmet need and should address medical, psychosocial and vocational needs.
4. Parents could benefit from peer-parent support groups to better support the autonomy development of their AYA and facilitate the inclusion of parents' personal experiences in the proposed plans.

References

1. Fonseca H. Viver com Adolescentes. 3rd ed. Barcarena: Editorial Presença; 2005.
2. Steinberg L. We know some things: adolescent–parent relationships in retrospect and prospect. J Res Adolesc. 2001;11:1–20.
3. Patterson J, Blum RW. Risk and resilience among children and youth with disabilities. Arch Pediatr Adolesc Med. 1996;150:6928.
4. Patterson J, Garwick A. The impact of chronic illness on families: a family systems perspective. Ann Behav Med. 1994;16(2):131–42.
5. Olson DH, Gorall DM. Circumplex model of marital and family systems. In: Walsh F, editor. Normal family processes. 3rd ed. New York: Guilford; 2003. p. 514–47.
6. Chaney JM, Peterson L. Family variables and disease management in juvenile rheumatoid arthritis. J Pediatr Psychol. 1989;14:389–403.
7. Akre C, Berchtold A, Suris JC. Parent-adolescent relationship in youths with a chronic condition. Child Care Health Dev. 2016;42(1):36–41.
8. Akre C, Suris JC. From controlling to letting go: what are the psychosocial needs of parents of adolescents with a chronic illness? Health Educ Res. 2014;29(5):764–72.
9. Heath G, Farre A, Shaw K. Parenting a child with chronic illness as they transition into adulthood: a systematic review and thematic synthesis of parents' experiences. Patient Educ Couns. 2017;100:76–92.

10. Babac A, von Friedrichs V, Litzkendorf S, Zeidler J, Damm K, Graf von der Schulenburg JM. Integrating patient perspectives in medical decision-making: a qualitative interview study examining potentials within the rare disease information exchange process in practice. BMC Med Inform Decis Mak. 2019;19(1):188. https://doi.org/10.1186/s12911-019-0911-z. PMID: 31533712; PMCID: PMC6751820
11. Griffin AC, Chung AE. Health tracking and information sharing in the patient-centered era: a Health Information National Trends Survey (HINTS) study. AMIA Annu Symp Proc. 2020;2019:1041–50. PMID: 32308901; PMCID: PMC7153080
12. Smith BM, Sharma R, Das A, Aboumatar H, Pitts SI, Day J, Holzhauer K, Bass E, Bennett WL. Patient and family engagement strategies for children and adolescents with chronic diseases: a review of systematic reviews. Patient Educ Couns. 2021;104(9):2213–23. https://doi.org/10.1016/j.pec.2021.02.026. Epub 2021 Feb 15. PMID: 33678498

Principles of Assessment in Adolescent and Young Adult Rheumatology Practice

6

Sharmila Jandial

Introduction

Musculoskeletal (MSK) presentations are common, ranking highly in the self-reported health problems amongst adolescents [1], presenting commonly to primary care [2] and result from a spectrum of causes (Table 6.1), which is different to adults. In many cases the course is self-limiting, but it is important to consider potentially life-threatening 'red flag' conditions (e.g. malignancy, sepsis, vasculitis) or MSK associations with chronic conditions (e.g. inflammatory bowel disease, cystic fibrosis, psoriasis). Examination tools such as a basic examination (pGALS) [3] and a more detailed regional MSK examination (pREMS) [4] facilitate a structured approach to support clinical decision making and should be interpreted in the context of general assessment, suspected 'red flags' and systemic enquiry (Table 6.2). The important issues to highlight are described below and further illustrated with clinical cases.

S. Jandial (✉)
Paediatric Rheumatology Newcastle upon Tyne Hospitals NHS Foundation Trust, Newcastle upon Tyne, UK
e-mail: sharmila.jandial@newcastle.ac.uk

C. Ciurtin, J. Hackett (eds.), *Adolescent and Young Adult Rheumatology In Clinical Practice*, In Clinical Practice,
https://doi.org/10.1007/978-3-031-82102-8_6

Table 6.1 Differential diagnosis of musculoskeletal pain

Differential diagnosis of joint pain
Life-threatening conditions Malignancy (leukaemia, lymphoma, bone tumour) Sepsis (septic arthritis, osteomyelitis) Nonaccidental injury
Joint pain with no joint swelling Hypermobility syndromes (patients sometimes report transient swelling) Complex regional pain syndromes (localized or widespread) Orthopaedic syndromes (e.g. slipped upper femoral epiphysis, Perthes' disease) Metabolic (e.g. hypothyroidism, lysosomal storage diseases) Referred pain from extra-articular causes (e.g. testicular torsion, inguinal hernia, urine infection, spinal tumour and nerve irritation)

Joint pain with joint swelling
JIA
Trauma (haemarthrosis)
Infection
  Septic arthritis and osteomyelitis (viral, bacterial [including Lyme disease], mycobacterial)
  Reactive arthritis (post-enteric, sexually acquired)
  Infection-related (rheumatic fever, vaccination-related)
Inflammatory bowel disease (Crohn's disease, ulcerative colitis)
Autoimmune rheumatic disease (systemic lupus erythematosus, scleroderma, dermatomyositis)—Joint swelling may be minimal (arthralgia > arthritis)
Sarcoidosis
Metabolic (e.g. osteomalacia [rickets], cystic fibrosis, mucopolysaccharidoses)
Haematological (haemophilia, haemoglobinopathy)
Tumour (benign/malignant)
Developmental/congenital (e.g. spondylo-epiphyseal dysplasia)
Chromosomal (e.g. Down's-related arthritis)

Table 6.2 General examination in the context of musculoskeletal disease

	Features	Context and comments
General observations	Overall impression of well-being Appearance, demeanour and interaction with parent or carer Features of dysmorphism (including faces and limbs/trunk/limb proportions) Height and weight plotted on a growth chart Pubertal status	An unwell AYA will require prompt admission and assessment for malignancy or sepsis Local safeguarding policies should be followed if concerns arise in the course of the consultation Faltering growth may be a sign of systemic or chronic disease, congenital syndrome or endocrine problem; Abnormal trunk and limb proportions may not be apparent until final skeletal height is achieved (e.g. marfanoid syndromes)
Skin inspection	Look for rashes including scalp and hair Overall feel of the skin, including colour and texture	Skin psoriasis—check extensor surfaces, scalp and if indicated natal cleft Skin elasticity and scars suggestive of heritable collagen disorders Evidence of self-harming behaviour may be on upper, non-dominant arms and thighs and should be handled sensitively; there may be reluctance to expose areas Malar butterfly rash—JSLE or JDM Violaceous heliotrope rash or Gottron's papules on the hands—JDM Evanescent macular salmon pink rash may be seen in systemic-onset JIA (often occurs with spikes of fever) and may demonstrate Koebner phenomenon Localized scleroderma may present with an isolated patch of pigmented skin (morphoea)—Systemic sclerosis is rare in childhood Vasculitis or livedo rash may occur in connective tissue disease (including JSLE or JDM)

(continued)

Table 6.2 (continued)

	Features	Context and comments
Nail examination	Nail pitting (psoriasis) Nail beds and capillaroscopy can be aided by magnification using a gel and ophthalmoscope or dermascope	Nail change of psoriasis may be subtle and the only manifestation of psoriasis Dilated, tortuous nail bed capillaries suggest active inflammation in the context of connective tissue disease
Ear, nose and throat examination	Cervical lymphadenopathy Oral mucosa, gums and teeth Ears and nose (bridge and mucosa) Parotid swelling if sicca features or suspicion of connective tissue disease or sarcoidosis	Significant cervical lymphadenopathy may occur in malignancy or multisystem disease Mouth ulcers—JSLE, inflammatory bowel disease and Bechet's disease. Perianal or genital examination may be required but should be handled sensitively, with a chaperone Dry mucous membranes, sometimes with poor dental dentition, may suggest Sjögren's syndrome (isolated or within mixed connective tissue disease) Poor dental hygiene is a concern, particularly in the immunosuppressed AYA, and may be more common in JIA with temporomandibular involvement or micrognathia ENT abnormalities are common in ANCA +ve vasculitis, e.g. saddle nose, sinusitis (granulomatosis with polyangiitis)
Cardiovascular	Blood pressure and pulses Presence of bruits Heart sounds	Hypertension in the context of rheumatic disease may signify renal involvement (e.g. vasculitic disease) Pericarditis is a feature of systemic-onset JIA and vasculitic disease Cardiac abnormalities are a feature of non-benign hypermobility syndromes (e.g. Marfan's and Ehlers–Danlos)

Respiratory	Lung fields Pulmonary function testing	Restrictive lung disease may be seen in connective tissue disease
Abdominal	Presence of tenderness/guarding Bruits Hepatosplenomegaly	Hepatosplenomegaly can be seen in multisystem disease, including SoJIA, vasculitis but also malignancy or inflammatory bowel disease Inflammatory bowel disease may coexist with inflammatory arthritis
Neurological	Full neurological examination of the lower limbs is always indicated with back pain Cranial nerve assessment in the context of headache Assessment of muscle strength	Abnormal neurological examination (such as altered sensation or hyper-reflexia) in back pain should lead to urgent imaging and expert assessment MRI ± angiography may be needed if cerebral vasculitis is suspected Reduced muscle strength is seen in JDM and mixed connective tissue disease
Eye	Acute red eye Reduced visual acuity Fundoscopy Slit lamp examination	In the AYA with JIA, chronic anterior uveitis may be asymptomatic and only detected by eye screening. Acute anterior uveitis may present with photophobia and a painful red eye as a feature of HLA-B27-related JIA/ERA Multisystem disease (e.g. Bechet's disease, sarcoidosis, vasculitis) may manifest with ocular involvement
Renal	Blood pressure Urinalysis	Haematuria is a feature of renal disease associated with ANCA +ve vasculitis JSLE-associated nephritis may present with hypertension and proteinuria Exclusion of UTI is important particularly if immunosuppressed

ANCA anti-neutrophil cytoplasmic antibodies, *ENT* ear, nose and throat, *ERA* enthesitis related arthritis*;* *JDM* juvenile dermatomyositis, *JIA* juvenile idiopathic arthritis, *JSLE* juvenile systemic lupus erythematosus, *UTI* urinary tract infection

The Impact of Growth

Normal variants (of age-related growth) in early childhood remain relevant to the AYA as persistent changes beyond accepted age ranges may present with functional problems (e.g. gait abnormality). Orthopaedic conditions (at the hip in particular) need to be excluded, e.g. persistent femoral anteversion presenting with intoeing, tarsal coalition and the painful nonmobile flat foot. Joint hypermobility is common and may be associated with nonspecific MSK pain (see Chap. 12).

Localised growth abnormalities also occur and may indeed become more severe in adolescence, e.g. scoliosis from a primary defect in the spine or secondary to leg malalignment from leg length inequality and valgus deformity at the knee (from chronic untreated arthritis), micrognathia and shortened digits.

Pattern Recognition

The spectrum of MSK pathology varies with age, such as causes of limp (Table 6.3). The differential diagnosis of the acute limp must include orthopaedic conditions; slipped upper femoral epiphysis is more common in adolescents (especially if overweight).

Chronic limp may result from a number of conditions including missed developmental dysplasia of the hip, or previous joint disease (e.g. Perthes, JIA or septic arthritis). Patterns of joint involvement and extra-articular features in JIA for the AYA differ from both adult rheumatoid arthritis and the younger child with JIA (see Chap. 7).

Table 6.3 Significant causes of limp

	4–10 years	11–16 years
Most common	Trauma Transient synovitis Perthes' disease	Trauma Osgood–Schlatter disease
Conditions requiring urgent intervention	Osteomyelitis Septic arthritis	Osteomyelitis Septic arthritis
	Nonaccidental injury Malignant disease (e.g. acute lymphocytic leukaemia)	Slipped upper femoral epiphysis Malignancy (e.g. bone tumours)
	Testicular torsion Appendicitis Inguinal hernia	
Other important conditions to consider at all ages	JIA Late presentation of developmental dysplasia of the hip Metabolic (e.g. rickets) Haematological disease (e.g. sickle cell anaemia) Reactive arthritis Lyme arthritis	

The History and the Physical Examination

The systematic enquiry into family and past history may be helpful (see Tables 6.1 and 6.2). A recent travel history (e.g. to an endemic area for Lyme disease) may be informative, and a sexual history is important in the adolescent with reactive arthritis and needs to be explored sensitively, acknowledging safeguarding concerns and the need for privacy and confidentiality. A medication history (e.g. response to NSAIDs, potential for drug-induced lupus), family history (e.g. autoimmune disease, muscle disease), social history and family dynamics may be also revealing. It is important to probe for symptoms suggestive of inflammatory joint or muscle disease (e.g. morning stiffness, gelling after rest, swelling) and discriminate against mechanical causes of pain (e.g. locking or giving way, pain worse on weight bearing or exercise). Conversely non-specific aches and pains are a feature of idiopathic pain syndromes (see Chap. 13).

Red flags (such as fever, malaise, anorexia, weight loss, bone pain, persistent night waking or raised inflammatory markers) are suggestive of serious potentially life-threatening conditions (e.g. sepsis or malignancy or multisystem disease), and a full general examination is needed. Additional clinical skills pending the clinical scenario include nailfold capillaroscopy or muscle strength testing (if connective tissue or muscle disease is suspected, respectively).

MSK history-taking can be misleading, even when taken by experienced clinicians, as the history alone may not identify sites of joint involvement [5]. It is important, therefore, that in all cases where MSK disease is suspected, a basic joint examination (such as pGALS; see later) is needed, as a minimum, to assess all joints. In the examination of AYA with learning disabilities and complex medical needs, joint problems can easily be overlooked; there is an association of inflammatory joint disease with chromosomal disorders (such as Down's syndrome or DiGeorge syndrome), and many complex genetic conditions (such as mucopolysaccharidoses) may present with or develop joint problems that can be indolent in older children/AYA [6].

pGALS and pREMS Musculoskeletal Examinations

The paediatric gait, arms, legs, spine (pGALS) assessment [3] is a simple, quick, evidence-based validated approach to MSK assessment in children based on the adult GALS (gait, arms, legs, spine) screen, with a series of simple manoeuvres. pGALS is useful to identify abnormal joints (e.g. inflammatory arthritis, orthopaedic problems at the hip, scoliosis). Following pGALS, the observer is directed to a more detailed examination of the relevant area(s) using the consensus approach to paediatric regional examination of the musculoskeletal system (called pREMS) [4]. This is based on the 'look, feel, move, function' principle similar to that of adult REMS for each joint or anatomical region, although there are differences reflecting pathologies from those observed in adults and the influence of growth and development; some tests (e.g. Schober's test for lumbosacral movement) are not reliable in younger adolescents; a history of inflammatory back symptoms in the presence of equivocal physical findings may necessitate imaging (magnetic resonance imaging—MRI) of the spine and sacroiliac joints (Chap. 15).

There is no absolute age 'cut-off' as to when to use pGALS or GALS or indeed pREMS or REMS. However, we would recommend that pGALS and pREMS be used in the younger adolescents and for those with chronic disease that started in childhood, given the differences in patterns of joint involvement in JIA and spectrum of pathology in AYA compared to adults. With the expansion of telemedicine, a virtual approach to pGALS has been developed although it is difficult to replicate the hands-on feeling of detecting subtle joint effusions, for example[7].

Along with general considerations in clinical consultations with AYA such as communication skills and respecting confidentiality (see Chap. 4), MSK clinical assessment also requires:

- An appropriate environment for AYA to be assessed. The appointment letter can explain that examination is important and suggest that appropriate clothing is brought to the appointment.
- Consideration of a chaperone (other than the accompanying parent/carer/friend/partner).

Full details of the examination techniques with demonstrations are provided on the Paediatric MSK Matters (PMM) website [8] and in Further Reading and Resources.

Training in Clinical Assessment of the AYA

Traditionally adult and paediatric clinical skills are taught independently, but it is important that all healthcare professionals have an appreciation of the additional complexity of the clinical assessment of AYA, as this group will present to primary care and either adult or paediatric services (see Chaps. 1, 2, 3, and 4). Acquisition of 'core' MSK clinical skills for paediatrics and adult practice [1,

6, 9, 10] needs to start within undergraduate education as the foundation for further postgraduate training.

Clinical Scenario to Illustrate Key Differences from Paediatric and Adult Clinical Assessment

Javeen is a 15-year-old boy, born in the UK with parents from India. He attends with his adult sister as his parents are at work and presents with a sore left ankle and foot for 2–3 weeks. He initially ascribed his symptoms to sport involvement although he cannot recall a specific injury. In the last week, his pain is present in the mornings and also later as the day progresses. He has felt more tired recently but has no other health concerns. There is no specific family history or past history of note. He has no history of red eyes.

On the MSK examination, he has difficulty walking on heel on the left side, and his left calf is slightly wasted. His lumbar spine appears restricted on forward flexion (he cannot reach his knees), and he has a nonmobile flat foot on the left, restricted midfoot movement and tenderness around the left heel. His spine has no tenderness, and he has a good range of movement with a normal Schober's measurement (15 cm increasing to 21 cm). Joint examination is otherwise normal, and he has no enthesitis and tender points elsewhere, nor skin abnormality.

Diagnosis

Javeen has enthesitis-related arthritis. He is HLA-B27 positive.

Learning Points

- With a pattern of oligo-JIA in adolescence, it is important to consider ERA.
- Enquire about family history (spondyloarthropathy, inflammatory bowel disease) and acute uveitis and check for enthesitis.
- The history of pain on heel walking suggests enthesopathy.
- Consider inflammatory joint disease with a nonmobile painful flat foot.

- Muscle wasting suggests prolonged disease duration and a more chronic aetiology.
- Schober's test is not reliable as an indicator of sacroiliac joint disease in AYA, and further imaging (MRI) may be needed and is the gold standard for sacroiliac inflammation detection.

Key Management Points

1. Musculoskeletal presentations are common during adolescence and young adulthood.
2. The impact of growth, localised and generalised, should be considered during clinical assessment of adolescents.
3. Pattern recognition for the AYA differs from both adult and archetypal paediatric diseases, and should be considered in the context of the young person's developmental stage.

Acknowledgement The current author would like to thank Professor Helen Foster and acknowledge her work on the previous edition of this chapter.

References

1. Goodman JE, McGrath PJ. The epidemiology of pain in children and adolescents—a review. Pain. 1991;46(3):247–64.
2. Tan A, Strauss VY, Protheroe J, et al. Epidemiology of paediatric presentations with musculoskeletal problems in primary care. BMC Musculoskelet Disord. 2018;19:40. https://doi.org/10.1186/s12891-018-1952-7.
3. Foster HE, Jandial S. pGALS—a simple examination of the musculoskeletal system. Pediatr Rheumatol Online. 2013;11:44.
4. Foster HE, Kay LJ, May CR, Rapley TR. pREMS—pediatric regional musculoskeletal examination for school aged children. Arthritis Care Res. 2011;63(11):1503–7.
5. Goff I, Rowan A, Bateman BJ, Foster HE. Poor sensitivity of musculoskeletal history in children. Arch Dis Child. 2012;97(7):644–6.
6. Chan MO, Sen E, Heasman P, Rapley T, Wraith E, Clayton E, Foster HE. Detecting joint abnormalities in children with mucopolysaccharidoses using pGALS. Pediatr Rheumatol Online J. 2014;12:32.

7. Shenoi S, Hayward K, Curran ML, et al. Telemedicine in pediatric rheumatology: this is the time for the community to embrace a new way of clinical practice. Pediatr Rheumatol. 2020;18:85. https://doi.org/10.1186/s12969-020-00476-z.
8. Smith N, Rapley T, Jandial S, English C, Davies B, Wyllie R, Foster HE. Paediatric musculoskeletal matters (pmm)—collaborative development of an online evidence based interactive learning tool and information resource for education in paediatric musculoskeletal medicine. Pediatr Rheumatol Online J. 2016;5;14(1):1.
9. Goff I, Wise E, Boyd D, Jandial S, Foster HE. Paediatric musculoskeletal medicine for primary care. Educ Prim Care. 2014;25:249–56.
10. Jandial S, Stewart J, Foster HE. What do medical students need to know about musculoskeletal medicine? BMC Med Educ. 2015;15:171.

Further Reading and Resources

BSR eLearning modules—https://rheumatologylearning.com—modules on adult JIA targeting educational needs of adult Rheumatology healthcare professionals.

Clinical skills resources for healthcare professionals hosted on Versus Arthritis https://www.versusarthritis.org/about-arthritis/healthcare-professionals/.

E-Learning for Healthcare. https://www.e-lfh.org.uk—modules on limp, normal Development and adolescent health issues.

EULAR/PReS Online course in Paediatric rheumatology https://www.eular.org/edu_online_course_paediatric.cfm.

EUTEACH—https://www.unil.ch/euteach/en/home.html—European Training in Effective Adolescent care and health.

Paediatric musculoskeletal matters[12] www.pmmonline.org. An online educational resources hosted by PReS.

pGALS app—a free resource. Available through app stores and in multiple languages.

Part II

Specific Autoimmune Rheumatic Conditions In Adolescence and Young Adulthood

Juvenile Idiopathic Arthritis in Adolescents and Young Adults

7

Kirsten Minden and Varvara Choida

Juvenile Idiopathic Arthritis

Juvenile idiopathic arthritis (JIA) is the most common chronic inflammatory rheumatic disease of adolescence and young adulthood. JIA encompasses all arthritides of unknown cause in childhood and adolescence and affects between 16 and 140 per 100,000 individuals in European populations [1]. Its prevalence is higher in adolescence than in childhood [2].

K. Minden (✉)
Department of Pediatric Respiratory Medicine, Immunology and Critical Care Medicine, Charité—Universitätsmedizin Berlin, Berlin, Germany

German Rheumatism Research Center, Epidemiology Unit, Berlin, Germany
e-mail: minden@drfz.de

V. Choida
Rheumatology Department, Homerton Healthcare NHS Foundation Trust, London, UK

Centre for Adolescent Rheumatology, Division of Medicine, University College London, London, UK
e-mail: v.choida@ucl.ac.uk

C. Ciurtin, J. Hackett (eds.), *Adolescent and Young Adult Rheumatology In Clinical Practice*, In Clinical Practice,
https://doi.org/10.1007/978-3-031-82102-8_7

Classification

All chronic arthritides of unknown cause occurring before the age of 16 are referred to as JIA according to the International League of Associations for Rheumatology (ILAR) criteria [3].

JIA thus represents a heterogeneous group of diseases with different clinical phenotypes, courses, and outcomes. Seven different JIA categories are currently differentiated based on clinical and laboratory features (Table 7.1). The JIA category distribution varies worldwide, among ethnic groups, and according to age [6]. For example, AYA are more likely to have polyarticular JIA and enthesitis-related-arthritis (ERA) than children. In view of the similarities between certain JIA categories, such as systemic JIA, rheumatoid factor (RF)-positive polyarthritis, and ERA with adult-onset Still's disease, rheumatoid arthritis and axial or peripheral spondyloarthritis, respectively in adults, there is a drive to review the ILAR criteria to facilitate the integration of these JIA categories and their adult-onset disease counterparts [7]. There is currently a lack of alignment between the classification criteria used for the diagnosis of spondyloarthritis in adults (developed by the Assessment of Spondyloarthritis International Society) and the JIA ILAR classification in children [8]. As a result, adolescents who meet the spondyloarthritis criteria will usually meet the ILAR classification criteria for ERA, psoriatic arthritis (PsA), or undifferentiated JIA. This has led to the emergence of the term juvenile spondyloarthritis with a view to harmonising the diagnosis and treatment of spondyloarthritis across ages. Despite some minor differences in the demographics and clinical presentation of systemic JIA and adult-onset Still's disease, these conditions are considered a continuum of the same disease and have been recently renamed as Still's disease [9].

Many young people will have ongoing care in adult clinics. They continue to have JIA and should not be reclassified in adulthood as having another type of inflammatory arthritis, because clinical phenotypes (with the exception of cases with systemic JIA, spondyloarthritis and RF-positive polyarthritis discussed above), genetic background, laboratory findings (e.g.,

Table 7.1 JIA categories and their specifics in adolescence and young adulthood

JIA category	Estimated relative frequency (in %)	Clinical features	To be considered in adult rheumatology
Oligoarthritis	35–45	Persistent oligoarthritis: <5 joints affected. Extended oligoarthritis: >4 joints affected. Most frequently affected joints: knee, ankle, elbow. Anterior asymptomatic uveitis in 15–20% of cases.	ANA can persist with inactive disease. Flares may occur after years of remission, uveitis activity may not correlate with arthritis activity. Insidious uveitis developing de novo in AYA is rare, but uveitis may flare after stopping MTX or adalimumab. Acute phase reactants are often normal in active disease.
Polyarthritis, RF- negative	15–25	>4 joints affected, often symmetric involvement of large and small joints. Anterior asymptomatic uveitis in about 10% of cases.	Can flare as oligoarthritis. Arthritis may present with increasing joint restrictions and without relevant swelling. Acute phase reactants can be normal in active disease, ANA can persist, anti- CCP antibodies are negative in >70%.
Enthesitis-related arthritis	15–25	Asymmetric oligoarthritis in 60–80% (especially of large joints of lower limb) and/or enthesitis in 50–70% of cases [8], HLA-B27-positivity in 50–70% of cases. Acute (symptomatic) anterior uveitis in about 10% of cases. Inflammatory back pain and/or sacroiliac joint tenderness in about one-third of the cases in early disease.	Axial disease and sacroiliitis are rare at disease onset, but progressively appear months to years after the onset (e.g. in more than half of AYA with JIA after at least 5 years of disease). Radiological alterations usually do not appear during adolescence, but incidence of defined ankylosing SpA increases over time (12–42% after 3–5 years, 19–90% after 9–11 years) [11].

(continued)

Table 7.1 (continued)

JIA category	Estimated relative frequency (in %)	Clinical features	To be considered in adult rheumatology
Psoriatic arthritis (PsA)	5–10	Arthritis (involvement of small joints, including distal interphalangeal joints) and psoriasis, dactylitis, nail abnormalities. Two different phenotypic subpopulations, depending on age at onset: (i) early-onset PsA (<6 years) similar to early-onset oligoarticular and polyarticular JIA; often with dactylitis and small joint involvement. (ii) later-onset PsA, more frequently with psoriasis, psoriatic nail changes, enthesitis, inflammatory back pain than with early-onset PsA. Anterior asymptomatic uveitis in 5–10% of cases with early PsA onset, symptomatic uveitis in late-onset PsA. Family history of psoriasis in first-degree relatives.	Psoriasis in only 50% of cases, rash may appear years after arthritis. Variable joint involvement, often polyarticular disease in adulthood.
Systemic JIA (or Still's disease)	3–7	Arthritis, fever, rash. Other manifestations: serositis, hepatosplenomegaly, lymphadenopathy. MAS in 6–10% of cases. No uveitis.	Systemic signs may be absent in adolescence/adulthood, a severe polyarthritis may then be present. MAS can occur at any stage of disease and can be triggered by infection or drugs.

Polyarthritis, RF- positive	2–5	>4 joints affected, often symmetric involvement (especially hands and feet, shoulders, and hips). Presence of RF IgM, anti-CCP antibodies. Mostly affects adolescent females. No uveitis.	High risk of progressive disease course and of relapse after DMARD withdrawal. Represents early onset of rheumatoid arthritis.
Other (undifferentiated) arthritis	2–5	Overlap between categories. Family history of psoriasis in first-degree relative. RF may be present. Uveitis (mostly asymptomatic) in 5–10% of cases.	

Legend: *ANA* antinuclear antibodies, *AYA* adolescents and young adults, *CCP* citrullinated cyclic peptides, *DMARD* disease modifying anti-rheumatic drugs, *Ig* immunoglobulin, *MAS* macrophage activation syndrome, *MTX* methotrexate, *RF* Rheumatoid factor, *SpA* spondyloarthritis

autoantibodies, inflammatory parameters), treatment responses and outcomes in JIA are different from adult-onset arthritis.

Presentation

About a third of all JIA cases start in adolescence. ERA, RF-positive polyarthritis and late onset of PsA have disease onset peaks in adolescence (Fig. 7.1). Clinical features of the different JIA categories are shown in Table 7.1. The juvenile form of SpA differs from that of adults, as it is characterised by a more peripheral pattern of arthritis with less frequent axial disease, at least at disease onset (Table 7.1) [10].

Two-thirds of AYA with JIA are female, and females predominate in all JIA categories, except in systemic JIA and ERA. AYA with JIA are usually ill on average for more than 5 years, which

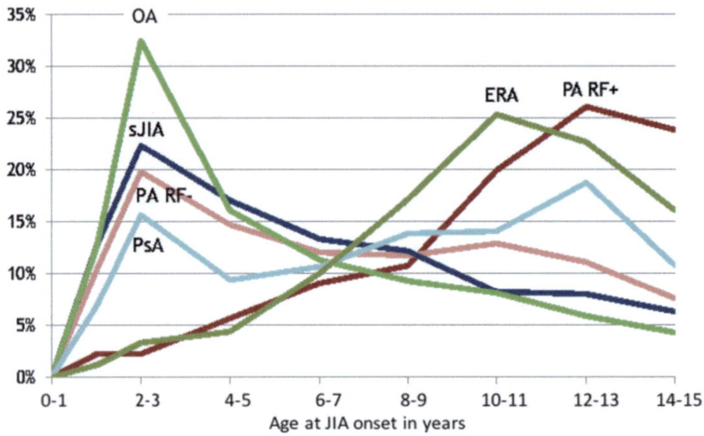

Fig. 7.1 Age at onset of selected categories of JIA: Data were derived from 8935 AYA with JIA recorded in the German paediatric rheumatologic database in 2016. Legend: *ERA* enthesitis-related arthritis, *OA* oligoarthritis, *PA RF* rheumatoid factor-negative polyarthritis, *PA RF+* rheumatoid factor-positive polyarthritis, *sJIA* systemic JIA, *PsA* psoriatic arthritis. (Figure modified after Hochberg, Rheumatology, 7e - 2-volume set, Elsevier, Atlanta, USA, Copyright © 2018)

burdens them in many ways [11]. Active disease and intensive treatment are associated with a reduced quality of life, due to pain, disease symptoms and limitations in physical function that lead to restricted participation in daily activities. Additionally, AYA experience potential side effects and psychosocial effects from treatments [12]. Pain has been identified as a major contributor to impaired quality of life for young people with JIA. Decreased pain thresholds have been reported in young adults with active and inactive disease, compared to controls [13], which might explain the persistence of pain in a subset of AYA with inactive disease. A 'treat-to-target' approach, irrespective of the treatment used, has demonstrated a reduction in pain levels [14]. Even though more than half have no functional limitations according to the Childhood Health Assessment Questionnaire (C-HAQ) [15], AYA report numerous functional limitations with far reaching consequences (Fig. 7.2). The inflammatory load of the disease often decreases over time.

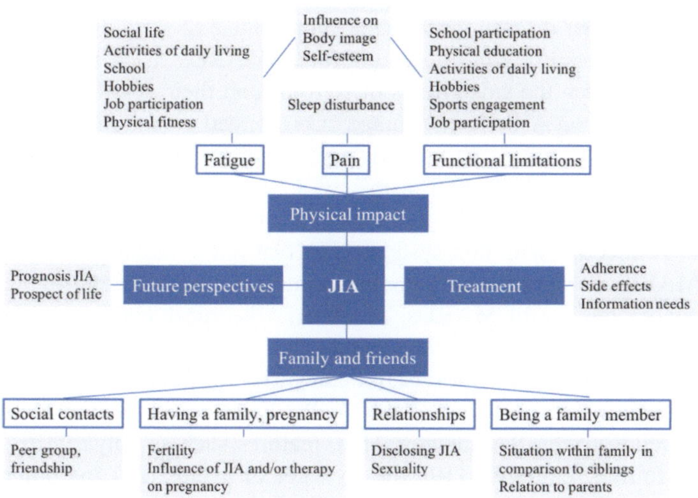

Fig. 7.2 Areas of life on which JIA has a special impact from AYA's point of view. (Figure modified according to Eyckmans et al. [16])

Management

Specialised rheumatology multidisciplinary teams are integral to optimal management of JIA. Treatment includes drug therapy, physical therapy, occupational therapy, and psychosocial support. Increasing evidence supports accelerated, early treatment pathways with a treatment goal of clinically inactive, or at least minimally active, disease. Such 'treat-to-target' approaches require standard evaluations of disease activity (see below).

Drug treatment is based on the use of non-steroidal anti-inflammatory drugs (NSAIDs), corticosteroids, conventional synthetic (cs), biologic (b) and targeted synthetic (ts) disease-modifying anti-rheumatic drugs (DMARDs). NSAIDs and intra-articular corticosteroids (IAC) are the mainstay of treatment for oligoarthritis, and are used in all JIA categories in addition to other therapies as needed. IACs are usually administered under general anesthesia in children; adolescents must gradually get used to injections under local or inhaled nitrous oxide anesthesia, which is a similar approach to adult practice. Systemic corticosteroid use has become uncommon and is limited to severe polyarticular disease for which a short course of steroids may be advisable as bridging therapy before DMARDs reach their full effect. Given the side effects of steroids and their possible negative effect on AYA's body image, a prolonged course of steroids should be avoided, particularly in the peripubertal phase when such side effects are often worse.

Methotrexate (MTX) is the most commonly used csDMARD in JIA. AYAs with non-systemic JIA that fail to respond to csDMARDs or discontinue them due to intolerance or side effects are candidates for bDMARDs. Nausea is the most common side effect of MTX and is more common in adolescents than young adults [17]. For the various JIA categories, different bDMARDs have become available (Table 7.2). The choice of treatment depends on the JIA category [18], features such as polyarthritis, sacroiliitis, enthesitis [19], the presence of uveitis [20] and other extra-articular manifestations. The most commonly used bDMARDs in non-systemic JIA are tumour necrosis factor

Table 7.2 Drug therapy for the various JIA categories and JIA-associated uveitis

	Persistent oligoarthritis	Polyarthritis (RF negative or positive), extended oligoarthritis	Enthesitis-related arthritis	Psoriatic arthritis	Systemic arthritis (or Still's disease)	JIA-associated uveitis
First-line	NSAIDs ± intra-articular corticosteroids.	csDMARDs: methotrexate, preferred over sulfasalazine, leflunomide and hydroxychloroquine; NSAIDs ± intra-articular corticosteroids (as adjunct therapy).	With sacroiliitis: NSAIDs Without sacroiliitis: NSAIDs, csDMARDs (methotrexate, sulfasalazine)	NSAIDs: if oligoarthritis/enthesitis present; csDMARDs are preferred for polyarthritis (methotrexate preferred over sulfasalazine, if active psoriasis)	NSAID (short trial if appropriate before bDMARD); Anakinra, canakinumab, tocilizumab (tapering of these treatments is recommended in inactive disease); Co-administration of steroids may be needed at the initial phase, although longer courses are not recommended anymore.	Topical cortico steroids (in selected complicated cases, systemic glucocorticoids can be used as short-term bridging therapy)

(continued)

Table 7.2 (continued)

	Persistent oligoarthritis	Polyarthritis (RF negative or positive), extended oligoarthritis	Enthesitis-related arthritis	Psoriatic arthritis	Systemic arthritis (or Still's disease)	JIA-associated uveitis
Second-line	csDMARDs (methotrexate, preferred over sulfasalazine, leflunomide and hydroxychloroquine).	TNFi, abatacept, tocilizumab, JAKi (tofacitinib, baricitinib).	TNFi (preferred over sulfasalazine/ methotrexate for AYA with enthesitis; TNFi preferred over sulfasalazine for AYA with sacroiliitis; methotrexate monotherapy not recommended for sacroiliitis; Secukinumab, JAKi (baricitinib).	TNFi, secukinumab, JAKi (tofacitinib, baricitinib), Ustekinumab	Switch to alternative option from first-line bDMARD treatments; Methotrexate is not recommended as monotherapy in AYA with JIA and systemic symptoms, but may be used in AYA with arthritis; Ciclosporin may be used as adjunct treatment for systemic symptoms/MAS; If MAS present, additional treatments that may be used include IVIG and etoposide	Methotrexate and mycophenolate mofetil

Third-line	TNFi, abatacept, tocilizumab.	Switch to alternative option from second-line treatments; If other options from second-line treatments are not suitable or effective, rituximab may be considered.	Switch to alternative option from second-line treatments.	Switch to alternative option from second-line treatments.	In cases of residual arthritis, additional options include TNFi, abatacept and other csDMARDs, JAKi.	TNFi (adalimumab> infliximab> golimumab; etanercept should not be used); If there is no response to the above TNFi, other bDMARDs (tocilizumab, abatacept, rituximab may be considered)

Legend: TNFi (TNF-α inhibitors): etanercept, adalimumab, certolizumab pegol, golimumab, infliximab), canakinumab and anakinra: IL-1 inhibitors, tocilizumab: IL-6 inhibitor, ustekinumab: IL-12/23- inhibitor, abatacept: T-cell co-stimulatory signal blocker, rituximab: anti-CD-20 monoclonal antibody, JAKi: Janus kinase inhibitors, secukinumab: IL-17 inhibitor, triamcinolone hexacetonide is the preferred corticosteroid for intra-articular injections, bDMARDs are often given in combination with methotrexate

(TNF)-α inhibitors (TNFi), although switching bDMARDs was required in 23% of JIA cases after a median duration of treatment of 1.3 years [21]. More recently, the approval of JAK inhibitors (JAKi) has provided an oral alternative for treatment escalation after MTX or bDMARD failure. However, the long-term safety profile of JAKi in AYA is still unclear. In older people with rheumatoid arthritis, the risk of cardiovascular events, venous thrombosis, and cancer was higher with JAKi (especially Tofacitinib) than with TNFi, risk about which AYA with JIA and their families should be informed [22]. There are ongoing clinical trials to test the efficacy of other bDMARDs and tsDMARDs in JIA that are already licensed in adults, such as sarilumab, secukinumab, ixekizumab, bimekizumab, guselkumab, risankizumab, apremilast, upadacitinib and filgotinib. There is a lack of head-to-head clinical trials comparing the efficacy of treatments in JIA. Additionally, there is a requirement to identify biomarkers to predict treatment response and develop effective strategies for tapering and discontinuing treatment.

Age-specific instruments should be used to measure treatment response and outcomes. Information about subjectively perceived health has to be collected from AYA, as parent-proxy ratings differ from self-assessments in terms of evaluation of functionality, pain, and global well-being [23].

Disease Status and Damage Measures

Core parameters to assess treatment response and disease activity include:

- Physician global assessment of disease activity (PGA, by visual analogue scale [VAS], numerical rating scale [NRS])
- Patient global assessment of well-being (by VAS, NRS)
- Functional ability up to the age of 17 by CHAQ (Childhood Health Assessment Questionnaire), from 18 years on by HAQ (Health Assessment Questionnaire)
- Active joint count (10, 27 or 71-joint count)

- Restricted joint count
  - Laboratory parameters (erythrocyte sedimentation rate [ESR], C-reactive protein [CRP])

An active joint is defined as a joint with either swelling, or with limited movement and pain or tenderness with movement. Due to the specific joint involvement, disease activity in young people should be assessed by the juvenile arthritis disease activity score (JADAS) instead of the Disease Activity Score assessing 28 joints used in adults with rheumatoid arthritis (DAS-28). The use of DAS-28 instead of JADAS can lead to underestimation of disease activity and thus to under-treatment [24]. The JADAS is a simple sum score and includes four measures: PGA; patient global assessment of well-being; ESR, normalized to a 0–10 scale; and a count of active joints (10, 27 or 71, resulting in three JADAS-versions) [25]. A simplified three-variable version that does not include the acute-phase reactant (clinical JADAS [cJADAS]) is also available. For AYAs with ERA, in addition, the Juvenile Spondyloarthritis Disease Activity Index (JSpADA) and its modifications (JSpADA6-no Schober, no CRP/ESR; JSpADA7-no Schober; and JSpADA7-no CRP/ESR) [26] as well as the Bath Ankylosing Spondylitis Disease Activity Index (BASDAI) are validated tools for disease activity assessment.

Ultrasound and magnetic resonance imaging (MRI) scans are increasingly used for diagnostic purposes (e.g. MRI imaging of sacroiliac joints), and to monitor disease activity in AYA with JIA. MRI can be performed without sedation in AYA and is the preferred option for the assessment of axial joints [27]. Ultrasound can also be used to guide intra-articular corticosteroid injections, or assess for tendonitis or enthesitis.

Damage or permanent alterations in joint structures or extra-articular organs/systems as a result of JIA or its treatment can be evaluated by the juvenile arthritis damage index (JADI). Instruments for assessing patient-reported outcomes are shown in Table 7.3.

AYA report more frequently about pain than children with JIA, but less often than adults with inflammatory joint disease. Approximately half of AYA with JIA report pain, and approximately 30% have functional limitation, as assessed by HAQ [15].

Table 7.3 Instruments for assessing AYA-reported outcomes

Patient-reported outcomes	Examples of instruments
Health-related quality of life (HRQoL)	**Ages 10–17 years:** Pediatric Quality of Life Inventory (PedsQL) Generic Core Module and PedsQL rheumatology module Child Health Questionnaire (CHQ) Quality of My Life Questionnaire (QoMLQ) Paediatric Rheumatology Quality of Life Scale (PRQL) Juvenile Arthritis Quality of Life Questionnaire (JAQQ) **Age > 17 years:** Medical Outcomes Short-Form 36 (SF-36)
Overall well-being	VAS/NRS
Pain	VAS/NRS
Fatigue	PedsQL Multidimensional Fatigue Scale (ages 10–18 years)
Multidimensional outcome	Juvenile Arthritis Multidimensional Assessment Report (JAMAR) (ages 10–18 years)

Morbidity and Extra-Articular Manifestations of JIA

Uveitis is the most frequent extra-articular manifestation of JIA. AYA with early onset of oligoarthritis, RF-negative polyarthritis, PsA, and ANA (antinuclear antibody) positivity are at particular risk for uveitis during the first 4 years of JIA. In these AYA, asymptomatic uveitis flares may even occur in adolescence/young adulthood. Uveitis screening should therefore also be carried out in AYA (usually every 6–12 months, depending on the risk factors). AYAs with ERA and late-onset PsA are at risk for both acute (symptomatic) anterior and chronic (asymptomatic) anterior uveitis; therefore, they require screening as well. Screening for uveitis should also be considered in AYA after DMARD treatment cessation [20].

Other extra-articular manifestations of ERA include inflammatory bowel disease, cardiac (e.g., aortic insufficiency or conduction disorders) and pulmonary manifestations (e.g., upper lobe fibrosis), of which, the last two are very rare. In RF-positive polyarthritis, less severe extra-articular manifestations (e.g., rheumatoid nodules) and severe (e.g., vasculitis, interstitial lung disease) may occur. Systemic JIA (sJIA), now called Still's Disease, as the name suggests, is associated with systemic manifestations (Table 7.1). More recently, lung disease has been recognised as a complication of sJIA, especially in patients treated with bDMARDs [28, 29]. AYA with sJIA should be screened for respiratory symptoms and clinical signs of lung disease (including clubbing) and if indicated, assessed with high-resolution computer tomography (HRCT) chest and lung function tests [4].

Macrophage activation syndrome (MAS) is a rare but life-threatening complication of JIA, most frequently seen in sJIA. The diagnosis is based on the clinical presentation, which almost always includes fever, laboratory parameters, and the presence of hemophagocytosis in bone marrow aspirate (its absence does not exclude MAS) [5]. It is important to exclude other triggers and mimics of this complication, such as infections, reactions to medications, and haematological or other malignancies [30].

Altogether, AYA with JIA are more likely to develop depressive symptoms and anxiety than their peers without a chronic illness. Young people who experience these symptoms have worse quality of life, with some evidence pointing to depression and anxiety symptoms having a greater impact on quality of life than other disease features, such as active joint count [31]. In addition, AYA are at increased risk of premature atherosclerosis and early-onset cardiovascular disease due to chronic inflammation, dyslipidemia, hypertension, insulin resistance, a physically inactive lifestyle, obesity, and tobacco smoking [32]. Thus, they require anticipatory guidance to promote cardiovascular health (see Key Management Points).

Finally, AYA with JIA may not have received certain live vaccinations in childhood according to the schedule due to concurrent immunosuppressive treatment, thus it is important to consider if and when these vaccinations can be administered at a later stage. In addition, AYA with JIA should be considered for vaccination against Varicella-Zoster VZV (where possible), influenza (non-live), pneumococcus, human papillomavirus (HPV), and COVID-19 [33].

Sexuality, Fertility and Pregnancy

Individuals with JIA show a similar attitude to sexual activity, contraception, and wish for children as their age and sex-matched peers in the general population.

Fertility is not impaired in females with JIA, but fecundity was found to be reduced.

Women with JIA have a higher rate of instrumental deliveries and a higher risk of unfavorable pregnancy and neonatal outcomes, such as preterm delivery, preeclampsia, and small for gestational age (SGA) infants [34]. Quiescent or minimal active JIA are not reactivated by pregnancy, and active disease at conception ameliorates in about 60% of pregnancies. Within a few weeks after delivery, disease activity increases or DMARD treatment is required in approximately as many cases as were treated before pregnancy [35].

Pregnancies in young people with JIA are often unplanned and occur during DMARD exposure. Developmentally appropriate counselling regarding contraception and pregnancy monitoring by an obstetrician and rheumatologist are important for AYA with JIA (see Chap. 19). There is limited data regarding the safety of bDMARDs and JAK inhibitors during pregnancy and breastfeeding. The treatment plan during pregnancy and breastfeeding should be individualised. MTX is contraindicated during pregnancy and breastfeeding, and AYA should be switched to another agent at least one month before planned conception. Sulfasalazine is safe during pregnancy and breastfeeding (only in full-term healthy infants). Sulfasalazine may cause oligospermia in men, but this is reversible after treatment cessation. The continuation of bDMARDs will depend on the agent and the disease activity of the person with JIA [36].

Prognosis

After 10 years of disease, less than 50% of AYA with JIA have achieved a drug-free remission [37]. The probability of drug-free remission varies significantly with disease-onset type, being best for systemic and oligoarticular JIA and worst for systemic and polyarticular JIA (Table 7.4).

Apart from drug-free remission, all other clinical outcomes have dramatically improved in the biologic treatment era. Most AYA have a good functional capacity. Articular damage (most often in hip, wrist, and temporomandibular joints) is the most important component of global damage. However, an arthroplasty is rarely needed in young adulthood (<2%).

The most frequent extra-articular damage components are

- ocular damage
- growth failure (linear growth failure in up to 10% and localised growth abnormalities, such as limb length discrepancies and micrognathia)
- muscle atrophy and decreased bone mass.

Ocular sequelae mainly develop as consequences of uveitis (in at least one-fifth of AYA with JIA) [41]. Complications most frequently include band keratopathy, cataract, posterior synechiae, maculopathy, and ocular hypertension. A significant visual loss results in 10–30% of young people with JIA. Blindness due to uveitis still occurs.

Reduced muscle mass and force contribute to bone loss. Abnormalities in body composition, i.e. a decreased lean body mass, an increased fat mass, and a reduced bone mineral density have been documented in AYA with JIA [42] (see Chap. 17).

The academic achievement of AYA with JIA is comparable to that of the general population. Conflicting data on employment rates exist, from transitioning into employment at an earlier age than peers without arthritis [43] to lower employment rates due to unemployment, longer training periods or early retirement. Young

Table 7.4 Long-term (≥7 years) outcomes of various JIA categories [15, 39–41]

JIA category	No drug-free remission, %	Functional limitations[a], %	Damage[b], %	Other possible adverse outcomes
Oligoarthritis, persistent	20–40	15–30	15	Persisting active uveitis, ocular sequelae, leg-length inequality
Oligoarthritis, extended	50–80	30–50	35	Persisting active uveitis, ocular sequelae, leg-length inequality
Polyarthritis, RF- negative	40–85	30–50	15–30	Linear growth failure, mandibular dysfunction, decreased bone mass
Enthesitis-related arthritis	60–85	30–50	15–30	Ankylosing spondylitis, hip damage
Psoriatic arthritis	50–80	30–50	10–50	Poorer physical health than oligo- or polyarthritis
Systemic JIA (or Still's disease)	20–40	15–60	25–40	Decreased bone mass, linear growth failure, hip damage, increased cardiovascular risk
Polyarthritis, RF- positive	60–100	50–70	30–100	Severe joint destruction

[a]Health Assessment Questionnaire >0
[b]Juvenile Arthritis Damage Index >0

people with JIA judge their quality of life still lower than age- and sex-matched controls, but in recent studies this is usually limited to physical health [44].

Summary

JIA in adolescence and young adulthood is characterised by specific clinical manifestations and requires a specific assessment and management. Rheumatologists need to be aware of the wide range of issues, including transitional care, sexual health and pregnancy, education and employment, potential adverse JIA outcomes and long-term comorbidities. A holistic life course approach to care for AYA is important to set the course for the future.

Specific points in the management of AYA with JIA are summarised in Key Management Points, and discussed further in Chaps. 20 and 21.

Key Management Points

1. Provide developmentally appropriate care and empower young people with JIA by embedding health education and health promotion in consultations.
2. Be alert to flares (arthritis, uveitis) with breaks of treatment or after pregnancy, taper or stop DMARDs only after about two years of clinically inactive disease
3. Be aware of possible co-morbidities, regularly assess, treat, if necessary, and avoid future cardiovascular risk factors by giving advice on a healthy lifestyle (e.g., sports, healthy eating, avoiding nicotine and overweight).
4. Provide anticipatory guidance, check vaccination status.
5. Provide counselling in regard to contraception and parenting
6. Provide a planned, coordinated transitional care and transfer to a developmentally appropriate, proactive (e.g., explorative, appointment reminiscent) service provision in adult rheumatology.

References

1. Minden K. Classification and epidemiology of juvenile idiopathic arthritis. In: Hochberg MCGE, Smolen JS, van der Heijde D, Weinblatt ME, Weisman MH, editors. Rheumatology. 8th ed. Philadelphia: Elsevier; 2022.
2. Lites TD, Foster AL, Boring MA, et al. Arthritis among children and adolescents aged <18 years—United States, 2017-2021. MMWR Morb Mortal Wkly Rep. 2023;72(29):788–92. https://doi.org/10.15585/mmwr.mm7229a3. Published Online First: 2023/07/20
3. Petty RE, Southwood TR, Manners P, et al. International League of Associations for Rheumatology classification of juvenile idiopathic arthritis: second revision, Edmonton, 2001. J Rheumatol. 2004;31(2):390–2. Published Online First: 2004/02/05
4. Fautrel B, Mitrovic S, De Matteis A, et al. EULAR/PreS recommendations for the diagnosis and management of Systemic Juvenile Idiopathic Arthritis (sJIA) and Adult Onset Still's Disease (AOSD) [abstract]. Ann Rheum Dis. 2024;83(12):1614–27.
5. Ravelli A, Minoia F, Davi S, et al. 2016 classification criteria for macrophage activation syndrome complicating systemic juvenile idiopathic arthritis: a European League Against Rheumatism/American College of Rheumatology/Paediatric Rheumatology International Trials organisation collaborative initiative. Arthritis Rheumatol. 2016;68(3):566–76. https://doi.org/10.1002/art.39332. Published Online First: 2015/09/01
6. Consolaro A, Giancane G, Alongi A, et al. Phenotypic variability and disparities in treatment and outcomes of childhood arthritis throughout the world: an observational cohort study. Lancet Child Adolesc Health. 2019;3(4):255–63. https://doi.org/10.1016/S2352-4642(19)30027-6. Published Online First: 2019/03/02
7. Martini A, Ravelli A, Avcin T, et al. Toward new classification criteria for juvenile idiopathic arthritis: first steps, pediatric rheumatology international trials organization international consensus. J Rheumatol. 2019;46(2):190–7. https://doi.org/10.3899/jrheum.180168.
8. Fisher C, Ciurtin C, Leandro M, et al. Similarities and differences between juvenile and adult Spondyloarthropathies. Front Med (Lausanne). 2021;8:681621. https://doi.org/10.3389/fmed.2021.681621. Published Online First: 2021/06/18
9. Antonio VV, Caggiano G, Lopalco HA et al. Still's disease continuum from childhood to elderly: data from the international AIDA Network Still's disease registry RMD Open 2023;9(4):e003578-10.1136/rmdopen-2023-003578
10. Goirand M, Breton S, Chevallier F, et al. Clinical features of children with enthesitis-related juvenile idiopathic arthritis / juvenile spondyloarthritis followed in a French tertiary care pediatric rheumatology centre.

Pediatr Rheumatol Online J. 2018;16(1):21. https://doi.org/10.1186/s12969-018-0238-9. Published Online First: 2018/04/04

11. Oen K, Tian J, Loughin TM, et al. Causal pathways to health-related quality of life in children with juvenile idiopathic arthritis: results from the ReACCh-Out cohort. Rheumatology (Oxford). 2021;60(10):4691–702. https://doi.org/10.1093/rheumatology/keab079. Published Online First: 2021/01/29
12. Wipff J, Sparsa L, Lohse A, et al. Impact of juvenile idiopathic arthritis on quality of life during transition period at the era of biotherapies. Joint Bone Spine. 2016;83(1):69–74. https://doi.org/10.1016/j.jbspin.2015.03.005.
13. Arnstad ED, Iversen JM, Uglem M, et al. Pain sensitivity in young adults with juvenile idiopathic arthritis: a quantitative sensory testing study. Arthritis Res Ther. 2020;22(1):262. https://doi.org/10.1186/s13075-020-02345-2.
14. Spekking K, Anink J, de Boer P, et al. Significant pain decrease in children with non-systemic juvenile idiopathic arthritis treated to target: results over 24 months of follow up. Pediatr Rheumatol. 2023;21(1):90. https://doi.org/10.1186/s12969-023-00874-z.
15. Glerup M, Rypdal V, Arnstad ED, et al. Long-term outcomes in juvenile idiopathic arthritis: eighteen years of follow-up in the population-based Nordic juvenile idiopathic arthritis cohort. Arthritis Care Res (Hoboken). 2020;72(4):507–16. https://doi.org/10.1002/acr.23853. Published Online First: 2019/02/15
16. Eyckmans L, et al. What does it mean to grow up with juvenile idiopathic arthritis? A qualitative study on the perspectives of patients. Clin Rheumatol. 2011;30:459–65.
17. Patil P, Parker RA, Rawcliffe C, et al. Methotrexate-induced nausea and vomiting in adolescent and young adult patients. Clin Rheumatol. 2014;33(3):403–7. https://doi.org/10.1007/s10067-013-2389-x. Published Online First: 2013/10/11
18. Onel KB, Horton DB, Lovell DJ, et al. 2021 American College of Rheumatology Guideline for the treatment of juvenile idiopathic arthritis: therapeutic approaches for oligoarthritis, temporomandibular joint arthritis, and systemic juvenile idiopathic arthritis. Arthritis Care Res (Hoboken). 2022;74(4):521–37. https://doi.org/10.1002/acr.24853. Published Online First: 2022/03/03
19. Ringold S, Angeles-Han ST, Beukelman T, et al. 2019 American College of Rheumatology/Arthritis Foundation guideline for the treatment of juvenile idiopathic arthritis: therapeutic approaches for non-systemic polyarthritis, sacroiliitis, and enthesitis. Arthritis Rheumatol. 2019;71(6):846–63. https://doi.org/10.1002/art.40884.
20. Angeles-Han ST, Ringold S, Beukelman T, et al. 2019 American College of Rheumatology/Arthritis Foundation guideline for the screening, monitoring, and treatment of juvenile idiopathic arthritis-associated uveitis.

Arthritis Care Res (Hoboken). 2019;71(6):703–16. https://doi.org/10.1002/acr.23871. Published Online First: 2019/04/26

21. Kearsley-Fleet L, Heaf E, Davies R, et al. Frequency of biologic switching and the outcomes of switching in children and young people with juvenile idiopathic arthritis: a national cohort study. Lancet Rheumatol. 2020;2(4):e217–e26. https://doi.org/10.1016/s2665-9913(20)30025-4. Published Online First: 2020/04/14
22. Sepriano A, Kerschbaumer A, Bergstra SA, et al. Safety of synthetic and biological DMARDs: a systematic literature review informing the 2022 update of the EULAR recommendations for the management of rheumatoid arthritis. Ann Rheum Dis. 2023;82(1):107–18. https://doi.org/10.1136/ard-2022-223357. Published Online First: 2022/11/15
23. Vanoni F, Suris JC, von Scheven-Gete A, et al. The difference of disease perception by juvenile idiopathic arthritis patients and their parents: analysis of the JAMAR questionnaire. Pediatr Rheumatol Online J. 2016;14(1):2. https://doi.org/10.1186/s12969-015-0063-3. Published Online First: 2016/01/07
24. Wu Q, Chaplin H, Ambrose N, et al. Juvenile arthritis disease activity score is a better reflector of active disease than the disease activity score 28 in adults with polyarticular juvenile idiopathic arthritis. Ann Rheum Dis. 2016;75(3):635–6. https://doi.org/10.1136/annrheumdis-2015-208462. Published Online First: 2015/12/31
25. Consolaro A, Giancane G, Schiappapietra B, et al. Clinical outcome measures in juvenile idiopathic arthritis. Pediatr Rheumatol Online J. 2016;14(1):23. https://doi.org/10.1186/s12969-016-0085-5. Published Online First: 2016/04/20
26. Srinivasalu H, Treemarcki EB, Rumsey DG, et al. Modified juvenile spondyloarthritis disease activity index in the Childhood Arthritis and Rheumatology Research Alliance (CARRA) registry. J Rheumatol. 2023;50(4):532–7. https://doi.org/10.3899/jrheum.220509. Published Online First: 2022/11/02
27. Hemke R, Herregods N, Jaremko JL, et al. Imaging assessment of children presenting with suspected or known juvenile idiopathic arthritis: ESSR-ESPR points to consider. Eur Radiol. 2020;30(10):5237–49. https://doi.org/10.1007/s00330-020-06807-8. Published Online First: 2020/05/14
28. Saper VE, Chen G, Deutsch GH, et al. Emergent high fatality lung disease in systemic juvenile arthritis. Ann Rheum Dis. 2019;78(12):1722–31. https://doi.org/10.1136/annrheumdis-2019-216040. Published Online First: 2019/09/29
29. Wobma H, Bachrach R, Farrell J, et al. Development of a screening algorithm for lung disease in systemic juvenile idiopathic arthritis. ACR Open Rheumatol. 2023;5(10):556–62. https://doi.org/10.1002/acr2.11600. Published Online First: 2023/09/09

30. Shakoory B, Geerlinks A, Wilejto M, et al. The 2022 EULAR/ACR points to consider at the early stages of diagnosis and management of suspected haemophagocytic lymphohistiocytosis/macrophage activation syndrome (HLH/MAS). Ann Rheum Dis. 2023;82(10):1271–85. https://doi.org/10.1136/ard-2023-224123. Published Online First: 2023/07/25
31. Fair DC, Rodriguez M, Knight AM, et al. Depression and anxiety in patients with juvenile idiopathic arthritis: current insights and impact on quality of life, a systematic review. Open Access Rheumatol. 2019;11:237–52. https://doi.org/10.2147/OARRR.S174408. Published Online First: 2019/12/07
32. Bohr AH, Fuhlbrigge RC, Pedersen FK, et al. Premature subclinical atherosclerosis in children and young adults with juvenile idiopathic arthritis. A review considering preventive measures. Pediatr Rheumatol Online J. 2016;14(1):3. https://doi.org/10.1186/s12969-015-0061-5. Published Online First: 2016/01/08
33. Jansen MHA, Rondaan C, Legger GE, et al. EULAR/PRES recommendations for vaccination of paediatric patients with autoimmune inflammatory rheumatic diseases: update 2021. Ann Rheum Dis. 2023;82(1):35–47. https://doi.org/10.1136/annrheumdis-2022-222574. Published Online First: 2022/06/21
34. Remaeus K, Johansson K, Askling J, et al. Juvenile onset arthritis and pregnancy outcome: a population-based cohort study. Ann Rheum Dis. 2017;76(11):1809–14. https://doi.org/10.1136/annrheumdis-2016-210879. Published Online First: 2017/07/01
35. Ursin K, Lydersen S, Skomsvoll JF, et al. Disease activity of juvenile idiopathic arthritis during and after pregnancy: a prospective multicenter study. J Rheumatol. 2018;45(2):257–65. https://doi.org/10.3899/jrheum.161410. Published Online First: 2017/12/03
36. Russell MD, Dey M, Flint J, et al. British Society for Rheumatology guideline on prescribing drugs in pregnancy and breastfeeding: immunomodulatory anti-rheumatic drugs and corticosteroids. Rheumatology (Oxford). 2023;62(4):e48–88. https://doi.org/10.1093/rheumatology/keac551. Published Online First: 2022/11/02
37. Shoop-Worrall SJW, Kearsley-Fleet L, Thomson W, et al. How common is remission in juvenile idiopathic arthritis: a systematic review. Semin Arthritis Rheum. 2017;47(3):331–7. https://doi.org/10.1016/j.semarthrit.2017.05.007. Published Online First: 2017/06/20
38. Nordal E, Zak M, Aalto K, et al. Ongoing disease activity and changing categories in a long-term nordic cohort study of juvenile idiopathic arthritis. Arthritis Rheum. 2011;63(9):2809–18. https://doi.org/10.1002/art.30426.
39. Dimopoulou D, Trachana M, Pratsidou-Gertsi P, et al. Predictors and long-term outcome in Greek adults with juvenile idiopathic arthritis: a 17-year continuous follow-up study. Rheumatology (Oxford).

2017;56(11):1928–38. https://doi.org/10.1093/rheumatology/kex265. Published Online First: 2017/11/01
40. Selvaag AM, Aulie HA, Lilleby V, et al. Disease progression into adulthood and predictors of long-term active disease in juvenile idiopathic arthritis. Ann Rheum Dis. 2016;75(1):190–5. https://doi.org/10.1136/annrheumdis-2014-206034. Published Online First: 2014/11/02
41. Del Giudice E, Simio C, Scala A, et al. Juvenile idiopathic arthritis-associated uveitis in the era of biological therapy: how the disease changed in more than 20 years of observation in a tertiary referral center in Rome (Italy). Int Ophthalmol. 2022;42(3):775–84. https://doi.org/10.1007/s10792-021-02043-1. Published Online First: 2021/10/21
42. Stagi S, Cavalli L, Signorini C, et al. Bone mass and quality in patients with juvenile idiopathic arthritis: longitudinal evaluation of bone-mass determinants by using dual-energy x-ray absorptiometry, peripheral quantitative computed tomography, and quantitative ultrasonography. Arthritis Res Ther. 2014;16(2):R83. https://doi.org/10.1186/ar4525. Published Online First: 2014/04/02
43. Jetha A, Theis KA, Boring MA, et al. Education and employment participation in young adulthood: what role does arthritis play? Arthritis Care Res (Hoboken). 2017;69(10):1582–9. https://doi.org/10.1002/acr.23175. Published Online First: 2016/12/21
44. Tollisen A, Selvaag AM, Aulie HA, et al. Physical functioning, pain, and health-related quality of life in adults with juvenile idiopathic arthritis: a longitudinal 30-year follow-up study. Arthritis Care Res (Hoboken). 2018;70(5):741–9. https://doi.org/10.1002/acr.23327. Published Online First: 2017/07/22

Systemic Lupus Erythematosus in Adolescence and Young Adulthood

8

Coziana Ciurtin, Stacy Ardoin, and Laura B. Lewandowski

Introduction

This chapter aims to address specific issues relating to systemic lupus erythematosus (SLE) in adolescents and young adults (AYA), referring primarily to challenges and particularities of disease management in this age group. SLE with onset before the age of 18 is called childhood-onset SLE (cSLE) or paediatric/juvenile SLE and has a peak of incidence at the time of puberty-onset [1]. Here we will mainly refer to particular aspects of management of cSLE during adolescence and young adulthood, rather than

C. Ciurtin (✉)
Centre for Adolescent Rheumatology, Division of Medicine, University College London, London, UK
e-mail: c.ciurtin@ucl.ac.uk

S. Ardoin
Nationwide Children's Hospital, Columbus, Ohio, USA
e-mail: Stacy.Ardoin@nationwidechildrens.org

L. B. Lewandowski
NIAMS, NIH, Bethesda, Maryland, USA
e-mail: laura.lewandowski@nih.gov

C. Ciurtin, J. Hackett (eds.), *Adolescent and Young Adult Rheumatology In Clinical Practice*, In Clinical Practice,
https://doi.org/10.1007/978-3-031-82102-8_8

exploring clinical features, diagnostic workup and treatment of cSLE, which have been covered in detail elsewhere (Chap. 23 in [2]). Specific guidelines, quality indicators and multidisciplinary care models for improved outcomes in cSLE, as well as recommendations towards 'treat to target' strategies provide helpful frameworks for a holistic, tailored, and optimised management of cSLE.

Epidemiology of cSLE in AYA

Approximately 15–20% of AYA with SLE experience the disease onset before the age of 18 years, with the highest incidence of cSLE being reported in girls aged 12–14 [1]. cSLE is more common and more severe in non-white children and adolescents [3, 4]. Disease onset peri-adolescence compared to younger age has been associated with increased severity and poorer outcomes [5].

Diagnosis of cSLE in AYA

The lack of awareness of the highly heterogeneous presentation of cSLE in AYA usually poses diagnostic challenges. The differential diagnosis of a young person with arthritis, fatigue, weight loss, and headaches is very broad, but includes cSLE as one of the rare causes of this presentation [4]. It is important to highlight that there are no specific classification criteria for cSLE. In practice, the adult SLE American College of Rheumatology (ACR) and the Systemic Lupus International Collaborating Clinics (SLICC) group classification criteria have been historically used as diagnostic criteria, although their main scope is that of defining homogeneous cohorts for research purposes. More recently, the ACR and the European Associations and Alliances of Rheumatology (EULAR) proposed novel classification criteria, which have also been tested in cSLE and found to have both lower performance [6] or improved specificity [7], based on various studies, highlighting the need for future research.

Impact of cSLE on Physical and Mental Health of AYA

Coming to terms with the diagnosis of a serious chronic disease is a challenge for AYA (see Chaps. 2 and 3). cSLE provides additional challenges based on the potential severity of the condition, uncertainty of long-term outcomes, and significant side effects of treatment. There are direct consequences of the inflammatory process associated with cSLE on AYA development, in addition to those related to the potentially irreversible impact of the disease on specific organ systems function.

AYA with cSLE have lower health-related quality of life and resilience compared to the general population [8]. A recent large integrative review of perceptions and experiences of AYA living with cSLE highlighted challenging symptoms related to disease severity, fatigue, depression, and anxiety; struggles with medication side-effects and adherence; limitations in taking part in sports or engaging in normal social life; lack of understanding from peers and family; as well as challenges in coping with the disease burden, and establishing optimal relationships with health providers and maintaining positivity, as the main themes [9].

AYA with cSLE desire independence and opportunity to negotiate goals towards achieving it, whilst acknowledging the need for adequate strategies for optimal communication between health providers delivering their care and improved self-management, to enable the attainment of disease control, preservation of adjusted personal goals, and protect social inclusion [10]. A study focused on adolescent health care needs in cSLE found that high-dose glucocorticoids and social marginalisation were associated with greater disease burden [11]. The integration of psychology and rheumatology services may support early identification of AYA at risk of poorer mental health outcomes and address their psychological needs [12].

General Management Considerations for cSLE in AYA

In addition to issues addressed as part of a developmentally appropriate assessment (see Chap. 4), there are other general health aspects which require specific attention in AYA with cSLE.

Adherence to long duration and complex medication regimens (see Chap. 21) is one of the major challenges in treating AYA with cSLE. While this is a challenge for adults with chronic illness as well, it can be even more challenging for adolescents who have not fully developed executive functioning [13]. Recent qualitative interviews assessing AYA with cSLE identified the following key factors affecting adherence: making sense of the treatment; contending with side effects of medications, lack of immediate benefit and regimen complexity; maintaining networks of support; and creating a ‘new normal’ [14].

Adherence to medications can be as low as 35%, with 44% of AYA self-reporting non-adherence to at least one medication prescribed for cSLE [15]. The main reasons identified were side effects (46%), difficulty remembering (33%) and paying for medications (25%). When AYA develop cSLE flares, the possibility of poor adherence should be considered.

Several strategies have been developed to improve adherence to medication, from text messaging or use of online self-management social media platform strategies to therapeutic recreational camps supporting improved adherence through peer modelling [16]. The use of an electronic pillbox to track adherence to medication could be an acceptable strategy for AYA with cSLE [17].

Sun avoidance education Sun protection needs to be provided and followed-up regularly for all AYA with cSLE. Young people were less compliant with reapplying sunscreen when sweating, using water-resistant sunscreen, applying sunscreen on the ears and dorsum of feet, and wearing sunglasses, mainly because they do not feel that sun protection is always necessary or dislike the texture of the topical formulations [18].

Vaccination AYA with cSLE are advised to have annual vaccines against influenza, and more recently COVID-19, as well as to be vaccinated against pneumococcus, meningococcus, and haemophilus influenzae, as they may be at particular risk for these infections. Non-live vaccines have been shown to be safe and are recommended in cSLE [19]. Vaccination against human papilloma virus (HPV) is particularly important, as there is an increased risk of persistent HPV infection, as well as precancerous cervical abnormalities in women with SLE [20]. For incomplete standard vaccine schedules in AYA with cSLE, the vaccination timing should be adjusted based on background immunosuppression therapy [19].

Sexual and Reproductive Health

Delayed puberty affects 1 in 10 adolescents with cSLE, with risk coming both from high disease activity and medication side effects. Although most adolescents do eventually enter puberty, the delay can affect bone health and final adult height.

Avoidance of unplanned pregnancy is important [21]. Pregnancy risks such as prematurity, preeclampsia, thrombotic risk, risk of developing nephritis, and other obstetric and fetal complications, as well as risk of disease flare during and after pregnancy are higher in cSLE and adult-onset SLE compared to general population [22]. In fact, the US Centers for Disease Control Medical Eligibility Criteria for Contraception identified SLE as one of 21 diseases for which unintended pregnancy imposes an unacceptable risk to health [23].

A recent exploration of the reproductive health needs of AYA with cSLE highlighted the lack of clear explanations related to the recommendation to avoid unplanned pregnancy, as well as the desire of young people to have their family members included in discussions with health professionals [24].

Teratogenicity from medications commonly used in cSLE is also a concern; however, being prescribed such medications has been associated with favourable odds for contraceptive advice provided by health care professionals to young women from age 15 [25].

Long-active contraception is considered the most effective option. While barrier methods are recommended for sexually active adolescents to prevent sexually transmitted diseases, they are less reliable to prevent unintended pregnancy. Combined hormonal contraceptives (CHCs) can be used safely, except in cases of active cSLE or in those at increased risk of thrombosis. Progestin-only contraceptives are good alternatives for AYA who have contraindications to CHCs, but they have a higher rate of break-through menstrual bleeding, potentially leading to discontinuation. Progestin-only implantable contraceptive methods are an excellent choice in cSLE.

The impact of contraception on the bone health has been investigated and concerns have been raised about the use of CHCs (including the ultralow-dose CHCs), as well as that of depot formulations (e.g. medroxyprogesterone acetate), which may have deleterious effects on bone health in very young adolescent females, but the mechanism is not completely elucidated [26]. Intrauterine devices (IUD), including hormone releasing IUDs, such as the levonorgestrel releasing device (Mirena coil) may be a good contraceptive choice as they are effective, well tolerated, associated with less complications and can be reversed. A single center study demonstrated that when offered comprehensive reproductive counseling, most AYA with cSLE choose long-acting reversible contraceptives such as an IUD [27]. Prospective studies of long acting reversible contraceptives in cSLE are lacking.

Decisions about the most appropriate contraception measures should be taken following assessing the risk profile of each adolescent or young woman with cSLE, and they should be revised periodically.

There are recognised age-related and dose-dependent fertility concerns with the use of cyclophosphamide therapy in cSLE. Adolescents have a lower risk for long term infertility, with highest rates in adults above age 32 or in those exposed to high cumulative doses of cyclophosphamide. Use of gonadotropin releasing hormone agonists during cyclophosphamide treatment as ovarian protection has been demonstrated to be safe [28].

Bone Health in AYA with cSLE

Potential negative consequences of cSLE and its treatments on bone health for AYA include osteoporosis (see Chap. 17) and avascular necrosis (AVN). AVN results from ischemic injury to bone causing subchondral necrosis and was found to affect 1/3 AYA with SLE in a recent meta-analysis [29]. The main risk factors were the use of steroid treatment early in disease course and at a high-dose, as well as more active organ involvement early in the disease course [29], suggesting that AVN could be particularly relevant to AYA with cSLE who have more severe disease at onset. Other possible contributing factors may be antiphospholipid antibodies, and active disease which leads to microvascular inflammation, although vitamin D deficiency had the strongest association with AVN in a cSLE cohort [30]. AVN most frequently affects the femoral head, but any bone as well as multi sites can be affected. Clinicians should have a high index of suspicion for AVN in AYA with persistent joint or bone pain. Radiographs may be initially normal, so magnetic resonance imaging (MRI) is required to ensure adequate sensitivity for early diagnosis of AVN.

Cardiovascular Health in AYA with cSLE

Cardiovascular disease (CVD) is a leading cause of morbidity and mortality in cSLE. AYA with cSLE were younger at the time of first CVD event (usually myocardial infarction) compared to adults with SLE, with CVD events identified at a median age of 16 years [31]. The degree of subclinical atherosclerosis in AYA with cSLE is heterogeneous and there are no reliable tests or scores able to identify AYA with high CVD-risk, despite evidence that longer cSLE duration, minority status, higher BMI, male sex, and abnormality in renal parameters have been associated with increase CVD-risk [31]. Clinicians caring for AYA with cSLE should therefore pay attention to modifiable risk factors for CVD, such as weight loss, control of renal disease and hypertension, and smoking/vaping cessation, as well as implement lipid lowering and diabetes control strategies, as relevant.

Neuropsychiatric manifestations in AYA with cSLE

Diagnosis of neuropsychiatric (NP) cSLE is challenging as AYA may have serologically inactive cSLE. Most AYA with cSLE experience NP events in the first 2 years of disease, and 30–70% of them present with more than one NP event, with an average of 2–3 events per disease course [32].

There is a wide range of NP manifestations, affecting both the central and peripheral nervous system. Objective NP manifestations such as stroke, neuropathies, seizures, chorea, or transverse myelitis are relatively easy to recognize clinically [32]. In contrast, headache, cognitive impairment, and mood disorders attributable to cSLE can be extremely difficult to diagnose, particularly in the adolescent population.

Testing for NP cSLE may include imaging, lumbar puncture to evaluate cerebrospinal fluid, and neuropsychological testing, depending on the clinical situation. Standard MRI is frequently performed, as it is readily available in most centres. The most reported features were nonspecific white matter hyperintensities (65%), and cerebral atrophy (88%) detected using T2- weighted/FLAIR MRI sequences [33]. As the NP cSLE diagnosis is generally attributed through multidisciplinary consensus, clinicians proposed a probability score, including variables, such as hallucinations, memory or sleep disturbance, and renal involvement, to facilitate diagnosis [33]. Attributing cognitive dysfunction to cSLE can be challenging in adolescents. Many adolescents have periods of struggling with academic performance or may describe difficulty with memory or other cognitive functions. The gold standard for diagnosis of neurocognitive abnormality is formal age and developmentally appropriate neurocognitive testing. Many cognitive tests have been adapted for use in young people [34]. In many clinical situations, school academic performance can be used as a reasonable proxy measure for cognitive ability.

Long-Term Outcomes, Educational Achievement, and Quality of Life

With improved treatments for cSLE, outcomes have also improved, with 10 and 15-year survival for young people with cSLE greater than 85% in most centres. Despite some progress, the standardised mortality rate in AYA with cSLE is still significantly increased, recently estimated at 7.2 (95% CI 3.3–14) compared to the general population [35]. Ethnic background influences outcomes, as AYA with non-white, Afro-American/Afro-Caribbean, or Hispanic backgrounds having worse outcomes, both in mortality and long-term damage [4, 36]. Compared with adults with SLE, AYA with cSLE accrue damage faster [36].

Health-related quality of life is poorer in children and youth with cSLE. The best predictors of disability were low annual income, arthritis, and higher pain scores, with 41% AYA with cSLE having at least low disability [37]. A recent study found that 44% of young adults with cSLE who completed education were unemployed, while in the employed group, 61% worked part-time and 51% were declared work disabled, due to cSLE damage [38].

Health care providers need to monitor for potential morbidities that can arise in AYA with cSLE, either disease-related or iatrogenic, including early CVD, osteoporosis, AVN, kidney damage, risk for infections, and possible increased risk of malignancy [39], as well as pay attention to the high prevalence of low mood in this patient group [11].

Youth with cSLE could be at increased risk for malignancy either due to exposure to immunosuppressive treatments or due to the disease itself. In a large registry-based study there was a small increased risk of cancer, with 14 invasive cancers reported overall in cSLE (standardized incidence ratio- SIR 4.13), and three of these being lymphomas (SIR 4.68) [40]. Studies in larger cohorts with longer follow-up are required.

Transition to Adulthood

Transition of care in AYA with cSLE is particularly complex for individuals on complicated medical treatment regimens and requires active involvement of multiple health care specialities, as it is usually the case with multi-system involvement (see Chap. 23). Early planning and coordination of transition of care are key for maintaining good disease control, minimising burden and ensuring improved long-term outcomes [10]. Successful transition requires close and reciprocal communication between pediatric and adult care teams, which can be supported by a transition document to bridge any gaps in communication.

Key Management Points

1. cSLE begins in adolescence in 15–20% of cases.
2. Diagnosis of cSLE should be considered in AYA who have a multisystem disease.
3. Treatment of AYA with cSLE and associated comorbidities can be complicated by challenges with adherence.
4. AYA with cSLE require developmentally appropriate and individualised management which can only be optimally delivered by multidisciplinary health care teams.

Acknowledgements The authors would like to thank Dr. Lori Tucker, Clinical Professor in Pediatrics and Division Head, Pediatric Rheumatology, University of British Columbia, Canada, for her contribution to the previous edition of this chapter.

References

1. Massias JS, Smith EMD, Al-Abadi E, Armon K, Bailey K, Ciurtin C, et al. Clinical and laboratory characteristics in juvenile-onset systemic lupus erythematosus across age groups. Lupus. 2020;29(5):474–81.
2. Ross E, Petty RML, Lindsley CB, Wedderburn L, Fuhlbrige RC, Mellins ED. Textbook of pediatric rheumatology. 8th ed; 2021. ISBN: 9780323636520

3. Lewandowski LB, Schanberg LE, Thielman N, Phuti A, Kalla AA, Okpechi I, et al. Severe disease presentation and poor outcomes among pediatric systemic lupus erythematosus patients in South Africa. Lupus. 2017;26(2):186–94.
4. Massias JS, Smith EM, Al-Abadi E, Armon K, Bailey K, Ciurtin C, et al. Clinical and laboratory phenotypes in juvenile-onset Systemic Lupus Erythematosus across ethnicities in the UK. Lupus. 2021;30(4):597–607.
5. Nelson MC, Chandrakasan S, Ponder L, Sanz I, Goldberg B, Ogbu EA, et al. Clinical determinants of childhood onset Systemic Lupus Erythematosus among early and peri-adolescent age groups. Children (Basel). 2022;9(12)
6. Smith EMD, Rasul S, Ciurtin C, Al-Abadi E, Armon K, Bailey K, et al. Limited sensitivity and specificity of the ACR/EULAR-2019 classification criteria for SLE in JSLE?-observations from the UK JSLE cohort study. Rheumatology (Oxford). 2021;60(11):5271–81.
7. Levinsky Y, Broide M, Kagan S, Goldberg O, Scheuerman O, Tal R, et al. Performance of 2019 EULAR/ACR classification criteria for systemic lupus erythematosus in a paediatric population-a multicentre study. Rheumatology (Oxford). 2021;60(11):5142–8.
8. Borgia RE, Ugarte-Gil MF, Vila LM, Reveille JD, McGwin G Jr, Alarcon GS. Health-related quality of life in adults with adolescent- and adult-onset systemic lupus erythematosus: a longitudinal study of a multiethnic US Cohort. Arthritis Care Res (Hoboken). 2023;75(7):1416–22.
9. Blamires J, Foster M, Napier S, Dickinson A. Experiences and perspectives of children and young people living with childhood-onset systemic lupus erythematosus-an integrative review. Children (Basel). 2023;10(6)
10. Jiang I, Major G, Singh-Grewal D, Teng C, Kelly A, Niddrie F, et al. Patient and parent perspectives on transition from paediatric to adult healthcare in rheumatic diseases: an interview study. BMJ Open. 2021;11(1):e039670.
11. DeCoste C, Moaf P, Mohamed I, Ng L, Ostojic-Aitkens D, Levy DM, et al. Adolescent health care needs and relationship to disease in patients with childhood-onset systemic lupus erythematosus. Arthritis Care Res (Hoboken). 2024;76(6):841–9.
12. Goldstein-Leever A, Bearer C, Sivaraman V, Akoghlanian S, Gallup J, Ardoin S. Increasing access to psychological services within pediatric rheumatology care. Pediatr Rheumatol Online J. 2023;21(1):51.
13. Harry O, Crosby LE, Smith AW, Favier L, Aljaberi N, Ting TV, et al. Self-management and adherence in childhood-onset systemic lupus erythematosus: what are we missing? Lupus. 2019;28(5):642–50.
14. Tan QEC, Gao X, Ang WHD, Lau Y. Medication adherence: a qualitative exploration of the experiences of adolescents with systemic lupus erythematosus. Clin Rheumatol. 2021;40(7):2717–25.
15. Semo-Oz R, Wagner-Weiner L, Edens C, Zic C, One K, Saad N, et al. Adherence to medication by adolescents and young adults with childhood-onset systemic lupus erythematosus. Lupus. 2022;31(12):1508–15.

16. Saez C, Nassi L, Wright T, Makris UE, Kramer J, Bermas BL, et al. Therapeutic recreation camps for youth with childhood-onset systemic lupus erythematosus: perceived psychosocial benefits. Pediatr Rheumatol Online J. 2022;20(1):39.
17. Harry O, Crosby LE, Mara C, Ting TV, Huggins JL, Modi AC. Feasibility and acceptability of an innovative adherence intervention for young adults with childhood-onset systemic lupus erythematosus. Pediatr Rheumatol Online J. 2020;18(1):36.
18. Suebsarakam P, Mairiang D. Accuracy and adequacy of photoprotection in pediatric systemic lupus erythematosus patients, and the effect of education on photoprotection: a prospective study. Pediatr Rheumatol Online J. 2023;21(1):123.
19. Jansen MHA, Rondaan C, Legger GE, Minden K, Uziel Y, Toplak N, et al. EULAR/PRES recommendations for vaccination of paediatric patients with autoimmune inflammatory rheumatic diseases: update 2021. Ann Rheum Dis. 2023;82(1):35–47.
20. Garcia-Carrasco M, Mendoza-Pinto C, Rojas-Villarraga A, Molano-Gonzalez N, Vallejo-Ruiz V, Munguia-Realpozo P, et al. Prevalence of cervical HPV infection in women with systemic lupus erythematosus: a systematic review and meta-analysis. Autoimmun Rev. 2019;18(2):184–91.
21. Rajendran A, Eudy AM, Balevic SJ, Clowse MEB. The importance of pregnancy planning in lupus pregnancies. Lupus. 2021;30(5):741–51.
22. Saavedra MA, Miranda-Hernandez D, Sanchez A, Morales S, Cruz-Dominguez P, Medina G, et al. Pregnancy outcomes in women with childhood-onset and adult-onset systemic lupus erythematosus: a comparative study. Rheumatol Int. 2016;36(10):1431–7.
23. Hoopes AJ, Simmons KB, Godfrey EM, Sucato GS. 2016 updates to US medical eligibility criteria for contraceptive use and selected practice recommendations for contraceptive use: highlights for adolescent patients. J Pediatr Adolesc Gynecol. 2017;30(2):149–55.
24. Carandang K, Mruk V, Ardoin SP, Huynh B, Clowse MEB, Berlan ED, et al. Reproductive health needs of adolescent and young adult women with pediatric rheumatic diseases. Pediatr Rheumatol Online J. 2020;18(1):66.
25. Chandramouli S, Alvarez C, Englund TR, Silverstein RG, Sheikh SZ. Teratogenic medication use associated with favourable odds of contraception counselling in a cohort of women with systemic lupus erythematosus at a large tertiary academic medical centre. Lupus Sci Med. 2022;9(1)
26. Hadji P, Colli E, Regidor PA. Bone health in estrogen-free contraception. Osteoporos Int. 2019;30(12):2391–400.
27. Al-Husayni N, Maslyanskaya S, Rubinstein TB, Coupey SM. Reproductive health care for female adolescents prescribed mycophenolate at a children's hospital: a 10-year retrospective cohort study. J Pediatr. 2023;253:252–8.

28. Kado R, McCune WJ. Ovarian protection with gonadotropin-releasing hormone agonists during cyclophosphamide therapy in systemic lupus erythematosus. Best Pract Res Clin Obstet Gynaecol. 2020;64:97–106.
29. Nevskaya T, Gamble MP, Pope JE. A meta-analysis of avascular necrosis in systemic lupus erythematosus: prevalence and risk factors. Clin Exp Rheumatol. 2017;35(4):700–10.
30. Gurion R, Tangpricha V, Yow E, Schanberg LE, McComsey GA, Robinson AB, et al. Avascular necrosis in pediatric systemic lupus erythematosus: a brief report and review of the literature. Pediatr Rheumatol Online J. 2015;13:13.
31. Ciurtin C, Robinson GA, Pineda-Torra I, Jury EC. Challenges in implementing cardiovascular risk scores for assessment of young people with childhood-onset autoimmune rheumatic conditions. Front Med (Lausanne). 2022;9:814905.
32. Appenzeller S, Pereira DR, Julio PR, Reis F, Rittner L, Marini R. Neuropsychiatric manifestations in childhood-onset systemic lupus erythematosus. Lancet Child Adolesc Health. 2022;6(8):571–81.
33. Labouret M, Trebossen V, Ntorkou A, Bartoli S, Aubart M, Auvin S, et al. Juvenile neuropsychiatric systemic lupus erythematosus: a specific clinical phenotype and proposal of a probability score. Lupus. 2024;9612033241229022
34. Kammeyer R, Ogbu EA, Cooper JC, Stolz E, Piquet AL, Fuhlbrigge RC, et al. Cognitive dysfunction in pediatric systemic lupus erythematosus: current knowledge and future directions. Child Neuropsychol. 2023;1-29
35. Moe SR, Haukeland H, Brunborg C, Botea A, Damjanic N, Wivestad GA, et al. Persisting mortality gap in systemic lupus erythematosus; a population-based study on juvenile- and adult-onset SLE in Norway 1999-2022. Rheumatology (Oxford). 2023;63(8):2109–17.
36. Smith EMD, Tharmaratnam K, Al-Abadi E, Armon K, Bailey K, Brennan M, et al. Attainment of low disease activity and remission targets reduces the risk of severe flare and new damage in childhood lupus. Rheumatology (Oxford). 2022;61(8):3378–89.
37. Hersh AO, Case SM, Son MB, Investigators CR. Predictors of disability in a childhood-onset systemic lupus erythematosus cohort: results from the CARRA Legacy Registry. Lupus. 2018;27(3):494–500.
38. Groot N, Kardolus A, Bijl M, Dolhain R, Teng YKO, Zirkzee E, et al. Effects of childhood-onset systemic lupus erythematosus on academic achievements and employment in adult life. J Rheumatol. 2021;48(6):915–23.
39. Ciurtin C, Robinson GA, Pineda-Torra I, Jury EC. Comorbidity in young patients with juvenile systemic lupus erythematosus: how can we improve management? Clin Rheumatol. 2022;41(4):961–4.
40. Bernatsky S, Clarke AE, Zahedi Niaki O, Labrecque J, Schanberg LE, Silverman ED, et al. Malignancy in pediatric-onset systemic lupus erythematosus. J Rheumatol. 2017;44(10):1484–6.

9 Juvenile Dermatomyositis in Adolescents and Young Adults

Christina Ann Boros

Introduction

Juvenile Dermatomyositis (JDM) is a systemic vasculopathy primarily affecting the skin and muscles, causing classic signs of rash and proximal muscle weakness. The incidence is approximately 3–4 per million children under the age of 18, with a female predominance: and an estimated female: male ratio of 2–5:1 [1]. It is difficult to assess the incidence and prevalence of idiopathic inflammatory myopathy (IIM) in adolescents and young adults (AYA) due to the paucity of published literature specifically addressing this age groups, but US and UK data report that 7% [2] and 10.5% [3] of cases were aged between 13 and 16 years at disease onset, respectively. JDM was diagnosed at a median age of 8 years in the Childhood Arthritis and

Christina Ann Boros: Published posthumously.

C. A. Boros (Deceased) (✉)
Women's and Children's Hospital, Adelaide, Australia

University of Adelaide, Adelaide, Australia
e-mail: christina.boros@adelaide.edu.au

C. Ciurtin, J. Hackett (eds.), *Adolescent and Young Adult Rheumatology In Clinical Practice*, In Clinical Practice,
https://doi.org/10.1007/978-3-031-82102-8_9

Rheumatology Research Alliance (CARRA) registry which started collecting data in 2019 [4].

A summary of the key differences between paediatric and adult disease are detailed in Table 9.1 [3–5].

Table 9.1 Differences between paediatric and adult idiopathic inflammatory myopathies IIM

Feature	Childhood IIM	Adult IIM
Rash	Could be present anywhere on the body, more likely to be ulcerative.	Distinctive skin rash in adult dermatomyositis; polymyositis may have no skin manifestations.
Muscle enzymes	Creatine kinase (CK)—less likely to be elevated in childhood IIM, so testing of other muscle enzymes: i.e. lactate dehydrogenase (LDH) and aspartate transaminase (AST) is needed.	CK is more likely to be elevated.
Interstitial lung disease	Less common, although 40% of young people with IIM have asymptomatic pulmonary function test abnormalities.	More common in adults with myositis and associated with poorer prognosis.
Calcinosis	More common in younger children; more typically a later sign associated with delayed diagnosis, a chronic course and/or inadequate treatment. It may manifest as subcutaneous plaques, nodules or large masses in muscle groups.	Very uncommon.

(continued)

Table 9.1 (continued)

Feature	Childhood IIM	Adult IIM
Major organ vasculopathy	More common.	Less common.
Association with malignancy	No clear association. Important to emphasise during disease education with the young person.	Dermatomyositis (DM) is considered to be a paraneoplastic syndrome in adults, and associated with triple the risk of all types of cancer reported, compared to the general population. Frequent association with the presence of anti- transcription intermediary factor 1 (TIF1)-γ autoantibodies, which are robustly linked with cancer-associated DM in adults. This association is not seen in JDM.
Polymyositis/ amyopathic phenotype	Less common.	More common.

Calcinosis

Risk factors for calcinosis include the presence of anti-nuclear matrix protein 2 (NXP2) and possibly that of anti-melanoma differentiation-associated gene 5 (MDA5) antibodies as well, in addition to higher initial levels of CK and prolonged elevation of muscle enzymes, and African American ethnicity [6]. Pathogenesis is uncertain, but is thought to involve local tissue trauma, active inflammation and dysregulation of proteins involved in calcium metabolism with calcium deposits occurring at sites of localised trauma or chronic mechanical stress. Calcinosis is particularly problematic when bridging joints and limiting movement or if ulcerating through overlying skin. Treatment is difficult and no specific therapy has been proven to be universally effective. Recent literature reported benefits in case series and case reports of JDM-associated calcinosis in adolescents with various therapeutic strategies, such as: abatacept (a fusion protein of cytotoxic T-lymphocyte antigen-4 and immunoglobulin that inhibits co-stimulation of T-cell activation), bisphosphonates (through inhibition of macrophage function and bone turnover), and Janus kinase (JAK) inhibitors (associated with a decrease in reactive oxygen species (ROS)-mediated mitochondrial calcium accumulation), as well as mycophenolate mofetil (that inhibits B- and T-cell proliferation by blocking DNA synthesis), rituximab (monoclonal antibody targeting CD20 on B-cells), sodium thiosulfate (a calcium chelating agent), tumour necrosis factor alpha (TNF-α) inhibitors (effective through suppression of local cytokine release), and tocilizumab (monoclonal antibody that binds the IL-6 receptor with role in dampening local inflammation). In some cases, these therapies led to a complete resolution of calcinosis; however, high quality studies are lacking and the selection of the best therapeutic strategy is still challenging [6].

Serology

Myositis specific antibodies in general tend to be associated with similar disease manifestations in childhood and adult IIMs, although with differing frequencies. However, children with antisynthetase antibodies are more likely to have overlapping myositis phenotypes, to present with falls and muscle atrophy, and less likely to have interstitial lung disease (ILD), mechanics' hands and Raynaud's phenomenon compared to adults with myositis. Children with anti-Mi-2 antibodies are more likely to exhibit V- or shawl-sign rashes, and have more cuticular overgrowth, whereas adults have a higher incidence of carpal tunnel syndrome [7].

Anti-NXP2 is found in 11–23% of children with myositis, but in only 1.6% of adult IIM patients. In JDM, anti-NXP2 antibody is strongly associated with the development of calcinosis, and a more severe disease course, with persistent disease activity and poor functional status [1, 2].The anti-MDA 5 antibody is associated with relatively mild muscle disease but more rash and a higher risk of ILD in children [8], as well as increase in calcinosis [6].

Pathophysiology

Although disease pathogenesis and genetic susceptibility are similar in adult and paediatric disease, childhood myositis is associated with more prevalent vasculopathy.

An internationally agreed standardised method to assess features and severity on muscle biopsy has enabled a more robust comparison of the pathophysiology between cases [9], and muscle biopsy scoring has also been predictive of JDM outcome [10, 11].

Classification of JDM

Recent progress has been achieved with the development of classification criteria for adult and juvenile IIM by EULAR/ACR in 2017, which opens opportunities for harmonized research in homogeneous JDM populations [12].

Management of JDM

Medical Treatment

The goals of treatment in IIM are to treat inflammation, restore function and ensure that growth and development are as normal as possible. Outcomes are improved with multidisciplinary care: the ideal team consists of a paediatric and adolescent rheumatologists up to age 19, and rheumatologists with expertise in young adult care from ages 19–24, in addition to rheumatology nurses, specialist physiotherapists, occupational therapists, and psychologists and social workers (as needed), all with age and developmentally-appropriate expertise. In addition, because of other potential organ and system involvement, multiple specialty experts (dermatologists, cardiologists, gastro-enterologists, chest physicians, bone specialists and surgeons, etc.) may also be involved in AYA care.

Early diagnosis and appropriate treatment lead to better disease control and quality of life, with the intensity of treatment determined by disease severity.

Consensus derived treatment pathways have now been developed by two main groups—CARRA [12, 13] and the Single Hub and Access point for paediatric Rheumatology in Europe consortium (SHARE) [14], in addition to the clinical practice guidance published the Paediatric Rheumatology Association of Japan [15]. The British Society of Rheumatology (BSR) is the first to publish treatment recommendations for IIM across the life span [16].

Treatment recommendations included induction with high dose oral or intravenous corticosteroids combined with methotrexate, based on evidence that the addition of methotrexate leads to better disease control than prednisolone alone. A combination of prednisolone and methotrexate, as opposed to prednisolone and cyclosporine A, has been recommended unanimously by all experts contributing to the BSR guideline as this has a more favourable toxicity profile [16].

Various conventional synthetic disease modifying anti-rheumatic drug (csDMARDs) (tacrolimus, azathioprine, methotrexate, ciclosporin, mycophenolate mofetil) can be used in combination with glucocorticoids early in the disease course to induce and maintain remission [16], as they are associated with steroid-sparing benefits.

For AYA with persistent active disease despite the use of csDMARDs, 'second-line' therapies, such as cyclophosphamide, rituximab, intravenous immunoglobulins G (IVIG) and abatacept, can be used.

The use of cyclophosphamide in severe JDM [17] had the greatest effect on global disease activity and skin involvement at 12 months after commencement, indicating sustained benefit.

Other biologics which have been used successfully to treat refractory myositis, including anti-TNF-α agents (infliximab, adalimumab, etanercept, and less commonly, golimumab) in JDM [18], as well as tocilizumab (IL-6 blockade), and in rarer cases, ustekinumab (IL12/23 blockade), eculizumab (complement C5 blockade), in addition to rituximab, which was the most frequently used, particularly in JDM cases with severe skin involvement [18, 19]. In addition, there is increasing interest in the potential of JAK inhibitors in refractory disease, particularly since JDM is now known to be an interferonopathy and that excess interferon (IFN) expression may drive the endothelial injury associated with JDM [20].

Other Management Strategies

Adjunctive treatment Exercise training, even in the setting of active disease, is also now well recognised to be beneficial.

Trigger avoidance Sun exposure is associated with flares of disease and sun exposure should be avoided. Additional care should also be taken with the use of medications which may increase photosensitivity throughout the disease course.

Disease activity and damage recording A consensus optimal dataset has recently been developed which includes 12 items to be completed at the initial visit, 56 to be completed at every clinic visit and 55 to be completed at baseline and every 12 months thereafter [21]. Disease trajectory analysis of JDM activity over time, particularly relevant for the care of AYA, revealed three trajectories: persistent active disease, persistent moderate disease, and high early disease activity with good response to treatment and long-term low disease activity [22].

Transitional care and planning As with all young people with chronic disease, AYA with JDM need effective transitional care (see Chap. 23) particularly in view of the different sub-specialist team involved in their care, as well as individual management needs.

Outcomes

Previous studies have suggested that only one third of children with IIM have a chronic disease course, but more recent evidence seems to contradict this, with increasing evidence that JDM is a chronic disease in 40–60% cases [22, 23]. The largest outcome study to date [23], which included 490 children and young people with JDM recruited from 27 European and South American centres and followed up for 2–25 years after diagnosis, found that most participants reported good quality of life, with few exhibiting severe muscle weakness or physical disability but, nonetheless, 40–60% of them had persistently active disease.

Mortality rates, though overall much reduced with modern treatment, are increased in JDM compared to the general population, particularly for those with overlapping myositis and anti-synthetase antibodies. A standardised mortality ratio (SMR) of 2.64 for JDM was reported in a US paediatric rheumatic disease registry, and a SMR of 8.3 (8 deaths) was reported for JDM and a SMR of 14.4 (17 deaths) for IMM overall were reported in a US juvenile myositis cohort [24].

Cardiovascular Health

IIM have been shown to be associated with an increased risk of cardiac involvement and atherosclerosis across the lifespan. The mechanisms thought to be causative of cardiac involvement are atherosclerosis and myocarditis [25]. Pericarditis has been reported in 12–15% of patients with JDM throughout the disease course [25]. Increased endothelial damage associated with high circulating levels of micro particles (increasing the risk of vaso-occlusive disease) and increased arterial stiffness during active disease are found in JDM [26]. These factors, combined with traditional cardiovascular risk factors, exposure to corticosteroids and chronic inflammation could well be contributors to early onset atherosclerosis in AYA with JDM.

In view of the above, anticipatory, developmentally appropriate guidance to promote cardiovascular health with respect to avoidance of nicotine, weight management, physical activity and dietary advice to ensure a normal lipid profile, is an important aspect of care for AYAs with JDM. Future research is required to support adequate identification of AYA with JDM at high cardiovascular risk, as well as support adequate management strategies [27].

Sexual and Reproductive Health

There is no published literature describing sexual health and fertility in AYA with JDM. Anticipatory guidance regarding contraception and safe sex practices is of particular importance for AYA on teratogenic medications. Chen et al., described pregnancy outcomes in women with rare autoimmune diseases including polymyositis/dermatomyositis [28]. The entire cohort included 409 births to 293 women with a median age of 33 years (range 16.7–45.9 years). Although most delivered healthy infants, they were at increased risk of adverse maternal and neonatal outcomes compared to healthy controls. A recent study highlighted that the reproductive needs of AYA with rheumatic diseases are not satisfactorily met during rheumatology consultations [29], leading to management recommendations published by ACR in 2020 [30]. Women with JDM should be monitored closely during pregnancy (see Chap. 19).

Vocational Outcomes

In a recent study investigating patient-reported long-term outcomes in IIM (n = 84), among respondents at school or in higher education, 13 out of 29 (44.8%) reported that their academic results were adversely affected by myositis, and that time missed, muscle weakness and fatigue were all significant contributors. Around two-thirds of respondents found that myositis had made it difficult to study. Fourteen of 50 (28%) reported career compromise caused by myositis; of these, 10/37 (27%) were employed and 4/13 (30.8%) were unemployed. Among 47 AYA aged 18–24, there were 21 (44.7%) who were employed; AYA in this study were twice as likely to be unemployed compared to the corresponding age group in the UK population (p = 0.001, OR 0.456, 95% CI 0.24, 0.84) [3].

Conclusions

JDM in AYA is rare, but recent studies demonstrate that chronic disease into adulthood is more common than previously recognised. JDM exhibits several important differences from adult onset disease in that it has a lower SMR, a better response to treatment and no known association with malignancy. However, skin disease is often worse and calcinosis and vasculopathy affecting other organ systems are more common in childhood. As with childhood onset systemic lupus erythematosus, increased cardiovascular risk has been demonstrated and so disease monitoring should include regular cardiovascular-risk assessment and counselling. Sun exposure should be limited with the careful use of photosensitising medications in order to prevent disease flare. AYA with JDM need careful and thorough transition plans with involvement of adult physicians in the process. Pregnancy in AYA with JDM also needs more intensive surveillance because of a higher incidence of adverse maternal and neonatal outcomes. More research is needed, and is supported by the evolving, multinational cohorts of patients using harmonised datasets, so that we can improve treatment, and thus outcomes for these young people.

Key Management Points

1. JDM is a rare disease which still requires vigilance to recognise early in the disease course.
2. AYA with JDM should be managed in centres where multidisciplinary care can be provided.
3. JDM is more often persistently active in the longer term than previously recognised, with significant associated organ-based and psychosocial morbidity.
4. Better understanding of disease phenotypes will provide the ability to personalise treatment and improve outcomes.

Acknowledgements This chapter has been published posthumously. Prof. Coziana Ciurtin, from the Centre for Adolescent Rheumatology, Division of Medicine, University College London, London, UK (email: c.ciurtin@ucl.ac.uk) reviewed and updated the chapter.

References

1. Papadopoulou C, Chew C, Wilkinson MGL, et al. Juvenile idiopathic inflammatory myositis: an update on pathophysiology and clinical care. Nat Rev Rheumatol. 2023;19:343–62. https://doi.org/10.1038/s41584-023-00967-9.
2. Pachman LM, Lipton R, Ramsey-Goldman R, Shamiyeh E, Abbott K, Mendez EP, et al. History of infection before the onset of juvenile dermatomyositis: results from the National Institute of Arthritis and Musculoskeletal and Skin Diseases Research Registry. Arthritis Rheum. 2005;53(2):166.
3. Boros C, McCann L, Ambrose N, Cortina-Borja M, Simou S, Pilkington C. Juvenile Dermatomyositis: what comes next? Arthritis Rheumatol. 2016;68(suppl 10)
4. Neely J, Ardalan K, Huber A, et al. Baseline characteristics of children with juvenile dermatomyositis enrolled in the first year of the new Childhood Arthritis and Rheumatology Research Alliance registry. Pediatr Rheumatol. 2022;20:50. https://doi.org/10.1186/s12969-022-00709-3.

5. Tansley S, Wedderburn LR. Comparing and contrasting clinical and serological features of juvenile and adult-onset myositis: implications for pathogenesis and outcomes. Curr Opin Rheumatol. 2015;27(6):601–7. https://doi.org/10.1097/BOR.0000000000000224. PMID: 26352731
6. Pinotti CS, Cannon L, Dvergsten JA, Wu EY. Calcinosis in juvenile dermatomyositis: updates on pathogenesis and treatment. Front Med (Lausanne). 2023;10:1155839. https://doi.org/10.3389/fmed.2023.1155839. PMID: 36936211; PMCID: PMC10017873
7. Rider LG, Shah M, Mamyrova G, Huber AM, Rice MM, Targoff IN, et al. The myositis autoantibody phenotypes of the juvenile idiopathic inflammatory myopathies. Medicine (Baltimore). 2013;92(4):223–43.
8. Tansley SL, Betteridge ZE, Gunawardena H, Jacques TS, Owens CM, Pilkington C, et al. Anti-MDA5 autoantibodies in juvenile dermatomyositis identify a distinct clinical phenotype: a prospective cohort study. Arthritis Res Ther. 2014;16(4):R138.
9. Varsani H, Charman SC, Li CK, Marie SK, Amato AA, Banwell B, et al. Validation of a score tool for measurement of histological severity in juvenile dermatomyositis and association with clinical severity of disease. Ann Rheum Dis. 2015;74(1):204–10.
10. Deakin CT, Yasin SA, Simou S, Arnold KA, Tansley SL, Betteridge ZE, et al. Muscle biopsy findings in combination with myositis-specific autoantibodies aid prediction of outcomes in juvenile dermatomyositis. Arthritis Rheumatol. 2016;68(11):2806–16.
11. Sag E, Demir S, Bilginer Y, Talim B, Haliloglu G, Topaloglu H, Ozen S. Clinical features, muscle biopsy scores, myositis specific antibody profiles and outcome in juvenile dermatomyositis. Semin Arthritis Rheum. 2021;51(1):95–100. https://doi.org/10.1016/j.semarthrit.2020.10.007. Epub 2020 Dec 22. PMID: 33360233
12. Lundberg IE, Tjärnlund A, Bottai M, Werth VP, Pilkington C, Visser M, Alfredsson L, Amato AA, Barohn RJ, Liang MH, Singh JA, Aggarwal R, Arnardottir S, Chinoy H, Cooper RG, Dankó K, Dimachkie MM, Feldman BM, Torre IG, Gordon P, Hayashi T, Katz JD, Kohsaka H, Lachenbruch PA, Lang BA, Li Y, Oddis CV, Olesinska M, Reed AM, Rutkowska-Sak L, Sanner H, Selva-O'Callaghan A, Song YW, Vencovsky J, Ytterberg SR, Miller FW, Rider LG; International Myositis Classification Criteria Project consortium, The Euromyositis register and The Juvenile Dermatomyositis Cohort Biomarker Study and Repository (JDRG) (UK and Ireland). 2017 European League Against Rheumatism/American College of Rheumatology classification criteria for adult and juvenile idiopathic inflammatory myopathies and their major subgroups. Ann Rheum Dis. 2017 ;76(12):1955–1964. doi: https://doi.org/10.1136/annrheumdis-2017-211468. Epub 2017 Oct 27. Erratum in: Ann Rheum Dis. 2018 Sep;77(9):e64. doi: https://doi.org/10.1136/annrheumdis-2017-211468corr1

13. Huber AM, Kim S, Reed AM, Carrasco R, Feldman BM, Hong SD, et al. Childhood arthritis and rheumatology research alliance consensus clinical treatment plans for juvenile dermatomyositis with persistent skin rash. J Rheumatol. 2017;44(1):110–6.
14. Enders FB, Bader-Meunier B, Baildam E, Constantin T, Dolezalova P, Feldman BM, et al. Consensus-based recommendations for the management of juvenile dermatomyositis. Ann Rheum Dis. 2017;76(2):329–40.
15. Kobayashi I, Akioka S, Kobayashi N, Iwata N, Takezaki S, Nakaseko H, Sato S, Nishida Y, Nozawa T, Yamasaki Y, Yamazaki K, Arai S, Nishino I, Mori M. Clinical practice guidance for juvenile dermatomyositis (JDM) 2018-update. Mod Rheumatol. 2020;30(3):411–23. https://doi.org/10.1080/14397595.2020.1718866.
16. Oldroyd AGS, Lilleker JB, Amin T, Aragon O, Bechman K, Cuthbert V, Galloway J, Gordon P, Gregory WJ, Gunawardena H, Hanna MG, Isenberg D, Jackman J, Kiely PDW, Livermore P, Machado PM, Maillard S, McHugh N, Murphy R, Pilkington C, Prabu A, Rushe P, Spinty S, Swan J, Tahir H, Tansley SL, Truepenny P, Truepenny Y, Warrier K, Yates M, Papadopoulou C, Martin N, McCann L. Hector Chinoy, for the British Society for Rheumatology Standards, Audit and Guidelines Working Group, British Society for Rheumatology guideline on management of paediatric, adolescent and adult patients with idiopathic inflammatory myopathy. Rheumatology. 2022;61(5):1760–8. https://doi.org/10.1093/rheumatology/keac115.
17. Deakin CT, Campanilho-Marques R, Simou S, Moraitis E, Wedderburn LR, Pullenayegum E, et al. Efficacy and safety of cyclophosphamide treatment in severe juvenile dermatomyositis shown by marginal structural modelling. Arthritis Rheumatology. 2018;
18. Campanilho-Marques R, Deakin CT, Simou S, et al. Retrospective analysis of infliximab and adalimumab treatment in a large cohort of juvenile dermatomyositis patients. Arthritis Res Ther. 2020;22:79. https://doi.org/10.1186/s13075-020-02164-5.
19. Sener S, Cam V, Ozen S, et al. Biologic drugs in the treatment of juvenile dermatomyositis: a literature review. Clin Rheumatol. 2024;43:591–602. https://doi.org/10.1007/s10067-023-06740-3.
20. Le Voyer T, Gitiaux C, Authier F-J, Bodemer C, Melki I, Quartier P, Aeschlimann F, Isapof A, Herbeuval JP, Bondet V, Charuel J-L, Frémond M-L, Duffy D, Rodero MP, Bader-Meunier B. JAK inhibitors are effective in a subset of patients with juvenile dermatomyositis: a monocentric retrospective study. Rheumatology. 2021;60(12):5801–8. https://doi.org/10.1093/rheumatology/keab116.
21. McCann LJ, Pilkington CA, Huber AM, Ravelli A, Appelbe D, Kirkham JJ, et al. Development of a consensus core dataset in juvenile dermatomyositis for clinical use to inform research. Ann Rheum Dis. 2018;77(2):241–50.

22. Nozawa T, Pullenayegum EM, Bell-Peter A, Marcuz J-A, Whitney K, Vinik O, Shupak R, Dover S, Feldman BM. Disease activity trajectories in juvenile dermatomyositis from childhood to adulthood. Rheumatology. 2024;63(SI2):SI129–35. https://doi.org/10.1093/rheumatology/keae027.
23. Ravelli A, Trail L, Ferrari C, Ruperto N, Pistorio A, Pilkington C, et al. Long-term outcome and prognostic factors of juvenile dermatomyositis: a multinational, multicenter study of 490 patients. Arthritis Care Res (Hoboken). 2010;62(1):63–72.
24. Huber AM, Mamyrova G, Lachenbruch PA, Lee JA, Katz JD, Targoff IN, et al. Early illness features associated with mortality in the juvenile idiopathic inflammatory myopathies. Arthritis Care Res (Hoboken). 2014;66(5):732–40.
25. Akgün G, Sözeri B, Başar EZ, et al. Cardiac evaluation of patients with juvenile dermatomyositis. Pediatr Res. 2024; https://doi.org/10.1038/s41390-024-03336-8.
26. Papadopoulou C, Hong Y, Krol P, Al Obaidi M, Pilkington C, Wedderburn LR, Brogan PA, Eleftheriou D. The vasculopathy of juvenile dermatomyositis: endothelial injury, hypercoagulability, and increased arterial stiffness. Arthritis Rheumatol. 2021;73(7):1253–66. https://doi.org/10.1002/art.41639. Epub 2021 May 28. PMID: 33393715
27. Ciurtin C, Robinson GA, Pineda-Torra I, Jury EC. Challenges in implementing cardiovascular risk scores for assessment of young people with childhood-onset autoimmune rheumatic conditions. Front Med (Lausanne). 2022;9:814905. https://doi.org/10.3389/fmed.2022.814905. PMID: 35237628; PMCID: PMC8883038
28. Chen JS, Roberts CL, Simpson JM, March LM. Pregnancy outcomes in women with rare autoimmune diseases. Arthritis Rheumatol. 2015;67(12):3314–23.
29. Carandang K, Mruk V, Ardoin SP, Huynh B, Clowse MEB, Berlan ED, Edens C. Reproductive health needs of adolescent and young adult women with pediatric rheumatic diseases. Pediatr Rheumatol Online J. 2020;18(1):66. https://doi.org/10.1186/s12969-020-00460-7. PMID: 32807193; PMCID: PMC7433038
30. Sammaritano LR, Bermas BL, Chakravarty EE, Chambers C, Clowse MEB, Lockshin MD, Marder W, Guyatt G, Branch DW, Buyon J, Christopher-Stine L, Crow-Hercher R, Cush J, Druzin M, Kavanaugh A, Laskin CA, Plante L, Salmon J, Simard J, Somers EC, Steen V, Tedeschi SK, Vinet E, White CW, Yazdany J, Barbhaiya M, Bettendorf B, Eudy A, Jayatilleke A, Shah AA, Sullivan N, Tarter LL, Birru Talabi M, Turgunbaev M, Turner A, D'Anci KE. 2020 American College of Rheumatology guideline for the management of reproductive health in rheumatic and musculoskeletal diseases. Arthritis Care Res (Hoboken). 2020;72(4):461–88. https://doi.org/10.1002/acr.24130. Epub 2020 Feb 26. PMID: 32090466

Systemic Vasculitis in Adolescence and Young Adulthood

10

Dilara Ünal, Hafize Emine Sönmez, and Seza Özen

Introduction

Systemic vasculitides in childhood are a group of disorders characterized by inflammation of vessel walls. The occurrence and prevalence of vasculitis among adolescents and young adults (AYA) remain unknown. Adolescence, as elaborated in Chaps. 1, 2 and 3, represents a distinctive phase of life, and enduring a suboptimal health status during this period may result in lifelong persistent effects. Considering the chronic and severe course of vasculitides, it is essential to acknowledge the challenges that arise during adolescence. Employing a multidisciplinary approach is crucial for effective management.

D. Ünal · S. Özen (✉)
Department of Pediatric Rheumatology, Hacettepe University Faculty of Medicine, Ankara, Turkey
e-mail: sezaozen@hacettepe.edu.tr

H. E. Sönmez
Department of Pediatric Rheumatology, Kocaeli University Faculty of Medicine, Kocaeli, Turkey

C. Ciurtin, J. Hackett (eds.), *Adolescent and Young Adult Rheumatology In Clinical Practice*, In Clinical Practice,
https://doi.org/10.1007/978-3-031-82102-8_10

Definitions and Classifications

The classification of vasculitides is primarily determined by the predominant size of the affected vessels. With the advancement of our understanding of etiopathogenesis, the nomenclature system for defining various forms of vasculitis was updated during the 2012 International Chapel Hill Consensus Conference (CHCC 2012) (Fig. 10.1) [1]. Descriptive names replaced eponyms in the classification of vasculitides, whenever possible. Consequently, Wegener's granulomatosis (WG), Churg–Strauss syndrome (CSS), and Henoch– Schönlein purpura (HSP) were renamed as granulomatosis with polyangiitis (GPA), eosinophilic GPA (EGPA), and immunoglobulin A vasculitis (IgAV), respectively.

Childhood vasculitides are classified according to the Ankara 2008 Consensus Conference criteria, which were endorsed by the European Allıance of Associations in Rheumatology/Paediatric Rheumatology International Trials Organisation/Paediatric Rheumatology European Society (EULAR/PRINTO/PRES) [2, 3] (Table 10.1). However, classification criteria for Kawasaki Disease (KD) and Behçet's Disease (BD) were not validated during the conference. Suspected individuals are classified as having

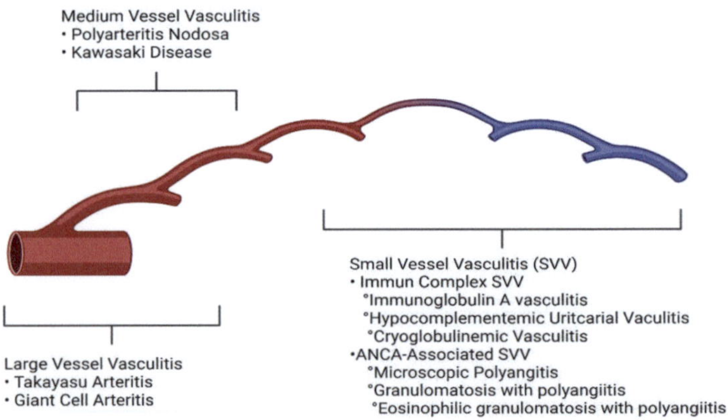

Fig. 10.1 Chapel Hill Consensus conferences 2012 classification criteria for systemic vasculitidis

Table 10.1 Ankara 2008 Consensus conference criteria for classification of childhood vasculitides

IgA vasculitis	Purpura or petechia (mandatory) with lower limb predominance, plus 1 of 4 criteria below: Abdominal pain Histopathology (predominant IgA deposit in a biopsy) Arthritis or arthralgia Renal involvement
Polyarteritis nodosa	Histopathology or angiographic abnormalities (mandatory) plus 1 of 5 criteria below: Skin involvement Myalgia/muscle tenderness Hypertension Peripheral neuropathy Renal involvement
Granulomatous polyangiitis	At least 3 of 6 criteria below: Histopathology (granulomatous inflammation) Upper airway involvement Laryngo-tracheo-bronchial stenosis Pulmonary involvement: chest X-ray or computer tomography (CT) showing presence of nodules, cavities, or fixed infiltrates Antineutrophil cytoplasmic antibody (ANCA) positivity Renal involvement
Takayasu arteritis	Angiography (conventional, CT or magnetic resonance imaging—MRI) of the aorta or its major branches and pulmonary arteries showing aneurysm/dilatation, narrowing, occlusion or thickened arterial wall (mandatory) plus 1 of 5 criteria below: Pulse deficit or claudication Four-limb blood pressure discrepancy >10 mmHg Bruits Hypertension (>95 percentile for height) Elevated acute phase reactants

Adapted from the Ankara 2008 criteria (EULAR/PRINTO/PRES)

KD based on the American Heart Association (AHA) criteria, which include unexplained fever lasting for more than 5 days and at least four of the following clinical findings: (A) bilateral non-exudative conjunctival injection, (B) changes in the oropharyngeal mucosa (fissured lips, strawberry tongue, or injected pharynx), (C) changes in peripheral extremities (erythema, edema of the hands and feet, or desquamation), (D) polymorphous rash, and (E) cervical lymphadenopathy [4]. The paediatric BD (PEDBD) group has proposed a new set of criteria to classify paediatric BD. According to PEDBD, a young person may be classified as having BD in the presence of three or more of the following criteria: (A) oral aphthosis (≥3 attacks per year), (B) genital aphthosis (typical with scars), (C) skin involvement (necrotic folliculitis, acneiform lesions, erythema nodosum), (D) neurological involvement (except isolated headaches), (E) ocular manifestations, and (F) vascular signs (venous thrombosis, arterial thrombosis, arterial aneurysms) [5].

Clinical and Laboratory Findings on Systemic Vasculitides

The clinical manifestations of systemic vasculitides may vary based on the predominant size of the involved vessels and the targeted organ systems. There is no specific diagnostic laboratory test for vasculitides, except for ANCA detection in serum in ANCA-associated vasculitides (Fig. 10.2).

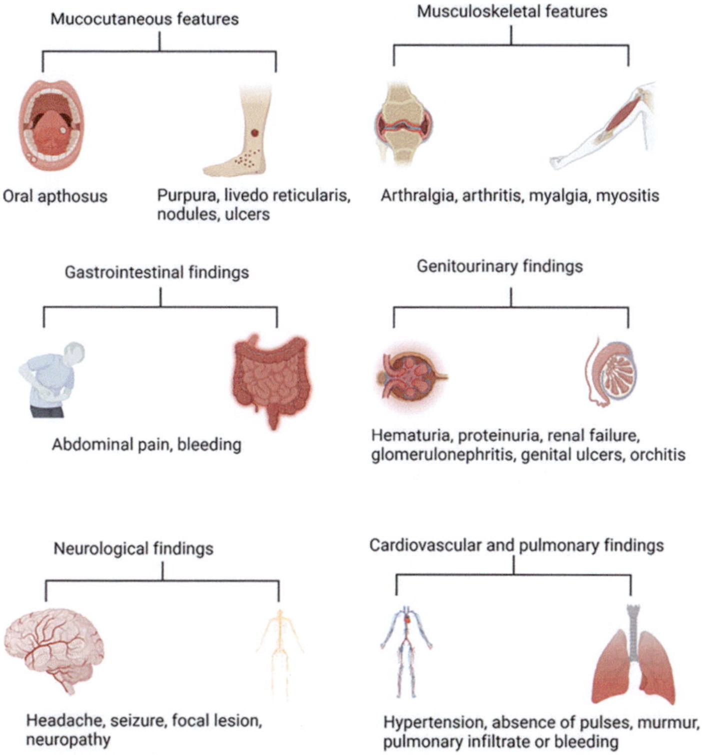

Fig. 10.2 Clinical findings indicative of systemic vasculitis

Predominantly Small Vessel Disease

Immunoglobulin A Vasculitis (IgAV)/Henoch-Schönlein Purpura (HSP)

Immunoglobulin A vasculitis (IgAV) is the most common systemic vasculitis of childhood, with an incidence of 3–29.9/100,000 [6]. It is predominantly observed in children under the age of 10. In childhood, IgAV mostly has a self-limiting course. The major clinical findings of IgAV include palpable purpura with lower limb predominance (Fig. 10.3a), arthritis/arthralgia, gastrointesti-

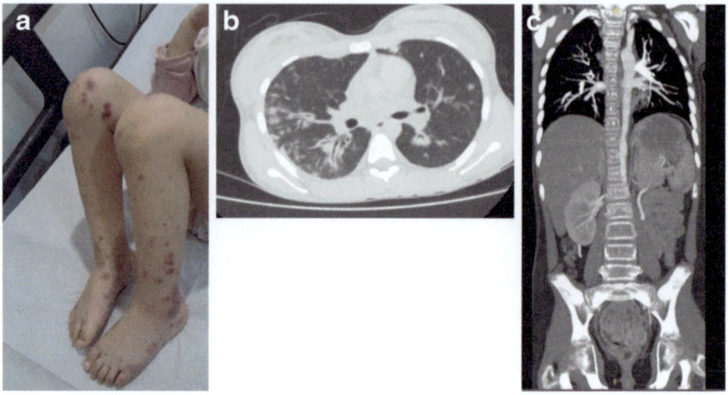

Fig. 10.3 Images relevant for various clinical manifestations of vasculitis. (**a**) Palpable purpura in a young person with IgAV. (**b**) CT image of diffuse alveolar haemorrhage in a young person with GPA. (**c**) MRI angiography of a young person with Takayasu arteritis

nal (GI) symptoms (abdominal pain, GI haemorrhage), and renal manifestations (haematuria, proteinuria, and IgA nephropathy). IgAV usually resolves on its own, however the early morbidity is defined by GI involvement, whereas long-term morbidity is defined by kidney involvement [7].

The diagnosis relies on clinical findings (Table 10.1). For the investigation of renal involvement, urinalysis and renal function tests should be assessed. Supportive treatment (appropriate analgesia, maintenance of hydration, nutrition, and electrolyte balance) is sufficient for most AYA with IgAV. However, corticosteroid (CS) treatment should be considered in young people with orchitis, cerebral vasculitis, pulmonary haemorrhage, and severe GI involvement [8]. The Single Hub and Access point for paediatric Rheumatology in Europe consortium (SHARE) recommendations suggest structured treatment plans for mild, moderate, and severe IgAV nephritis [8].

Antineutrophil Cytoplasmic Antibody (ANCA) Associated Vasculitis

ANCA-associated vasculitis (AAV) (GPA, microscopic polyangiitis [MPA], EGPA) is a group of vasculitides characterised by small/medium-sized vessel inflammation and the presence of myeloperoxidase (MPO)- or proteinase 3 (PR3)-ANCA autoantibodies. Similar to the adult literature, in paediatrics, GPA is the most frequent type of AAV, followed by MPA and EGPA [9].

The incidence of paediatric-onset GPA is estimated to range between 0.02 and 0.64/100,000 per year. GPA is characterised by granulomatous inflammation of the upper and lower respiratory tracts, necrotizing and pauci-immune glomerulonephritis, and vasculitis that involves multiple organs. GPA is most commonly associated with cytoplasmic ANCA and antibodies to PR3 [10]. GPA may have a severe presentation in childhood with early aggressive ear-nose and throat involvement (subglottic stenosis and nasal septal perforation) [11]. Pulmonary involvement in GPA ranges from asymptomatic lung nodules to life- threatening diffuse alveolar haemorrhage (Fig. 10.3b). Renal manifestations of childhood GPA contribute to significant morbidity. Presentation can vary: from urinary sediment abnormalities or mild renal dysfunction to acute kidney injury requiring renal replacement therapy [12].

Childhood MPA peaks in early adolescence and has a higher prevalence in females. MPA onset is insidious and often presents with constitutional symptoms of fever, weight loss, myalgias, and arthralgias. This disease commonly manifests as a component of pulmonary–renal syndrome. Pulmonary involvement often manifests as chronic cough, hemoptysis, chest pain, or anaemia because of pulmonary haemorrhage. Renal involvement is very common and presents with hypertension, hematuria, and proteinuria [13, 14].

EGPA is defined as necrotizing vasculitis that often involves the respiratory tract, characterised by eosinophil-rich necrotizing granulomatous inflammation [14]. EGPA typically presents with late-onset asthma, nasal polyps, lung infiltration, eosinophilia, and frequent episodes of non-infectious rhinitis and sinusitis. Cardiomyopathy has a higher prevalence in paediatric populations than in adults, which could explain the higher mortality rate in children [15]. The presence of ANCA is less common in AYA with EGPA than in adults [14]. Renal disease is generally mild [16].

There is no consensus on the treatment of paediatric AAV specifically. The treatment of AAV is generally divided into two stages: remission induction followed by a longer period of maintenance of remission. Corticosteroids (CS) and cyclophosphamide (CYC) or rituximab are used for remission induction in AYA with AAV [17]. Azathioprine (AZP), and rituximab, along with low-dose CS, are the primary treatments used to maintain remission. For AYA with non-severe EGPA, the American College of Rheumatology (ACR) recommended initiating treatment with mepolizumab (humanised monoclonal antibody that antagonises IL-5) and CS over methotrexate (MTX) or AZP.

In addition, a recent trial demonstrated that avacopan, a complement C5 receptor inhibitor, could facilitate the reduction of CS doses, bringing forward a possible steroid-sparing role of this new therapy [18].

Predominantly Medium Vessel Disease

Polyarteritis Nodosa (PAN)

Polyarteritis nodosa (PAN) is a primary systemic necrotizing vasculitis, manifesting as inflammatory lesions of medium-sized vessels. Deficiency of adenosine deaminase 2 (DADA2) may perfectly mimic PAN, which is caused by loss-of-function mutations in the *ADA2* gene, formerly called *CECR1* [19]. This condition leads to necrotizing vasculitis involving medium-sized arteries [20, 21]. However, young individuals with DADA2 often present with strokes and may have accompanying immune dysregulation or varying degrees of cytopaenia [22].

PAN is usually characterised by constitutional symptoms such as malaise, fever, weight loss, and a variety of skin manifestations including livedo reticularis, subcutaneous nodules, and necrotic lesions. Furthermore, arthralgia, arthritis, myalgia, renal involvement (haematuria, proteinuria, and hypertension), and neurological features (focal defects, hemiplegia, visual loss, mononeuritis multiplex, and organic psychosis) and gastrointestinal involvement may occur [19].

ANCA is consistently negative. Typical histopathological findings of PAN involve fibrinoid necrosis of predominantly medium-sized arterial walls. Characteristic angiographic features may reveal aneurysms in the renal, coeliac, mesenteric, or other arteries. While conventional angiography is considered the gold standard, CT angiography has emerged as an alternative, non-invasive technique for detecting vasculitic lesions [17].

The conventional treatment approach for PAN includes CS and CYC for remission induction, along with either AZP or MTX in combination with low-dose CS for maintenance treatment [17]. EULAR has elaborated treatment recommendations for adults with PAN, that may be extrapolated for children as well [23].

Kawasaki Disease (KD)

Kawasaki disease (KD) primarily affects children and is exceptionally rare in adolescence. KD is acute childhood vasculitis that leads to coronary artery aneurysms in approximately 25% of untreated cases. The current standard therapy for KD involves a single administration of 2 g/kg intravenous immunoglobulin (IVIG) combined with acetylsalicylic acid (ASA) [4]. In cases where coronary abnormalities are present, low-dose ASA should be continued indefinitely [4]. It should be emphasized that during the COVID outbreak, adolescents presented with KD-like features, which are now recognised as a new clinical entity, called multisystem inflammatory syndrome in children (MIS-C), or paediatric inflammatory multisystem syndrome (PIMS/PIMS-TS).

Predominantly Large Vessel Disease

Takayasu Arteritis (TA)

Takayasu arteritis (TA) is a chronic, granulomatous vasculitis that targets large vessels, notably the aorta and its major branches (Fig. 10.3c) [24]. The condition is primarily identified among adolescents, with the median age of diagnosis being 11.8 years for children [25]. At the time of diagnosis, the most prevalent findings included arterial hypertension (82%), headache (31%), fever (29%), dyspnea (23%), and weight loss. MRI angiography, and CT angiography, are used to assess the extent of involvement and vessel wall inflammation [26].

Steroids remain the cornerstone of TA therapy. Immunosuppressive agents or biologics may be prescribed for remission induction, and maintenance treatment may involve a lower dose of CS along with MTX [17]. EULAR proposed treatment recommendations for adults, which include biologics, including interleukin 6 and tumour necrosis factor alpha (TNF-α) blockade [27]. SHARE recommendations advocate for treatment strategies for children depending on the extent of involvement [28]. Surgical interventions may be necessary to address the destructive impact of the disease on large vessels [29].

Variable Vessel Disease

Behçet's Disease (BD)

Behçet's disease (BD) manifests as vasculitis with variable vessel involvement characterized by multisystemic manifestations. The disease can affect vessels of all sizes, including both arteries and venules. Involvement may extend to the central nervous system, musculoskeletal system, GI tract, heart, lungs, and kidneys [30]. Approximately 5–10% of individuals with BD experience disease onset during childhood, with the usual presentation occurring in adolescence.

It is crucial to acknowledge that in evaluating genital aphthosis in this age group, sexually transmitted infections should also be considered (see below).

Table 10.2 Differential diagnosis of vasculitis

Infections
Malignancy (lymphoma, leukaemia)
Substance use (cocaine, marijuana)
Systemic autoimmune/inflammatory diseases (systemic lupus erythematosus causing secondary vasculitis, juvenile dermatomyositis, and sarcoidosis)
Monogenic Vasculitis: DADA2 or SAVI (STING-associated vasculopathy with onset in infancy, associated with neonatal-onset systemic inflammation, interstitial lung disease (ILD), and severe cutaneous vasculopathy located in acral regions, including fingers, toes, ears, and nose).
Primary immune deficiency syndromes (Wiscott-Aldrich syndrome, interleukin-12 receptor beta-1 deficiency, recombination-activating 1 or 2 gene defects, etc.)

The treatment approach for BD typically depends on the site and severity of the involvement. Mild oral or genital ulcers are often managed with topical therapies, including CS- or lidocaine-containing creams, sucralfate suspension, and colchicine. For refractory cases, recommendations include AZP, interferon alpha, and TNF-α antagonists. A controlled trial has highlighted the efficacy of apremilast (phosphodiesterase type-4 inhibition) for oral ulcers [31].

Differential Diagnosis of Vasculitis

Several diseases that mimic systemic vasculitides must be excluded (Table 10.2). In AYA, it is crucial to exclude substance use, particularly illegal drugs, and sexually transmitted diseases.

Specific Issues in Adolescents Diagnosed with Vasculitis

Successful treatment significantly depends on adherence to treatment, especially for AYA, which requires a multidisciplinary approach that frequently involves psychologists and other members of the multidisciplinary team (MDT) (refer to Chaps. 22 and

23). AYA should undergo evaluation not only for disease activity, but also for the overall burden of the disease and that of treatment side effects. For instance, although the use of CS is the mainstay treatment for remission induction and maintenance in systemic vasculitides, AYA undergoing long-term CS treatment face the risk of serious side effects, including Cushing syndrome, growth suppression, osteoporosis (refer to Chap. 17), metabolic effects, immunosuppression, glaucoma, hypertension, and mood disorders. Gonadal toxicity is a frequently encountered long-term consequence of CYC, and the risk is heightened after puberty. Intravenous administration of CYC is associated with a lower total cumulative dose compared with daily oral administration, thus CYC should be given intravenously, preferably as a low-dose regimen [32]. Luteinizing hormone-releasing hormones may offer protection against CYC-induced ovary damage [33].

In developed countries, KD is the most prevalent cause of acquired heart disease and myocardial ischemia in young adults. Regular follow-up by cardiologists is essential [4]. Ongoing inflammation may result in early atherosclerosis and coronary artery disease (CAD). Beyond KD, the association between CAD and vasculitis in childhood is rare, although studies in adults have shown an elevated risk of CAD among individuals with rheumatic diseases. Encouraging cardiovascular health is equally crucial, involving guidance and support on the significance of physical activity, weight management, and abstaining from nicotine and/or other drug use.

Providing proactive guidance on sexual and reproductive health is essential for all AYA with vasculitis. Human papillomavirus (HPV) infections are the most prevalent sexually transmitted infections globally. Although HPV vaccination is advised for girls and boys during adolescence, there is a gap in data regarding the safety of vaccination for children with vasculitides or those undergoing immunosuppressive treatments. Contraception plays a pivotal role in reproductive health. According to adult studies, it is well established that women with vasculitides experience increased rates of pregnancy complications, including pregnancy loss and preterm birth [34] (see Chap. 20). The use of oestrogen-containing contraceptives may be challenging because of thrombotic susceptibility.

The establishment of an effective transition program is crucial for facilitating the smooth transfer of adolescents to adult clinics (the reader is referred to Chap. 23). A recent study from Canada showed favourable outcomes, as reflected by the continuity of follow-up and no increased risk of relapse when using a standard transition model [35]. Transition programs address both medical and psychosocial aspects during this critical period. The evolving landscape of paediatric vasculitis care relies on ongoing multidisciplinary collaboration, promising advancements in diagnostics, treatments, and support systems. Sustaining this collaborative momentum is essential for navigating the complexities of these conditions and providing the best possible care for AYA and their families [36].

Summary

In conclusion, specific vasculitides tend to be more prevalent or severe during adolescence and young adulthood. It is essential to consider the impact of the disease burden and that of certain treatment side effects may be more troublesome in young individuals.

Key Management Points

1. Systemic vasculitides have a broad differential diagnosis in childhood and adolescence.
2. Depending on the type of vasculitides, some AYA require long-term treatment and regular follow-ups.
3. The management of systemic vasculitides in AYA should be holistic, as well as age and developmentally-appropriate, to minimise the risk of disease and treatment-related long-term complications.

References

1. Jennette JC, Falk RJ, Bacon PA, Basu N, Cid MC, Ferrario F, et al. 2012 revised International Chapel Hill consensus conference nomenclature of vasculitides. Arthritis Rheum. 2013;65(1):1–11.
2. Ozen S, Pistorio A, Iusan SM, Bakkaloglu A, Herlin T, Brik R, et al. EULAR/PRINTO/PRES criteria for Henoch-Schonlein purpura, childhood polyarteritis nodosa, childhood Wegener granulomatosis and childhood Takayasu arteritis: Ankara 2008. Part II: final classification criteria. Ann Rheum Dis. 2010;69(5):798–806.
3. Ruperto N, Ozen S, Pistorio A, Dolezalova P, Brogan P, Cabral DA, et al. EULAR/PRINTO/PRES criteria for Henoch-Schonlein purpura, childhood polyarteritis nodosa, childhood Wegener granulomatosis and childhood Takayasu arteritis: Ankara 2008. Part I: overall methodology and clinical characterisation. Ann Rheum Dis. 2010;69(5):790–7.
4. McCrindle BW, Rowley AH, Newburger JW, Burns JC, Bolger AF, Gewitz M, et al. Diagnosis, treatment, and long-term management of Kawasaki disease: a scientific statement for health professionals from the American Heart Association. Circulation. 2017;135(17):e927–e99.
5. Kone-Paut I, Shahram F, Darce-Bello M, Cantarini L, Cimaz R, Gattorno M, et al. Consensus classification criteria for paediatric Behcet's disease from a prospective observational cohort: PEDBD. Ann Rheum Dis. 2016;75(6):958–64.
6. Piram M, Maldini C, Biscardi S, De Suremain N, Orzechowski C, Georget E, et al. Incidence of IgA vasculitis in children estimated by four-source capture-recapture analysis: a population-based study. Rheumatology (Oxford). 2017;56(8):1358–66.
7. Hu YC, Yang YH, Chiang BL. Immunoglobulin A vasculitis: The clinical features and pathophysiology. Kaohsiung J Med Sci. 2024;40:612–20.
8. Ozen S, Marks SD, Brogan P, Groot N, de Graeff N, Avcin T, et al. European consensus-based recommendations for diagnosis and treatment of immunoglobulin A vasculitis—the SHARE initiative. Rheumatology. 2019;58(9):1607–16.
9. Jariwala M, Laxer RM. Childhood GPA, EGPA, and MPA. Clin Immunol. 2020;211:108325.
10. Iudici M, Quartier P, Terrier B, Mouthon L, Guillevin L, Puéchal X. Childhood-onset granulomatosis with polyangiitis and microscopic polyangiitis: systematic review and meta-analysis. Orphanet J Rare Dis. 2016;11(1):141.
11. Iudici M, Pagnoux C, Quartier P, Büchler M, Cevallos R, Cohen P, de Moreuil C, Guilpain P, Le Quellec A, Serratrice J, Terrier B, Guillevin L, Mouthon L, Puéchal X, French Vasculitis Study Group. Childhood- versus adult-onset ANCA-associated vasculitides: a nested, matched case-

control study from the French Vasculitis Study Group Registry. Autoimmun Rev. 2018;17(2):108–14.

12. Cabral DA, Canter DL, Muscal E, Nanda K, Wahezi DM, Spalding SJ, et al. Comparing presenting clinical features in 48 children with microscopic polyangiitis to 183 children who have granulomatosis with polyangiitis (Wegener's): an ARChiVe Cohort Study. Arthritis Rheumatol. 2016;68(10):2514–26.
13. Sacri AS, Chambaraud T, Ranchin B, Florkin B, See H, Decramer S, et al. Clinical characteristics and outcomes of childhood-onset ANCA-associated vasculitis: a French nationwide study. Nephrol Dial Transplant. 2015;30(Suppl 1):i104–12.
14. Plumb LA, Oni L, Marks SD, Tullus K. Paediatric anti-neutrophil cytoplasmic antibody (ANCA)-associated vasculitis: an update on renal management. Pediatr Nephrol. 2018;33(1):25–39.
15. Calatroni M, Oliva E, Gianfreda D, Gregorini G, Allinovi M, Ramirez GA, et al. ANCA-associated vasculitis in childhood: recent advances. Ital J Pediatr. 2017;43(1):46.
16. Eleftheriou D, Gale H, Pilkington C, Fenton M, Sebire NJ, Brogan PA. Eosinophilic granulomatosis with polyangiitis in childhood: retrospective experience from a tertiary referral centre in the UK. Rheumatology (Oxford). 2016;55(7):1263–72.
17. de Graeff N, Groot N, Brogan P, Ozen S, Avcin T, Bader-Meunier B, et al. European consensus-based recommendations for the diagnosis and treatment of rare paediatric vasculitides—the SHARE initiative. Rheumatology (Oxford). 2019;58(4):656–71.
18. Matsuo Y, Miyabe Y. Avacopan for the treatment of ANCA-associated vasculitis. N Engl J Med. 2021;384(21):e81.
19. Sonmez HE, Armagan B, Ayan G, Barut K, Batu ED, Erden A, et al. Polyarteritis nodosa: lessons from 25 years of experience. Clin Exp Rheumatol. 2019;37 Suppl 117(2):52–6.
20. Zhou Q, Yang D, Ombrello AK, Zavialov AV, Toro C, Zavialov AV, et al. Early-onset stroke and vasculopathy associated with mutations in ADA2. N Engl J Med. 2014;370(10):911–20.
21. Navon Elkan P, Pierce SB, Segel R, Walsh T, Barash J, Padeh S, et al. Mutant adenosine deaminase 2 in a polyarteritis nodosa vasculopathy. N Engl J Med. 2014;370(10):921–31.
22. Ozen S, Batu ED, Taskiran EZ, Ozkara HA, Unal S, Guleray N, et al. A monogenic disease with a variety of phenotypes: deficiency of adenosine deaminase 2. J Rheumatol. 2020;47(1):117–25.
23. Mukhtyar C, Guillevin L, Cid MC, Dasgupta B, de Groot K, Gross W, et al. EULAR recommendations for the management of primary small and medium vessel vasculitis. Ann Rheum Dis. 2009;68(3):310–7.
24. Grayson PC, Ponte C, Suppiah R, Robson JC, Gribbons KB, Judge A, et al. 2022 American College of Rheumatology/EULAR classification criteria for Takayasu arteritis. Ann Rheum Dis. 2022;81(12):1654–60.

25. Eleftheriou D, Varnier G, Dolezalova P, McMahon AM, Al-Obaidi M, Brogan PA. Takayasu arteritis in childhood: retrospective experience from a tertiary referral centre in the United Kingdom. Arthritis Res Ther. 2015;17:36.
26. Aeschlimann FA, Yeung RSM, Laxer RM. An Update on Childhood-Onset Takayasu Arteritis. Front Pediatr. 2022;10:872313.
27. Hellmich B, Agueda A, Monti S, Buttgereit F, de Boysson H, Brouwer E, et al. 2018 update of the EULAR recommendations for the management of large vessel vasculitis. Ann Rheum Dis. 2020;79(1):19–30.
28. de Graeff N, Groot N, Brogan P, Ozen S, Avcin T, Bader-Meunier B, et al. European consensus-based recommendations for the diagnosis and treatment of rare paediatric vasculitides—the SHARE initiative. Rheumatology (Oxford). 2020;59(4):919.
29. Keser G, Aksu K. What is new in management of Takayasu arteritis? Presse Med. 2017;46(7–8 Pt 2):e229–e35.
30. Sota J, Rigante D, Lopalco G, Emmi G, Gentileschi S, Gaggiano C, et al. Clinical profile and evolution of patients with juvenile-onset Behcet's syndrome over a 25-year period: insights from the AIDA network. Intern Emerg Med. 2021;16(8):2163–71.
31. Hatemi G, Melikoglu M, Tunc R, Korkmaz C, Turgut Ozturk B, Mat C, et al. Apremilast for Behcet's syndrome—a phase 2, placebo-controlled study. N Engl J Med. 2015;372(16):1510–8.
32. Miller JJ 3rd, Williams GF, Leissring JC. Multiple late complications of therapy with cyclophosphamide, including ovarian destruction. Am J Med. 1971;50(4):530–5.
33. Clowse ME, Behera MA, Anders CK, Copland S, Coffman CJ, Leppert PC, Bastian LA. Ovarian preservation by GnRH agonists during chemotherapy: a meta-analysis. J Womens Health. 2009;18(3):311–9.
34. Machen L, Clowse ME. Vasculitis and pregnancy. Rheum Dis Clin North Am. 2017;43(2):239–47.
35. Mulla I, Yeung RSM, Noone DG, Bell-Peter A, Pagnoux C. Paediatric-to-adult transition experience in vasculitis: report of a model of care and outcomes. Clin Exp Rheumatol. 2022;40(4):772–8.
36. Foster A. Vasculitis in pediatrics unique challenges and emerging treatments. J Vasc. 2023;9(6):210.

Childhood Onset Sjögren Disease in Adolescence and Young Adulthood

11

Edoardo Marrani, Muthana Al Obaidi, and Coziana Ciurtin

Introduction

Childhood-onset Sjögren's disease (cSjD) is a rare but significant rheumatic condition caused by autoimmune infiltration of exocrine glands. The condition has been well described in adults, and defined as an "autoimmune epithelitis", in which the gradually progressing immune-mediated destruction of the exocrine glands, affecting predominantly the salivary and lacrimal glands, results in cumulative damage [1]. Once a critical threshold of parenchymal destruction is reached, the characteristic symptoms of the disease—ocular and oral dryness—develop.

E. Marrani
Pediatric Rheumatology Unit, Meyer Children's Hospital IRCCS, Firenze, Italy
e-mail: edoardo.marrani@meyer.it

M. Al Obaidi
Great Ormond Street Hospital for Children, London, UK
e-mail: Muthana.alobaidi@gosh.nhs.uk

C. Ciurtin (✉)
Centre for Adolescent Rheumatology, Division of Medicine, University College London, London, UK
e-mail: c.ciurtin@ucl.ac.uk

C. Ciurtin, J. Hackett (eds.), *Adolescent and Young Adult Rheumatology In Clinical Practice*, In Clinical Practice,
https://doi.org/10.1007/978-3-031-82102-8_11

In recent years, cSjD has garnered significant attention from researchers as a distinct and clinically relevant condition affecting adolescents and young adults (AYA), with a potential detrimental impact on quality of life (QoL). The aim of this chapter is to explore the characteristics of cSjD in AYA, with particular focus on the challenges and unique aspects of managing the disease in this age group. A comprehensive description of the clinical features, diagnostic workup, and treatment of cSjD is beyond the scope of this chapter, as they have been addressed elsewhere [2].

Epidemiology and Pathogenesis of cSjD in AYA

Sjögren's disease (SjD) is the most common systemic connective tissue disease in adults [3]. cSjD is diagnosed before 18 years of age in only 1% of cases [4], and has a peak of incidence after puberty and a female sex predominance (female: male ratio = 4:1) [4, 5].

Non-white children and adolescents often have disease onset at a younger age [4] while data on comparative manifestations and severity between ethnic groups in childhood are lacking. In almost 10% of cases, cSjD is associated with another connective tissue disorder, in particular systemic lupus erythematosus [6].

The exact pathogenesis of cSjD remains unknown. In adult SjD, activated mucosal epithelial cells are believed to play a key role in initiating the inflammatory cascade. These cells may react to environmental stimuli, mainly viral infections, and contribute to the activation of the innate and adaptive immune systems. The key role of lymphocytes in maintaining and amplifying the inflammatory process is reflected by the presence of autoantibodies and immune complexes, and by the lymphocytic infiltrate in the exocrine glands, leading to the formation of germinal centre-like structures and to potential malignant transformation [1, 2].

Emerging evidence suggests that cSjD is characterised by significant molecular heterogeneity and immune dysregulation driven by unique immune cell subpopulations, which could have implications for personalised treatment strategies [7].

Clinical Presentation

In children and AYA, cSjD manifests with a heterogeneous clinical spectrum, ranging from mild glandular symptoms to severe systemic involvement.

In adults, the predominant phenotype is characterised by a combination of dry mouth and eyes, fatigue, and joint pain, with these symptoms being present in over 80% of cases [1]. Unlike its adult counterpart, cSjD often presents with recurrent inflammation of the salivary glands, rather than the more common symptoms of sicca syndrome.

Moreover, extraglandular manifestations and systemic involvement are more common than in adult-onset disease. The extraglandular involvement is a direct consequence of lymphocytic infiltration of epithelia in various organs (e.g., leading to interstitial nephritis, autoimmune primary biliary cholangitis, obstructive bronchiolitis) or immune-complex deposition (e.g. palpable purpura, cryoglobulinaemia-associated glomerulonephritis, interstitial pneumonitis, peripheral neuropathy). Antibodies against Sjögren's syndrome–related antigen A (anti-SSA) are present in two-thirds of adults with SjD, often associated with anti-SSB antibody positivity, while rheumatoid factor is present in approximately half of individuals with SjD [1].

Contrary to the classical depiction of SjD as a predominantly "sicca" condition, a large cohort study showed that clinical phenotypes and disease evolution depend on the age at diagnosis, with more severe phenotypes being seen in younger individuals, although this study did not specifically differentiate between cSjD and adult-onset SjD [8]. Individuals with early-onset SjD phenotypes form a distinct subset with a high prevalence of antinuclear antibodies (ANA), anti-SSA, anti-SSB, and rheumatoid factor. This group also exhibits higher disease activity, reflected by higher disease activity in several domains (glandular, lymphadenopathy, cutaneous, constitutional, and biological), estimated using the validated European Alliance of Associations for Rheumatology (EULAR) Sjögren's syndrome disease activity index (ESSDAI). Over time, sicca symptoms, articular manifestations, and pulmonary complications become more prominent in SjD [8].

In AYA, the clinical phenotype often mirrors that of early-onset adult SjD [9, 10]. Recurrent parotitis may be the initial symptom prompting rheumatological consultation [11]. Compared to older adults, AYA often present with systemic symptoms such as fever, involuntary weight loss, and night sweats, along with extraglandular manifestations like cytopaenias, vasculitis, neuromyelitis optica spectrum disorder, or diffuse lymphadenopathies [6, 12, 13]. In some cases, mucosa-associated lymphoid tissue (MALT) lymphoma might be the first presentation of cSjD [14].

Unmet Need for Development and Validation of cSjD-Specific Classification Criteria

In 2016, a joint initiative by the American College of Rheumatology (ACR) and EULAR developed data-driven classification criteria for adult-onset SjD to identify homogeneous study populations for future research. The ACR/EULAR criteria emphasise dryness symptoms, particularly dry eyes and mouth [15], but these symptoms may be absent in at least one-third of children and adolescents [5, 6, 12]. Despite being intended for classification, these criteria are often used to diagnose the disease in adults [16]. However, they showed reduced sensitivity in AYA due to the heterogeneity of clinical manifestations at disease onset in young people. As there are no validated diagnostic or classification criteria for cSjD, paediatric rheumatologists often rely on clinical judgement and experience, along with employing adult criteria, to diagnose cSjD [17, 18]. This reliance, coupled with the limited number of cSjD cases managed by individual physicians, raises concerns about under-diagnosis.

Therefore, the differential diagnosis of an adolescent with symptoms suggestive of a systemic connective tissue disease should include cSjD, as early recognition is crucial for optimised management. While there is no definitive test for cSjD, minor or major salivary or lacrimal gland biopsy to assess for focal lymphocytic sialadenitis or dacryoadenitis, in addition to imaging techniques (such as sialography, ultrasound and magnetic resonance imaging—MRI) may be indicated, as these investigations can exclude other disease mimickers and facilitate diagnosis [19–21]. Recent efforts have been made to establish diagnostic tools and scoring system to assist classification and long-term monitoring of AYA with cSjD, but they require further research and validation [22, 23]. Additionally, paediatric rheumatology specialists from Japan initially proposed and subsequently revised clinical practice recommendations for cSjD, which also include a diagnostic guidance algorithm based on clinical and serological findings, which require further testing in larger and ethnically diverse populations [24].

General Management Considerations for cSjD in AYA

Given its rarity and complexity, a multidisciplinary approach within specialist centres to address both the glandular and systemic components of the disease is crucial in the management of AYA with cSjD. Collaboration among paediatricians, rheumatologists, ophthalmologists, dentists and oral health specialists, radiologists, and other health care professionals is essential for comprehensive care of AYA with cSjD [25]. Treatment goals are to reduce symptoms, prevent long-term damage, and manage systemic involvement, aiming to ultimately preserve QoL.

The management of AYA with cSjD should rely on the regular monitoring for both glandular and extraglandular manifestations, as symptoms of the disease might accrue over time and complications need to be mitigated against.

Regular follow-up with dental and ophthalmology services is crucial to monitor and manage oral and ocular health. Preventative measures, including topical fluoride treatments and regular eye exams, are recommended to mitigate complications of sicca syndrome (dry eyes and mouth). Moreover, despite the absence of patient-reported complaints of dryness, a significant proportion of AYA with cSjD has objective exocrine gland secretory dysfunction [22].

Although the risk of MALT-associated lymphoma is not known in AYA with cSjD, this is a well-known rare but potentially severe complication of SjD in adults [10].

Patient education is of utmost importance to ensure adherence to treatment and to enhance patient empowerment in managing their condition effectively. As adolescence and young adulthood are critical developmental phases in life, psychological support should be offered to young people with cSjD, along with specific support to prevent any impact of the disease on educational, vocational or employment opportunities.

Vaccination status should be assessed periodically [26] and vaccination against influenza and pneumococcal infections should be offered, especially in AYA requiring immunosuppression. As some individuals with SjD are at risk for varicella zoster infection [27], vaccination should be recommended in selected cases, with a preference for inactivated VZV vaccine. Age appropriate vaccination against human papilloma virus (HPV) for both sexes is also recommended.

Therapeutic Approaches for Glandular and Extraglandular Manifestations in cSjD

The treatment of SjD involves a combination of topical and systemic treatments tailored to the individual's age, clinical features, severity of manifestations, impact on QoL, comorbidities, and other considerations (e.g. pregnancy, see Chap. 19) [28, 29]. However, evidence for the most appropriate treatment and management strategies for cSjD is limited, and most treatment recommendations are extrapolated from studies conducted in adult populations, which do not consider the specific needs or disease particularities of AYA [30, 31]. Furthermore, no licensed systemic immunomodulatory agents are available for cSjD.

In clinical practice, a combination of topical treatments, systemic immunomodulatory agents, and supportive strategies have been used in AYA with cSjD [17, 18, 24].

Sicca symptoms may be managed with topical therapies, such as: preservative-free artificial tears or ocular gels/ointments for ocular dryness; saliva substitutes or non-pharmacological glandular stimulation (e.g., sugar-free acidic candies, xylitol, or sugar-free chewing gum) for oral dryness; and moisturisers and lubricants for vaginal dryness [28, 29]. In severe or refractory cases, pharmacological interventions such as topical cyclosporine A, and autologous or allogeneic serum eye drops can be used to address ocular dryness, and oral pilocarpine or cevimeline to enhance exocrine gland secretion overall, and they are all recommended for adult populations and have been also used in AYA with cSjD [28, 29]. Recent advances in techniques such as sialendoscopy have shown promise in managing persistent glandular symptoms and improving long-term outcomes, including in the paediatric population [32].

However, several limitations, such as the lack of standardised age-specific cutoffs for glandular function tests, the absence of paediatric-reported outcomes tailored for younger individuals, and the absence of clinical trials comparing different therapeutic approaches, may present significant challenges in evaluating the disease severity and determining appropriate management strategies for dryness in AYA with cSjD [31].

According to two recent surveys conducted by the Childhood Arthritis Research Alliance (CARRA) and the Pediatric Rheumatology European Society (PReS) Sjögren Interest group, systemic treatment is most commonly initiated to treat severe extraglandular involvement (such as arthritis, lung disease, renal disease, central nervous system or cutaneous involvement), or in cases of recurrent and symptomatic parotitis refractory to non-steroidal anti-inflammatories and short courses of oral steroids. However, significant variation in practice patterns, medication use and definition of response to treatment was observed, depending on the manifestation being treated and the clinician's experience [17, 18].

When analysing the results from the CARRA survey, recurrent parotitis was most commonly treated with a variable combination of hydroxychloroquine, corticosteroids, methotrexate, and mycophenolate mofetil. Systemic manifestations were commonly treated with a combination of hydroxychloroquine, corticosteroids, and conventional or biologic disease-modifying anti-rheumatic drugs [17].

Physicians with higher self-reported experience in cSjD or who managed a larger caseload yearly were more likely to prescribe biologics, including abatacept, belimumab, and rituximab [17]. Due to the lack of long-term studies focusing on the natural history and potential complications of cSjD, these treatments have been adopted based on expertise with their use in other paediatric autoimmune conditions or in adults with SjD despite an unclear benefit/risk ratio. Thus, data on the long-term treatment response and prognosis of cSjD are required to support cSjD management recommendations [31].

Impact of cSjD on Physical Health and QoL Based on Clinical Manifestations

SjD has a significant impact on the QoL of affected individuals. The QoL could potentially be affected in AYA due to a combination of multiple detrimental factors, including fatigue, pain/articular involvement, ocular and oral dryness with impact on eating and speaking, pruritus, impaired oral health, sexual dysfunction due to vaginal dryness, impaired sleep, pulmonary manifestations, which can also affect the physical and psychological well-being [33].

In cSjD, the clinical features considered by treating physicians to impact QoL were fatigue, dry eye, parotitis, dry mouth, and pain [17].

While dryness symptoms might exert the highest negative impact on QoL later in life [8], these symptoms might be absent in AYA in 30–70% of cases [6, 34]. Constitutional and articular symptoms, however, might directly impact the QoL of AYA [4].

Constitutional symptoms, such as fever, weight loss, and malaise, are extremely frequent in cSjD (11–70%) [5, 6], and have a detrimental effect on QoL by reducing school attendance, leisure activities, and relationships with peers.

Articular symptoms, such as arthritis and arthralgia, are extremely frequent in cSjD, with a prevalence ranging from 26.5% [4] to 80% [5]. Arthritis may be found in up to a quarter of these AYA with cSjD [6], while muscular complaints are reported with a lower frequency (0–17%) [5, 34]. When evaluated, fatigue is reported in 40–60% of cSjD cases [5, 12, 34].

However, until now, no studies have addressed the direct impact of cSjD on QoL in adolescence or early adulthood.

Patient Education and Lifestyle Change

Patient empowerment and self-management education should be encouraged, as this has been identified as a key issue in SjD. Written or online educational materials should be offered to AYA [28], and digital tools might be preferred by this age group [35]. Additionally, participation in peer-to-peer support initiatives and patient associations (https://www.sjogreneurope.org) should be encouraged [28].

Coping strategies and lifestyle changes might help AYA with cSjD better manage their symptoms and maintain a higher QoL. Exercise should be encouraged as regular practice might help reduce SjD-associated fatigue [28]. Regular oral and eye health care, including the use of lubricants, masticatory stimulation, and adequate hydration, is essential for maintaining oral and ocular health. Regular dental evaluations should be encouraged to prevent tooth decay, erosion, and loss [28, 29].

AYA with cSjD should be advised to avoid environmental triggers that can worsen symptoms of dry eyes, such as low humidity, drafts from air conditioners or fans, smoke, dust, or excessive makeup. Smoking cessation is strongly recommended for all AYA with cSjD.

Sexual and Reproductive Health

Sexuality development during adolescence and young adulthood significantly impacts the QoL and relationships later in life. It is well known that chronic conditions can negatively affect psychosexual development. SjD has been shown to significantly reduce sexual QoL due to a combination of physical symptoms, such as vaginal dryness, and psychosocial factors [36].

Despite the absence of studies specifically assessing sexual life in AYA with cSjD, an overall impaired sexual life is also reported in premenopausal women with SjD. In cSjD, the prevalence of vaginal dryness varies from 5% to 57% [5, 6].

As the positivity for anti-SSA antibodies, and to a lesser extent anti-SSB and anti-U1-RNP (anti U1-ribonucleoprotein), is associated with pregnancy risk of developing foetal congenital heart block and neonatal lupus erythematosus [37], female AYA with cSjD should be educated to minimise the risk of unplanned pregnancy.

Furthermore, SjD should be regarded as a high-risk pregnancy condition associated with comorbidities and potentially adverse maternal and foetal outcomes [38].

Thus, female of childbearing age should be counselled regarding contraceptive methods, and pregnancy planning should be conducted to prevent complications related to the disease itself and mitigate against the potential negative effects of immunosuppressive medications, such as methotrexate, mycophenolate mofetil, leflunomide, which are contraindicated in pregnancy. The impact of timing of B cell depletion therapy on pregnancy plans and newborn vaccinations should also be considered [28] (see Chap. 19).

Long-Term Outcomes in cSjD

Although SjD has historically been considered a "benign" condition with no significant impact on life expectancy, studies conducted on adults with SjD have shown increased cardiovascular morbidity, a higher risk of hospitalisation for infections, neurological disease, and malignancies [39]. Additionally, there has been a significant increase worldwide in the age-standardised mortality rate in recent years [40].

The presence of a systemic inflammatory state, as indicated by the presence of cryoglobulins and a high ESSDAI score, is associated with an increased mortality risk [39]. cSjD could be associated with systemic involvement, with high ESSDAI score being documented in 17–30% of cases at presentation [4, 12, 34], associated with high prevalence of extraglandular manifestations, and signs of marked B-cell activation (such as hypocomplementemia, rheumatoid factor positivity, hypergammaglobulinemia, autoantibody positivity, and the presence of cryoglobulinemia) [4–6, 8].

Therefore, despite the absence of long-term studies on the prognosis of cSjD, AYA with cSjD should be monitored regularly as studies focusing on early-onset SjD (defined as disease onset before 35 years of age) have shown a trend towards worsening ESSDAI scores over time [9] and a higher risk of developing lymphoma [10].

At the same time, early therapeutic intervention aiming to reduce the inflammatory burden in children and AYA with cSjD might potentially prevent the development of complications and exert a beneficial impact on the long-term prognosis [34]. Further studies are needed to confirm the existence of a therapeutic "window of opportunity" and to determine the best therapeutic strategies for cSjD.

Transition to Adulthood in cSjD

The transition of care of young people with any childhood-onset chronic rheumatic disease is a key process with implications in determining their long-term prognosis [41]. However, the available guidelines do not provide specific indications for the transition of care in cSjD [25, 29], so the broad joint EULAR/PReS recommendations are used in clinical practice [42].

Despite the existence of such guidelines, their implementation is inconsistent across centres, leading to wide variability in transition of care programs [43]. No study has specifically addressed the efficacy of established transition of care programs specifically for cSjD, and this population may be under-represented in existing studies [44].

As an overall principle, due to the complexity and heterogeneity of this condition, the transition of care for cSjD should involve transfer from paediatric rheumatology services to adult centres specialised in connective tissue diseases, where a multidisciplinary approach in cSjD management should be offered. Further studies are required to evaluate the specific requirements and highlight the unmet needs of transitional care of AYA with cSjD.

Key Management Points

1. In children and adolescents with cSjD), recurrent parotitis may be the initial symptom prompting rheumatological consultation, while systemic symptoms are common overall, compared to older adults.
2. A multidisciplinary approach, along with educational and psychological support for adolescents and their families/caregivers, is cornerstone in managing cSjD.
3. Regular monitoring of both glandular and extraglandular manifestations and their impact on QoL is warranted to minimise the risk of damage accrual and promptly treat potential severe complications.
4. Hydroxychloroquine is frequently used to manage parotitis and other systemic manifestations, despite limited evidence supporting its efficacy. Corticosteroids are recommended only for short-term therapy during acute exacerbations and severe systemic involvement. In refractory cases, immunosuppressive agents such as methotrexate, mycophenolate mofetil, leflunomide, and biologics may be considered. Local treatments such as artificial tears and saliva substitutes may reduce disease burden, and if insufficient, pilocarpine or cevimeline or topical ocular cyclosporine A can be added.
5. Additional relevant issues for AYA include transition to adult care, contraception and pregnancy planning, and vaccinations to minimise infectious risks.

References

1. Mariette X, Criswell LA. Primary Sjögren's syndrome. N Engl J Med. 2018;378(10):931–9.
2. Randell RL, Lieberman SM. Unique aspects of pediatric Sjögren disease. Rheum Dis Clin North Am. 2021;47(4):707–23.
3. Narváez J, Sánchez-Fernández SÁ, Seoane-Mato D, Díaz-González F, Bustabad S. Prevalence of Sjögren's syndrome in the general adult population in Spain: estimating the proportion of undiagnosed cases. Sci Rep. 2020;10(1):10627.

4. Ramos-Casals M, Acar-Denizli N, Vissink A, Brito-Zerón P, Li X, et al. Childhood-onset of primary Sjögren's syndrome: phenotypic characterization at diagnosis of 158 children. Rheumatology (Oxford). 2021;60(10):4558–67.
5. Marino A, Romano M, Giani T, Gaggiano C, Costi S, et al. Childhood Sjogren's syndrome: an Italian case series and a literature review-based cohort. Semin Arthritis Rheum. 2021;51(4):903–10.
6. Basiaga ML, Stern SM, Mehta JJ, Edens C, Randell RL, et al. Childhood Sjögren syndrome: features of an international cohort and application of the 2016 ACR/EULAR classification criteria. Rheumatology (Oxford). 2021;60(7):3144–55.
7. Kim MC, De U, Borcherding N, Wang L, Paek J, Bhattacharyya I, et al. Single-cell transcriptomics unveil profiles and interplay of immune subsets in rare autoimmune childhood Sjögren's disease. Commun Biol. 2024;7(1):481.
8. Retamozo S, Acar-Denizli N, Horváth IF, Ng WF, Rasmussen A, et al. Influence of the age at diagnosis in the disease expression of primary Sjögren syndrome. Analysis of 12,753 patients from the Sjögren Big Data Consortium. Clin Exp Rheumatol. 2021;39 Suppl 133(6):166–74.
9. Anquetil C, Hachulla E, Machuron F, Mariette X, Le Guern V, et al. Is early-onset primary Sjögren's syndrome a worse prognosis form of the disease? Rheumatology (Oxford). 2019;58(7):1163–7.
10. Goules AV, Argyropoulou OD, Pezoulas VC, Chatzis L, Critselis E, et al. Primary Sjögren's syndrome of early and late onset: distinct clinical phenotypes and lymphoma development. Front Immunol. 2020;11:594096.
11. Schiffer BL, Stern SM, Park AH. Sjögren's syndrome in children with recurrent parotitis. Int J Pediatr Otorhinolaryngol 2020;129:109768. doi: https://doi.org/10.1016/j.ijporl.2019.109768. Epub 2019 Nov 6.
12. Legger GE, Erdtsieck MB, de Wolff L, Stel AJ, Los LI, et al. Differences in presentation between paediatric- and adult-onset primary Sjögren's syndrome patients. Clin Exp Rheumatol. 2021;39 Suppl 133(6):85–92.
13. Gong Y, Liu H, Li G, Zhang T, et al. Childhood-onset primary Sjögren's syndrome in a tertiary center in China: clinical features and outcome. Pediatr Rheumatol Online J. 2023;21(1):11. Published 2023 Jan 27.
14. Tesher MS, Esteban Y, Henderson TO, Villanueva G, Onel KB. Mucosal-associated Lymphoid Tissue (MALT) Lymphoma in Association with pediatric primary Sjogren syndrome: 2 cases and review. J Pediatr Hematol Oncol. 2019;41(5):413–6.
15. Shiboski CH, Shiboski SC, Seror R, Criswell LA, Labetoulle M, et al. 2016 American College of Rheumatology/European League against rheumatism classification criteria for primary Sjögren's Syndrome: a consensus and data-driven methodology involving three international patient cohorts. Arthritis Rheumatol. 2017;69(1):35–45.

16. Van Nimwegen Jf, Van Ginkel Ms., Arends S Et Al.: Validation of the ACR-EULAR criteria for primary Sjögren's syndrome in a Dutch prospective diagnostic cohort. Rheumatology 2018; 57: 818–825
17. Randell RL, Stern SM, Van Mater H, Schanberg LE, Lieberman SM, et al. Pediatric rheumatologists' perspectives on diagnosis, treatment, and outcomes of Sjögren disease in children and adolescents. Pediatr Rheumatol Online J. 2022;20(1):79.
18. Melo Gomes S, Marrani E, Sahin S, Jelusic M, et al. Childhood-onset Sjögren disease in current practice: an international survey study. Abstract accepted at the 31st annual Pediatric Rheumatology European society (PReS) Meeting, September 2024
19. Yokogawa N, Lieberman SM, Sherry DD, Vivino FB. Features of childhood Sjögren's syndrome in comparison to adult Sjögren's syndrome: considerations in establishing child-specific diagnostic criteria. Clin Exp Rheumatol. 2016;34(2):343–51. Epub 2016 Jan 20
20. Ciurtin C, Cho Y, Al-Obaidi M, Jury EC, Price EJ. Barriers to translational research in Sjögren's syndrome with childhood onset: challenges of recognising and diagnosing an orphan rheumatic disease. Lancet Rheumatol. 2021 Feb;3(2):e138–48.
21. Hammenfors DS, Valim V, Bica B, Pasoto SG, et al. Juvenile Sjögren's syndrome: clinical characteristics with focus on salivary gland ultrasonography. Arthritis Care Res (Hoboken). 2020;72(1):78–87.
22. Zeng W, Thatayatikom A, Winn N, Lovelace TC, Bhattacharyya I, et al. The Florida Scoring System for stratifying children with suspected Sjögren's disease: a cross-sectional machine learning study. Lancet Rheumatol. 2024;6(5):e279–90.
23. Ciurtin C, Jury EC. A new tool for stratifying children with suspected Sjögren's disease. Lancet Rheumatol. 2024;6(5):e255–6.
24. Tomiita M, Kobayashi I, Itoh Y, Inoue Y, Iwata N, et al. Clinical practice guidance for Sjögren's syndrome in pediatric patients (2018)—summarized and updated, Mod Rheumatol, Volume 31, Issue 2, 4 March 2021, Pages 283–293
25. Treemarcki EB, Lieberman SM, Basiaga ML, Orrock J, Edens C, et al. Opportunities in childhood Sjogren's disease-results from collaborative roundtable discussions. Rheumatology (Oxford). 2024:keae258.
26. Jansen MH, Rondaan C, Legger G, Minden K, Uziel Y, et al. Efficacy, immunogenicity and safety of vaccination in Pediatric Patients With Autoimmune Inflammatory Rheumatic Diseases (pedAIIRD): a systematic literature review for the 2021 update of the EULAR/PRES recommendations. Front Pediatr. 2022;10:910026.
27. Goulabchand R, Makinson A, Morel J, Witkowski-Durand-Viel P, Nagot N, et al. Hospitalizations for infections in primary Sjögren's syndrome patients: a nationwide incidence study. Ann Med. 2022;54(1):2672–80.

28. Price EJ, Benjamin S, Bombardieri M, Bowman S, Carty S, et al. British Society for Rheumatology guideline on management of adult and juvenile onset Sjögren disease. Rheumatology (Oxford). 2024:keae152.
29. Ramos-Casals M, Brito-Zerón P, Bombardieri S, Bootsma H, De Vita S, et al. EULAR-Sjögren Syndrome Task Force Group. EULAR recommendations for the management of Sjögren's syndrome with topical and systemic therapies. Ann Rheum Dis. 2020;79(1):3–18.
30. Doolan G, Faizal NM, Foley C, Al-Obaidi M, et al. Treatment strategies for Sjögren's syndrome with childhood onset: a systematic review of the literature. Rheumatology (Oxford). 2022;61(3):892–912.
31. Ciurtin C, Price E. A viewpoint on therapeutic approaches and unmet needs in the management of young people with Sjögren disease. touchREVIEWS in RMD. 2024;3(1):31–6.
32. Drew K, Kronlage R, Cha S, Thatayatikom A, Schrepfer T. Long-term efficacy of sialendoscopy in treating childhood Sjögren's disease with chronological monitoring by salivary gland ultrasonography: a novel approach. Pediatr Rheumatol Online J. 2023;21(1):83.
33. Mardale DA, Opriş-Belinski D, Bojincă V, Bojincă M, Mazilu D, et al. The physical and psychosocial impact of fatigue among patients with Sjogren's syndrome: a systematic review. J Clin Med. 2024;13(6):1537.
34. Iwata N, Tomiita M, Kobayashi I, Inoue Y, Nonaka Y, Okamoto N, Umebayashi H, Hara R, Ito Y, Sato Y, Mori M. Utility of the EULAR Sjögren syndrome disease activity index in Japanese children: a retrospective multicenter cohort study. Pediatr Rheumatol Online J. 2020;18(1):73.
35. McCallum C, Campbell M, Vines J, Rapley T, Ellis J, Deary V, Hackett K. A smartphone app to support self-management for people living with Sjögren's syndrome: qualitative co-design workshops. JMIR Hum Factors. 2024;11:e54172.
36. Hsu CW, Lee JT, Koo M. Sexual dysfunction in women with primary Sjögren's syndrome: a systematic review and meta-analysis. Sex Med Rev. 2024:qeae009.
37. Brito-Zerón P, Pasoto SG, Robles-Marhuenda A, Mandl T, Vissink A, et al. Autoimmune congenital heart block and primary Sjögren's syndrome: characterisation and outcomes of 49 cases. Clin Exp Rheumatol. 2020;38 Suppl 126(4):95–102.
38. Yang Y, Huang XX, Huo RX, Lin JY. Impact of Sjögren's syndrome on maternal and fetal outcomes following pregnancy: a systematic review and meta-analysis of studies published between years 2007–2022. Arch Gynecol Obstet. 2024;309(4):1135–49.
39. Brito-Zerón P, Flores-Chávez A, Horváth IF, Rasmussen A, Li X, et al. Mortality risk factors in primary Sjögren syndrome: a real-world, retrospective, cohort study. EClinicalMedicine. 2023;61:102062.

40. Scherlinger M, Mertz P, Sagez F, Meyer A, et al. Worldwide trends in all-cause mortality of auto-immune systemic diseases between 2001 and 2014. Autoimmun Rev. 2020;19(6):102531.
41. Hersh A, von Scheven E, Yelin E. Adult outcomes of childhood- onset rheumatic diseases. Nat Rev Rheumatol. 2011;7:290–5.
42. Foster HE, Minden K, Clemente D, et al. EULAR/PReS standards and recommendations for the transitional care of young people with juvenile-onset rheumatic diseases. Ann Rheum Dis. 2017;76(4):639–46.
43. Marrani E, Zajc Avramovic M, Marinello D, et al. Challenges in the transition of care for rare connective tissue diseases: results from the 2023 ERN-ReCONNET Transition of Care Task Force survey. Abstract accepted at the 31st annual Pediatric Rheumatology European society (PReS) Meeting, September 2024
44. Walter M, Kamphuis S, van Pelt P, de Vroed A, Hazes JMW. Successful implementation of a clinical transition pathway for adolescents with juvenile-onset rheumatic and musculoskeletal diseases. Pediatr Rheumatol Online J. 2018;16(1):50.

12 Hypermobility in Adolescence and Young Adulthood

Ellie Potts and Sophia Mavrommatis

Introduction

Distinguishing potentially advantageous hypermobility from that which is troublesome to adolescents and young adults (AYA) i.e. problematic, causing pain and fatigue during or after activities, is often challenging. There is a broad spectrum of joint flexibility within the normal population [1–3], and joints and soft tissues normally become less flexible with age. With the onset of puberty, hormonal changes have an impact upon joint flexibility and function of surrounding muscles (see Chap. 1). The tendency for AYA to develop pain and fatigue with hypermobility may change throughout adolescence and young adulthood. This relates to growth and hormonal influences on the musculoskeletal system,

E. Potts (✉)
Department of Paediatric and Adolescent Rheumatology, Evelina London Children's Hospital, Guy's and St Thomas' NHS Foundation Trust, London, UK
e-mail: ellie.potts@gstt.nhs.uk

S. Mavrommatis
Department of Adolescent & Young Adult Rheumatology, University College London NHS Foundation Trust, London, UK
e-mail: sophia.mavrommatis@nhs.net

C. Ciurtin, J. Hackett (eds.), *Adolescent and Young Adult Rheumatology In Clinical Practice*, In Clinical Practice,
https://doi.org/10.1007/978-3-031-82102-8_12

as well as changing exercise patterns and demands of young people.

Pain has a reduced impact upon function in high performing athletes who combine flexibility with extreme strength and agility. Similarly, the overall aim in management of problematic hypermobility is to help the AYA regain control over flexible joints and improve function despite pain. A goal-based practical approach helps AYA to rehabilitate to better cope with physical challenges they may face. This chapter will discuss both assessment and rehabilitation.

Terminology

Problematic hypermobility may be referred to using several different terms. The most common of these are hypermobility syndrome, joint hypermobility syndrome, benign joint hypermobility syndrome (to distinguish from hypermobility due to an underlying connective tissue or genetic disorder), Ehlers-Danlos syndrome hypermobility type (EDS-HT), generalised joint laxity, generalised joint hypermobility and, most recently, hypermobility spectrum disorders [4]. These terms are used in paediatric, adolescent and adult populations. For simplicity this chapter will use the umbrella term hypermobility (HM) to refer to all these conditions.

Diagnosis

Initially described in the 1960s using the Berlin nosology (1988) and latterly the Villefranche nosology (1998), the criteria for diagnosis of HM have evolved over time. In 2017 an updated EDS classification was proposed including HM [4]. Since then, there has been a drive to make the old terminology obsolete and replace HM previously classified as non-genetically proven EDS-HT with the term hypermobility spectrum disorders [4].

It is important to differentiate HM from other heritable connective tissue disorders which may present with hypermobile joints. These include the Ehlers-Danlos spectrum (arthrochalasia, classical and vascular), Marfan's syndrome, Stickler's syndrome, osteogenesis imperfecta, skeletal dysplasias, velocardiofacial syndrome, Loeys-Dietz syndrome and trisomy 21. These conditions have clinical features distinguishing them from HM, and the majority are identified at an early age. Skeletal dysplasia is one potential exception in which isolated joint hypermobility can present in younger years, prior to progressive joint squaring with loss of range of movement (ROM), particularly at the hips, knees, shoulders, elbows and spine, during adolescence.

The fundamental distinction of problematic HM from increased joint flexibility is based upon:

- The presence of pain and/or fatigue during/after activity with relation to joint flexibility
- Intermittent joint swelling, lasting for only a few hours or days
- Poor muscular control around a flexible joint

Presenting symptoms of HM in AYA are frequently isolated to the knees, shoulders, spine or hands. The incidence may rise around the transition from primary to secondary school and during the AYA years. These are typically periods of increased physical activity during daily life, through attendance at larger schools or work, as well as the demands of sports and physical education at a time when muscle strength and control are less developed and coordinated. Since the speed of bone growth exceeds that of muscle, there is typically a lag period in muscle lengthening, or muscles may tighten with overuse. This is commonly seen with knee and lumbar spine flexibility in AYA.

Muscles need to be strong and fit to carry out their roles of power, stability and endurance in multidirectional movements. Young people with HM often have muscle weakness [5], which may be associated with fatigue [6]. The presence of pain is linked to the severity of fatigue. These adversely impact upon health-related quality of life [7].

Flexibility reduces with age. A young person who is hypermobile at the beginning of puberty may lose flexibility with skeletal and muscular maturity. The growing young person can have fluctuating symptomatology linked to their activity, joint range and muscular control during this period. Ongoing reassessment of the AYA's needs is pivotal in their rehabilitation, alongside reassurance by specific discussion of typical changes young people may experience.

Scoring Systems

The classification of HM in clinical practice is based upon several scoring systems (Table 12.1). Historically the main scoring system in clinical practice is the Beighton scale (1973) [8]. As with all classifications, there are some challenges and limitations.

Although the most widely used, there are shortcomings in the validity of the *Beighton scale* [8–11]. When tested in the paediatric population, scores did not correlate with post-activity pain, suggesting other factors may be at play [8]. The reproducibility of the test is modest with a kappa score of 0.75–0.8 at most joints, falling to 0.6 at the fifth finger and elbows [8]. Assessment is limited to the sagittal plane, and the score fails to assess other key joints including the shoulder, which is commonly associated with pain and/or instability in the hypermobile adolescent and adult. A self-reported Beighton scale has been validated in adults aged 20–66, although this has lower reproducibility and is yet to be validated in adolescents [9]. Despite these limitations, the score is clinically useful provided it is applied in a consistent manner using a cut-off ≥5/9 to diagnose HM.

The *Brighton criteria* were devised to further classify HM. It expands upon true joint-related flexibility to include the contribution from skin elasticity, arthralgia and extra-articular features [12]. This uses a lower Beighton cut-off than the current consensus (≥4/9), carrying a risk of overdiagnosis. Currently only validated in the adult population, it has good reliability and validity of the musculoskeletal manifestations. The skin signs are less clear (kappa = 0.63) [12].

Lower Limb Hypermobility Assessment Score (LLHAS) assesses the physiological and accessory ROM of hips, knees, ankles and feet. It has excellent intra- and inter-rater reliability in 5–16-year-

Table 12.1 Scoring systems for hypermobility

Tool	Description	Advantages	Limitations
Beighton scale [8–12]	9-point ROM scale Hands (4 points) Knees (2 points) Elbows (2 points) Spine (1 point) Cut-off ≥5/9	Simplicity Widespread clinical use	Lacks clear, validated instructions Overlooks problem areas (hips, feet and shoulders)
Brighton criteria [12]	2 major criteria, 8 minor criteria 2 major criteria Or one major and ≥2–4 minor criteria	Validated in adults with good reliability	Skin criteria unreliable Not validated in adolescents or children
Lower limb hypermobility assessment score (LLHAS) [13]	Accessory and physiological ROM Hips Knees Ankles Feet Cut-off ≥7/11	Reliable in children and AYA	Variable sensitivity and specificity Small sample size
Upper limb hypermobility assessment tool (ULHAT) [14]	Accessory and physiological ROM Shoulders Elbows Hands Cut-off ≥7/12	Valid in later AYA population	Validated in predominantly Caucasian population Small sample size

olds using a cut-off ≥7/11, but variable sensitivity and specificity. The same has been shown in young adults (aged 20–30 years) with improved specificity and moderate sensitivity [13].

Like the LLHAS, the *Upper Limb Hypermobility Assessment Tool (ULHAT)* is relatively new but has been shown to identify those with likely or known hypermobility. The recommended cut-off of ≥7/12 best distinguishes those with upper limb hypermobility from those without. It did not reach significance when correlating and discriminating between age and ethnicity, and further work is needed to validate in the younger adolescent population and wider ethnicities and assess inter-rater reliability [14].

Hypermobility Rehabilitation of the AYA

A functional and practical approach to symptom management is essential for AYA with problematic HM. It is often helpful to list current problems and how best to address them, prior to discussing the concept of HM. Treatment should include interdisciplinary management looking at education (including nutrition); physical and occupational therapies to address functional, physical and fatigue-related issues; psychological intervention to facilitate pain and mood management; and in some cases surgical intervention with appropriate and timely rehabilitation.

Physical and Functional Management

To date there is limited specific evidence for the management of adolescents with musculoskeletal pain secondary to HM. However, one can extrapolate evidence from the management of children, adults and sports training principles. As with all RMD, it is important to consider bone mineral density development in adolescence (see Chap. 17) promoting weight bearing exercise. Exercising into the hypermobile range reduces pain-related psychosocial factors with HM [7].

Adolescents with increased hypermobility may have impaired balance particularly in the non-dominant leg and shorter hamstrings. Balance and functional movement control exercises should be part of an effective rehabilitation programme. This is a prelude to plyometrics and power-based dynamic balance work.

Muscle strengthening aims to provide the young person with sufficient strength and endurance to carry out activities they enjoy. Combining progressive muscle strengthening to maintain joint flexibility and function is essential. Current evidence supports a 6–8-week programme [7]. Pacing will gradually and effectively build up stamina to cope with every day, as well as higher-demand activities and sports. Analysis and paced reintegration of functional activities with a stronger fitter body enable the AYA to positively approach both school and the workplace.

Even in high-level sports, people who are hypermobile and well trained have an increased tendency to injury and reinjure, especially during competition. The frequency of training is key as there is a risk of overtraining increasing injury (see Chap. 16). This further highlights the need for young people with HM to carefully maintain their strength and stamina, even during periods of wellness.

Psychological Management

Evidence confirms a link between anxiety and mood in those with HM [15, 16]. The causative factors are unknown; however, the impact of mood on musculoskeletal pain should not be underestimated. Holistic management is vital, especially in the complex AYA years. Goal setting, education and pain management are useful to support the young person achieve their targets. The use of activity and developmentally appropriate outcome measures are fundamental to determining effectiveness of treatment. Goal-based outcomes, where individuals identify the support they need to reach their goals, improve rehabilitation adherence [17]. Since AYA brain development continues into the mid-20s (see Chap. 1), it is essential that management during these years adapts as the young person and their needs develop.

Surgical Management

Surgery is generally not warranted in HM, with the exception of specific indications such as stabilisation of a recurrently dislocating joint. It is important that surgical planning forms part of an MDT approach and that appropriate postsurgical rehabilitation is carried out to ensure the best outcomes [18].

Issues Specific to AYA

Studies looking at long-term disability in AYAs with HM-related disorders support multifaceted rehabilitation, but as yet provide limited insight into long-term prognostic factors [16]. The body goes through many changes between adolescence and young adulthood, and symptoms of HM in the early years may resolve or indeed evolve over time. Adolescent-specific issues tend to be complex, due to the effects of rapid transformation physically and psychologically.

Muscles hypertrophy without hyperplasia during adolescence, reaching normal adult cross-sectional muscle fibre area by the end of puberty. In young men testosterone causes an increase in muscle bulk and consequently strength, which can impact upon joint flexibility. These changes in muscle composition and fibre type lend boys towards strength and girls towards endurance activities. Females are more dependent upon training to improve power, thus influencing the type of treatment they may need to overcome the challenges of HM in adulthood.

There are many different risk factors for pain in HM postulated. A large population-based study of 6000 adolescents identified obesity to be a risk factor for pain in hypermobile girls but not when looking at those with a Beighton score ≥6/9 [1]. Other studies suggest a potential link to those with a more sedentary lifestyle [16]. AYA change rapidly; hence further work is needed to tease this out.

Conclusion

Hypermobility-related problems are common. They require interdisciplinary, goal-oriented rehabilitation which focuses upon eventual self-management for the individual young person.

Key Management Points

1. Problematic hypermobility may resolve or evolve through AYA.
2. Strengthening, endurance and plyometrics are essential tools in rehabilitation.
3. Functional activities and a goal-based approach offer the young person control over their treatment and provide useful steps to achieving their targets.
4. Work towards self-management.

References

1. Clinch J, Deere K, Sayers A, Palmer S, Riddoch C, Tobias JH and Clark EM. Epidemiology of generalized joint laxity (hypermobility) in fourteen-year-old children from the UK: a population-based evaluation. Arthritis Rheum. 2011;63(9):2819–27.
2. Morris SL, O'Sullivan PB, Murray KJ, Bear N, Hands B, and Smith AJ. Hypermobility and musculoskeletal pain in adolescents. J Pediatr. 2017;181:213–21. Elsevier Inc.
3. Sobhani-Eraghi A, Motalebi M, Sarreshtehdari S, Molazem-Sanandaji B, Hasanlu Z. Prevalence of joint hypermobility in children and adolescents: a systematic review and meta-analysis. J Res Med Sci Off J Isfahan Univ Med Sci [Online]. 2020;25(1):104. https://doi.org/10.4103/jrms.JRMS_983_19.
4. Castori M, Tinkle B, Levy H, Grahame R, Malfait F, Hakim A. A framework for the classification of joint hypermobility and related conditions. Am J Med Genet C: Semin Med Genet. 2017;175(1):148–57. https://doi.org/10.1002/ajmg.c.31539.
5. Jindal P, Narayan A, Ganesan S, MacDermid JC. Muscle strength differences in healthy young adults with and without generalized joint hypermobility: a cross-sectional study. BMC Sports Sci Med Rehabil. 2016;8(1):12. https://doi.org/10.1186/s13102-016-0037-x.
6. Voermans NC, Knoop H, Bleijenberg G, van Engelen BG. Fatigue is associated with muscle weakness in Ehlers-Danlos syndrome: an explorative study. Physiotherapy [Online]. 2011;97(2):170–4. https://doi.org/10.1016/j.physio.2010.06.001.
7. Engelbert RHH, Juul-Kristensen B, Pacey V, de Wandele I, Smeenk S, Woinarosky N, Sabo S, Scheper MC, Russek L, Simmonds JV. The evidence-based rationale for physical therapy treatment of children, adoles-

cents, and adults diagnosed with joint hypermobility syndrome/ hypermobile Ehlers Danlos syndrome. Am J Med Genet Part C: Semin Med Genet [Online]. 2017;175(1):158–67. https://doi.org/10.1002/ajmg.c.31545.

8. Juul-Kristensen B, Schmedling K, Rombaut L, Lund H, Engelbert RHH. Measurement properties of clinical assessment methods for classifying generalized joint hypermobility-a systematic review. Am J Med Genet C: Semin Med Genet. 2017;175(1):116–47. https://doi.org/10.1002/ajmg.c.31540.
9. Cooper DJ, Scammell BE, Batt ME, Palmer D. Development and validation of self-reported line drawings of the modified Beighton score for the assessment of generalised joint hypermobility. BMC Med Res Methodol. 2018;18(1):11. https://doi.org/10.1186/s12874-017-0464-8.
10. Singh H, McKay M, Baldwin J, Nicholson L, Chan C, Burns J, Hiller CE. Beighton scores and cut-offs across the lifespan: cross-sectional study of an Australian population. Rheumatology. 2017;56(11):1857–64. https://doi.org/10.1093/rheumatology/kex043.
11. Malek S, Reinhold EJ, Pearce GS. The Beighton Score as a measure of generalised joint hypermobility. Rheumatol Int. 2021;41(10):1707–16. https://doi.org/10.1007/s00296-021-04832-4.
12. Grahame R, Bird HA, Child A. The revised (Brighton 1998) criteria for the diagnosis of benign joint hypermobility syndrome (BJHS). J Rheumatol. 2000;27(7):1777–9.
13. Meyer KJ, Chan C, Hopper L, Nicholson LL. Identifying lower limb specific and generalised joint hypermobility in adults: validation of the Lower Limb Assessment Score. BMC Musculoskelet Disord. 2017;18(1):514. https://doi.org/10.1186/s12891-017-1875-8.
14. Nicholson LL, Chan C. The Upper Limb Hypermobility Assessment Tool: a novel validated measure of adult joint mobility. Musculoskelet Sci Pract. 2018;35:38–45. https://doi.org/10.1016/j.msksp.2018.02.006.
15. Scheper MC, Juul-Kristensen B, Rombaut L, Rameckers EA, Verbunt J, Engelbert RH. Disability in adolescents and adults diagnosed with hypermobility-related disorders: a meta-analysis. Arch Phys Med Rehabil. 2016;97(12):2174–87. https://doi.org/10.1016/j.apmr.2016.02.015.
16. Bulbena A, Baeza-Velasco C, Bulbena-Cabré A, Pailhez G, Critchley H, Chopra P, Mallorquí-Bagué N, Frank C, Porges S. Psychiatric and psychological aspects in the Ehlers-Danlos syndromes. Am J Med Genet C: Semin Med Genet [Online]. 2017;175(1):237–45. https://doi.org/10.1002/ajmg.c.31544.
17. Law D and Jacobs J. Goals and goal based outcomes (GBOs): some useful information. 3rd ed. London: CAMHS Press; 2015.
18. Vavken P, Tepolt FA, Kocher MS. Open inferior capsular shift for multidirectional shoulder instability in adolescents with generalized ligamentous hyperlaxity or Ehlers-Danlos syndrome. J Shoulder Elb Surg. 2016;25(6):907–12. https://doi.org/10.1016/j.jse.2015.10.010.

Chronic Musculoskeletal Pain in Adolescents and Young Adults

13

Jacqui Clinch

The new International classification of Diseases (ICD) 11 classification still defines chronic pain as persistent or recurrent pain for at least 3 months. Chronic primary pain is a concept originating from the idea that conditions associated with chronic pain should be acknowledged in their own right, even if a clear understanding of the underlying aetiology or pathophysiology is missing. From a paediatric MSK pain perspective, the relevant categories within Chronic Primary Pain are chronic primary MSK pain and complex regional pain syndrome. Persistent pain in conjunction with a rheumatologic disease: e.g. Juvenile Idiopathic Arthritis (JIA), Juvenile Dermatomyositis or Chronic Nonbacterial Osteomyelitis, would fall into the Chronic Secondary Pain category [1].

It is important to remember that pain is a normal sensation but becomes disabling when persistent and associated with suffering.

In AYA, MSK pains account for up to 64% of all the pains presenting to medical setting [2]; a recent systematic review that included all studies evaluating those under 19 years showed a prevalence of 25.7% [3]. A separate Canadian study found that

J. Clinch (✉)
Bristol Royal Hospital for Children, Bristol, UK

Young Person's Pain Service, Bath Centre for Pain Services, Royal National Hospital for Rheumatic Diseases, Bath, UK
e-mail: Jacqui.Clinch@uhbw.nhs.uk; Jacqui.Clinch@UHBristol.nhs.uk

C. Ciurtin, J. Hackett (eds.), *Adolescent and Young Adult Rheumatology In Clinical Practice*, In Clinical Practice,
https://doi.org/10.1007/978-3-031-82102-8_13

there were 28.6 million health professional visits over a nine-year period for chronic MSK pain for people under the age of 25 years, equivalent to an average of 3.2 million visits per year across the USA [4]. Current evidence regarding epidemiology of pain in AYA is summarised in Table 13.1 and associated features of chronic pain in Table 13.2.

Table 13.1 Epidemiology of pain in AYA

Type of pain	Prevalence	References
Primary Chronic Widespread Pain (CWP)—significant proportion musculoskeletal, sometimes referred to as juvenile fibromyalgia	4.3–8.5% in adolescents 14.3% in 18–25 year olds	[2, 5, 6]
Complex Regional Pain Syndrome (CRPS)	Prevalence in adults is 26 per 100,000 person years. In paediatrics it is estimated at 1.2 per 100,000 5–15 year olds	[7, 8]
Chronic back pain	Low back pain, mid-back and neck pain are reported as problematic in AYA	See Chap. 15
Persistent joint pain following previous or controlled inflammation (secondary chronic widespread pain)	In JIA persistent pain is a significant problem for many young people. A significant minority progress to develop MSK pain as young adults not directly related to control of their JIA	[9, 10]; Also see Chap. 7
MSK pain associated with joint laxity/hypermobility	Hypermobility, as currently defined, is present in 19.8% of the normal UK adolescent population. There is a relationship between localised knee pain and significant hypermobility (Beighton score 6 or above), but not CWP.	[11, 12]; Also see Chap. 12

Table 13.2 Factors associated with chronic pain in AYA

Age at onset—The incidence of chronic widespread MSK pain peaks in older adolescence [13].
Physical disabilities—Adolescents and adults with physical disabilities have a higher prevalence of chronic MSK pain [14].
Gender—Girls more frequently have chronic pain than boys, regardless of the location of the pain, and this discrepancy increases with age [13].
Socioeconomic—Low income and low educational backgrounds have higher incidence of chronic pain conditions [15].
Psychological factors—Several emotional and cognitive factors influence the perception, expression and response to pain in children and AYA [16].
Family history—Parental chronic pain has been identified as a strong correlation for pain in their child [17].
Sleep—A bidirectional relationship between sleep and chronic pain, with higher levels of disrupted sleep being associated with higher reports of pain which can have a prolonged impact [18].
Injury—often cited as a trigger for CRPS in AYA [19].
Joint laxity/hypermobility—association with localised joint pain (loading joints) but not chronic widespread pain [20].

Clinical Features of Chronic Musculoskeletal Pain

MSK pain often starts in a localised area of the body. The pain can intensify and radiate to other areas. It can be associated with a reluctance to mobilise and avoidance of movement. In adults, avoidance and fear of pain (and thus movement) can reduce fitness and further increase pain. In children and AYA this occurs in a MSK system that is still developing. As discrete pains multiply and continue, the young person may avoid contact with, or use of, an area of the body affected, and this can then lead to muscular spasms and abnormalities of posture and gait. As gait alters, the resultant asymmetry can lead to other vulnerable sites (including lower lumbar, anterior knee, and lateral aspect of pelvis) taking an altered load and causing further discomfort. Over time, affected limbs may adopt flexed positions and tendons may tighten, further exaggerating imbalance and pain.

A young person who is more anxious (including those who are neurodiverse) is at more risk of developing the fixed painful limb positioning.

Associated symptoms and signs of chronic pain in AYA

- Hypervigilance and pain sensitivity that is greater than expected from a given physical trigger [21]
- Perceived thermodysregulation—more common in adolescent girls. Limbs may be cool and mottled [22]
- Autonomic dysfunction—pain is a powerful stressor and can heighten sympathetic system activity with tachycardia, hyperventilation (compounded with panic attacks), cold sweats, blurred vision, abdominal pain and extreme pallor [21]
- MSKl disequilibrium—these young people are often still growing, and MSK pain can have lasting effects on the final positioning. Proprioceptive signals from the joints are reduced and the limb held in a rigid, fixed position. As gait alters, the resultant asymmetry can lead to other vulnerable sites (including lower lumbar, anterior knee, and lateral aspect of pelvis) taking an altered load and causing further discomfort. Over time, affected limbs may adopt flexed positions, and tendons tighten, further exaggerating imbalance and pain.

Effect of AYA with Chronic Pain on the Family

Chronic MSK pain, irrespective of its trigger, can be associated with persistent and recurrent distress, disability, adult attention, widespread family disruption and a tendency to catastrophize. AYA with MSK chronic pain report sleep disturbance, disordered mood, appetite disruption, low feelings (depression is often masked in this population), social isolation, and unwelcome dependency on parents. AYA with chronic pain report that they are less socially developed on virtually every metric than their peers [23].

Specific AYA Musculoskeletal Pain Conditions

Chronic Widespread Pain (CWP)/Juvenile Fibromyalgia [24]

This describes generalised, widespread pain, often located over muscles and joints, and with significant pain associated disability. The onset of pain in CWP is often gradual. There may have been an initial insult or trauma but often there is no trigger. There may be areas of allodynia (profound hypersensitivity to light touch) but often an absence of the autonomic changes (including reduced cutaneous perfusion, localised swelling, shiny stretched appearance) seen in more localised pain conditions.

What is striking in young people with diffuse pain is the associated fatigue, poor sleep pattern, and extremely low mood. It is widely believed, however, that low mood in adolescents is reactive (to the pain-associated disability) rather than a primary depression. This is in contrast to adults with fibromyalgia where primary depression is frequently seen. Menstrual cycling has been shown to affect fibromyalgia-related symptoms in nearly 50% of adult patients and this may be relevant in the adolescent female population.

Complex Regional Pain Syndrome (CRPS)

Rheumatologists frequently encounter patients presenting with CRPS and the diagnosis and treatment continues to court controversy. The diagnosis of CRPS remains a clinical one. There may be precipitating trauma. In AYA the lower limb is much more commonly involved than the upper limb. The pain is usually out of proportion to the inciting event and accompanied by allodynia. AYA most often describe the pain as burning and describe sensations akin to dysaesthesia. Autonomic changes are present; these include swelling, reduced cutaneous perfusion and thermodynamic instability. As this is present on the background of a developing MSK system, limbs can become distorted, and feet/hands held in seemingly fixed and often flexed positions. Cutaneous blood flow often reduces; the affected limb develops a purplish hue with other colour changes that can cause concern to the AYA and family. The skin takes on a shiny, stretched appearance, with coarse hairs developing in patches.

In adults the updated Budapest Criteria [25] are used to robustly diagnose CRPS. Whilst not validated in young people, these are useful in providing guidance.

Early recognition and multidisciplinary management are critical in improving outcome and preventing resistant CRPS, but even AYA with delayed diagnosis can still have complete functional restoration. Recurrence rates in the same or other locations appear higher than in adults (described in up to 30%), but response to re-initiation of treatment seems to be effective [26].

The Practical Approach to Chronic Pain in AYA [27]

Diagnosis

The goals of history taking are to exclude serious possible causes of pain with main differential diagnoses being trauma, inflammation, infection and malignancy. Physical examination is key (see Chap. 6) and once these are excluded the next steps are to identify key problems, build a trusting relationship with the young person (and family), and, if possible, identify a treatment plan. Assessment and treatment should be delivered by a multidisciplinary team and focus on rehabilitation and self management.

The Assessment of Chronic Pain

MSK pain intensity in AYA has long been measured using simple severity measurement tools, such as the visual analogue scale. These give a subjective measure of the pain intensity according to the AYA and/or pain perceived by their carer. While useful measures, they give no indication of the impact of pain on the young person. Multidisciplinary tools that have been validated in JIA-related chronic pain and the more general paediatric pain population include:

- Bath Adolescent Pain Questionnaire (BAPQ) for measuring the impact of pain on (i) adolescents with chronic pain and (ii) The Bath Adolescent Pain—Parental Impact Questionnaire (BAP-PIQ) [28]
- Pediatric Quality of Life Inventory TM (PEDsQL)—short quality of life score to assess impact. This has adolescent and young adult versions [29]

There are now also electronic, digital and multidimensional pain assessment tools which young people can use to record pain remotely. These can provide data that informs healthcare professionals' clinical assessment, communication and management of pain in this group [30].

Rehabilitation and Self-Management: Multidisciplinary Team Delivery of Physical, Psychological, Pharmacological Therapy and Education

The primary treatment approach to AYA with chronic MSK pain is one of symptom management and psychosocial rehabilitation. A dedicated team that works consistently with the adolescent and family will facilitate communication, ensure effective delivery of therapy, reduce iatrogenic influences and enable goals to be reached earlier [31]. Most approaches to rehabilitation share common features that include education, symptom control, behavioural science and physical therapy. Early recognition and intervention in an outpatient or inpatient setting is key and, in most cases, leads to a more favourable outcome. Including parents and, where possible tailoring interventions for them, is important. By changing parent behaviour and responses to their young person's pain, the young person achieves more optimal outcomes [32].

Education

A critical first step in rehabilitation is to offer, reoffer, and reinforce an understanding of how one's body may be working to maintain pain. Education about pain may be difficult to grasp because there is a dominant cultural view of pain in joints and muscles as a warning sign that a disease process or abnormality is present, and there is often a need for the AYA and family (and physician), to identify a cause. Education can play a valuable role as a fear reduction strategy, providing information to counter beliefs that they have a unique medical complication, or that their symptoms are related to an underlying mysterious disease. Rhetorical devices (metaphors, stories, examples, pictures) that counter the often rigid thinking can be helpful. Explaining the fascinating case of phantom limb experiences can also be helpful, to introduce flexibility and challenge the idea that brain signals must signify peripheral damage [33].

Pharmacotherapy

Many analgesics, given in different modalities, have been used for young people with chronic musculoskeletal pain, Recent Cochrane reviews [34] evaluating data on paracetamol, opioids, antidepressants and anticonvulsants concluded that there were insufficient data in all groups for meaningful analysis. Worryingly young people are turning to increasing amounts of over-the-counter medications and recreational substances to alleviate pain. When considering analgesia, it is sensible to follow the WHO guidelines [35] and, if considering opiates, to use these with very frequent reviews as part of a multidisciplinary approach.

Psychological Therapies

Psychological interventions, often devised around a CBT model (with tailored variations), are shown to have a larger impact on function than any pharmacological interventions to date.

It is widely understood that, when directing the rehabilitation of AYA with chronic MSK pain, proactively including dedicated psychology is key [36, 37].

Physical Therapies

Physical activity and exercise are crucial components in the management of chronic MSK pain however, most of the recommendations are based on adult populations and there are limited studies that robustly evaluate the effect of physiotherapy in childhood pain conditions. There are no standardised guidelines for exercise or treatment protocols for CYP with chronic MSK pain [38].

In conditions such as CRPS, early intensive physiotherapy (including desensitisation) with behavioural support can occasionally provide dramatic reversal of the presenting signs and symptoms for some young people [39], but more often this is a more paced, interdisciplinary journey. The aim is accelerated mobilisation, but this is hindered if the diagnosis is delayed and access to appropriate physical and psychological rehabilitation is limited. Increase of activity should be gradual and consistent. With MSK pains the more active the MSK system becomes, the more likely the muscle spasms and tightening are to be reduced. Proprioception improves and any autonomic changes subside. Where possible the AYA should work to devise his or her own 'fitness plan'. Using a local gym rather than a hospital physiotherapy gym allows them to start to return to a more normal environment [40]. Working in this consistent and paced manner can be extremely hard for the AYA and their parents. The pain invariably continues at the beginning (if not throughout) and motivation is poor. Parental anxiety is high and there is a fear that damage will be done. Psychological support during this time is important.

Natural History and Long-Term Outcomes

Although there is a high prevalence of chronic MSK pain in children and AYA, studies concerning outcomes and predictive factors for persistence and recurrence of pain are scarce. Despite general understanding that chronic pain syndromes in children and AYA are often reversible with interdisciplinary interventions, psychological morbidity can be significant. As a young person enters young adult life with MSK pain, anxiety disorders are particularly prevalent [41].

Early multidisciplinary input (including CBT) has been associated with improved outcomes, and this is improved if the parents are involved in the rehabilitation process [42].

Across MSK pain conditions, female gender, older age group (11+), coexistence of psychosomatic symptoms, having high disability index, and multisite pain are associated with long-term persistence of pain [43].

Key Management Points

1. Untreated complex AYA MSK pain is common and personally, socially, and financially burdensome for individuals, families, and societies.
2. Ensure an early, thorough history and physical MSK examination to rule out new or sub optimally treated pathology in children with chronic MSK pain.
3. Evaluate the impact of the pain on the AYA and family (not just the level of pain) so that rehabilitation can be tailored.
4. Involve a multidisciplinary team early (ideally in joint clinics) to facilitate cohesive working and the introduction of psychological and physical therapies.
5. Evidence shows that early dedicated therapy can significantly improve the outcome of chronic MSK pain during adolescence and young adulthood.
6. Key areas for further research include evaluating the physiology of adolescent musculoskeletal pain, the role of parents, and evaluating the efficacy of pharmacological interventions in AYA.

References

1. Nicholas M, Vlaeyen JWS, Rief W, Barke A, Aziz Q, Benoliel R, Cohen M, Evers S, Giamberardino MA, Goebel A, Korwisi B, Perrot S, Svensson P, Wang SJ, Treede RD, IASP Taskforce for the Classification of Chronic Pain. The IASP classification of chronic pain for ICD-11. Pain. 2019;160(1):28–37.
2. Deere KC, Clinch J, Holliday K, McBeth J, Crawley EM, Sayers A, et al. Obesity is a risk factor for musculoskeletal pain in adolescents: findings from a population-based cohort. Pain. 2012;153(9):1932–8.
3. Chambers CT, Dol J, Tutelman PR, Langley CL, Parker JA, Cormier BT, Macfarlane GJ, Jones GT, Chapman D, Proudfoot N, Grant A, Marianayagam J. The prevalence of chronic pain in children and adolescents: a systematic review update and meta-analysis. Pain. 2024;165(10):2215–34.
4. Feldman DE, Nahin RL. National estimates of chronic musculoskeletal pain and its treatment in children, adolescents and young adults in the United States: data from the 2007–2015 national ambulatory medical care survey. J Pediatr. 2021;233:212–9.
5. Kang Y, Trewern L, Jackman J, McCartney D, Soni A. Chronic pain: definitions and diagnosis. BMJ. 2023;381:e076036. https://doi.org/10.1136/bmj-2023-076036.
6. Hoftun GB, Romundstad PR, Zwart JA, et al. Chronic idiopathic pain in adolescence-high prevalence and disability: the young HUNT Study 2008. Pain. 2011;152(10):2259–66.
7. Weiss JE, Stinson JN. Pediatric pain syndromes and noninflammatory musculoskeletal pain. Pediatr Clin N Am. 2018;65(4):801–26.
8. De Mos M, de Bruijn AG, Huygen FJ, Dieleman JP, Stricker BH, Sturkenboom MC. The incidence of complex regional pain syndrome: a population based study. Pain. 2007;2007(129):12–20.
9. Hanns L, Cordingley L, Galloway J, Norton S, Carvalho LA, Christie D, Sen D, Carrasco R, Rashid A, Foster H, Baildam E, Chieng A, Davidson J, Wedderburn LR, Hyrich K, Thomson W, Ioannou Y. Depressive symptoms, pain and disability for adolescent patients with juvenile idiopathic arthritis: results from the Childhood Arthritis Prospective Study. Rheumatology (Oxford). 2018;57(8):1381–9. https://doi.org/10.1093/rheumatology/key088.
10. Rashid A, Cordingley L, Carrasco R, Foster HE, Baildam EM, Chieng A, Davidson JE, Wedderburn LR, Ioannou Y, McErlane F, Verstappen SMM, Hyrich KL, Thomson W. Patterns of pain over time among children with juvenile idiopathic arthritis. Arch Dis Child. 2018;103(5):437–43.
11. Clinch J, Deere K, Sayers A, Palmer S, Palmer S, Riddoch C, et al. Epidemiology of generalized joint laxity (hypermobility) in fourteen-year-old children from the UK. Arthritis Rheum. 2011;63:2819–27.

12. Tobias J, Deere K, Clinch J. Hypermobility and mechanical pain. Arthritis Rheum. 2013;65(4):1107–15.
13. King S, Chambers CT, Huguet A, et al. The epidemiology of chronic pain in children and adolescents revisited: a systematic review. Pain. 2011;152(12):2729–38.
14. Dario AB, Kamper SJ, O'Keeffe M, et al. Family history of pain and risk of musculoskeletal pain in children and adolescents: a systematic review and meta-analysis. Pain. 2019;160(11):2430–9.
15. Andias R, Silva AG. The onset of chronic musculoskeletal pain in high school adolescents: associated factors and the role of symptoms of central sensitization. Phys Ther. 2022;102(4):pzab286. https://doi.org/10.1093/ptj/pzab286.
16. Eccleston C, Crombez G, Scotford A, Clinch J, Connell H. Adolescent chronic pain: patterns and predictors of emotional distress in adolescents with chronic pain and their parents. Pain. 2004;108(3):221–9.
17. Higgins KS, Birnie KA, Chambers CT, Wilson AC, Caes L, Clark AJ, et al. Offspring of parents with chronic pain: a systematic review and meta-analysis of pain, health, psychological, and family outcomes. Pain. 2015;156(11):2256–66.
18. Valrie CR, Bromberg MH, Palermo T, Schanberg LE. A systematic review of sleep in pediatric pain populations. J Dev Behav Pediatr. 2013;34(2):120–8. https://doi.org/10.1097/DBP.0b013e31827d5848.
19. Fisher E, Monsell F, Clinch J, Eccleston C. Who develops chronic pain after an acute lower limb injury? A longitudinal study of children and adolescents. Pain. 2024;165(11):2507–16. https://doi.org/10.1097/j.pain.0000000000003274.
20. Tobias JH, Deere K, Palmer S, Clinch J. Joint hypermobility is a risk factor for musculoskeletal pain during adolescence: findings of a prospective cohort study. Arthritis Rheum. 2013;65(4):1107–15.
21. Ocay DD, Ye DL, Larche CL, Potvin S, Marchand S, Ferland CE. Clusters of facilitatory and inhibitory conditioned pain modulation responses in a large sample of children, adolescents, and young adults with chronic pain. Pain Rep. 2022;7(6):e1032.
22. Geisser ME, Casey KL, Brucksch CB, Ribbens CM, Appleton BB, Crofford LJ. Perception of noxious and innocuous heat stimulation among healthy women and women with fibromyalgia: association with mood, somatic focus, and catastrophizing. Pain. 2003;102(3):243–50.
23. de la Vega R, Racine M, Sánchez-Rodríguez E, Tomé-Pires C, Castarlenas E, Jensen MP, Miró J. Pain extent, pain intensity, and sleep quality in adolescents and young adults. Pain Med. 2016;17(11):1971–7.
24. Kashikar-Zuck S, Ting TV. Juvenile fibromyalgia: current status of research and future developments. Nat Rev Rheumatol. 2014;10(2):89–96.
25. Harden NR, McCabe CS, Goebel A, et al. Complex regional pain syndrome: practical diagnostic and treatment guidelines, 5th edition. Pain Med. 2022;23(Suppl 1):S1–S53. https://doi.org/10.1093/pm/pnac046.

26. Weissmann R, Uziel Y. Pediatric complex regional pain syndrome: a review. Pediatr Rheumatol Online J. 2016;14(1):29.
27. Raja SN, Carr DB, Cohen M, Finnerup NB, Flor H, Gibson S, Keefe FJ, Mogil JS, Ringkamp M, Sluka KA, Song XJ, Stevens B, Sullivan MD, Tutelman PR, Ushida T, Vader K. The revised international association for the study of pain definition of pain: concepts, challenges, and compromises. Pain. 2020;161(9):1976–82.
28. Jordan A, Eccleston C, McCracken LM, Connell H, Clinch J. The Bath Adolescent Pain—Parental Impact Questionnaire (BAP-PIQ): development and preliminary psychometric evaluation of an instrument to assess the impact of parenting an adolescent with chronic pain. Pain. 2008;137:478–87.
29. Varni JW, Burwinkle TM, Seid M, Skarr D. The PedsQL 4.0 as a pediatric population health measure: feasibility, reliability, and validity. Ambul Pediatr. 2003;3(6):329–41.
30. Connelly M, Lee RR. Technology to assess and treat pain in pediatric rheumatology. Rheum Dis Clin N Am. 2022;48(1):31–50.
31. Bruce BK, Ale CM, Harrison TE, Bee S, Luedtke C, Geske J, Weiss KE. Getting back to living: further evidence for the efficacy of an interdisciplinary pediatric pain treatment program. Clin J Pain. 2017;33(6):535–42.
32. Gauntlett-Gilbert J, Jordan A. Fear, boldness, and caution: parent effects on how children manage chronic pain. Pain. 2020;161(6):1127–8.
33. Harrison LE, Pate JW, Richardson PA, Ickmans K, Wicksell RK, Simons LE. Best-evidence for the rehabilitation of chronic pain part 1: pediatric pain. J Clin Med. 2019;8(9):1267.
34. Eccleston C, Fisher E, Cooper TE, et al. Pharmacological interventions for chronic pain in children: an overview of systematic reviews. Pain. 2019;160(8):1698–707.
35. World Health Organisation. Guidelines on the management of chronic pain in children (who.int). Dec 2020. https://www.who.int/publications/i/item/9789240017870.
36. Cohen EM, Morley-Fletcher A, Mehta DH, Lee YC. A systematic review of psychosocial therapies for children with rheumatic diseases. Pediatr Rheumatol. 2017;15(1):6.
37. Pielech M, Vowles KE, Wicksell R. Acceptance and commitment therapy for pediatric chronic pain: theory and application. Children. 2017;4(2):10.
38. Booth J, Moseley GL, Schiltenwolf M, Cashin A, Davies M, Hübscher M. Exercise for chronic musculoskeletal pain: a biopsychosocial approach. Musculoskeletal Care. 2017;15(4):413–42.
39. Cucchiaro G, Craig K, Marks K, Cooley K, Cox TKB, Schwartz J. Short- and long-term results of an inpatient programme to manage Complex Regional Pain Syndrome in children and adolescents. Br J Pain. 2017;11(2):87–96.

40. Klein S, Chui K, Clinch J, Liossi C. Musculoskeletal pain in children and young people. In: Twycross A, Stinson J, Zempsky WT, Jordan A, editors. Managing pain in children and young people. Hoboken: John Wiley & Sons Ltd.; 2024. p. 147–69. https://doi.org/10.1002/9781119645641.ch9.
41. Cunningham NR, Jagpal A, Tran ST, et al. Anxiety adversely impacts response to cognitive behavioral therapy in children with chronic pain. J Pediatr. 2016;171:227–33.
42. Gauntlett-Gilbert J, Connell H, Clinch J, et al. Acceptance and values-based treatment of adolescents with chronic pain: outcomes and their relationship to acceptance. J Pediatr Psychol. 2013;38(1):72–81.
43. Holden S, Roos EM, Straszek CL, et al. Prognosis and transition of multi-site pain during the course of 5 years: results of knee pain and function from a prospective cohort study among 756 adolescents. PLoS One. 2021;16(5):e0250415. https://doi.org/10.1371/journal.pone.0250415.

Systemic Autoinflammatory Diseases and Their Management During Adolescence and Young Adulthood

14

Kerstin Nott and Eileen Baildam

Introduction

The concept of autoinflammation was introduced in 1999. Since then, more than 50 genes have been identified in hereditary autoinflammatory disorders (https://infevers.umai-montpellier.fr/web/), and there are detailed descriptions of a growing number of polygenic "complex" syndromes and acquired syndromes.

The rarity of Systemic Autoinflammatory Diseases (SAIDs) can lead to delayed recognition throughout adolescence and into adulthood (Table 14.1) [1]. Some resolve in childhood, but more require long-term care into adult life [2].

The E-Merge project [3] merged epidemiological and clinical data from three large European registries, Eurofever [4], JIR-cohort and AID-Net, with a total coverage of 7825 cases from 278

K. Nott (✉)
Southampton Children's Hospital, University Hospital Southampton NHS Foundation Trust, Southampton, UK
e-mail: kerstin.nott@uhs.nhs.uk; kerstinnott@doctors.org.uk

E. Baildam
The Alexandra Hospital, Cheshire, UK

C. Ciurtin, J. Hackett (eds.), *Adolescent and Young Adult Rheumatology In Clinical Practice*, In Clinical Practice,
https://doi.org/10.1007/978-3-031-82102-8_14

Table 14.1 Demographics and characteristics of individuals with systemic autoinflammatory diseases presented in three registries [3]

	JIR cohort (n = 1897)	Eurofever (n = 4552)	AID-Net (n = 1375)
Number of participating countries	13	42	2
Number of different types of SAIDs recorded	18	32	10
Male/female ratio	50/50	49/51	50/50
Children (<18y)/adult ratio	78/22	83/17	96/2 (2 unknown)
Age at diagnosis, in years	7 (0.6–72)	11 (0.2–66)	6 (0.2–56)
Number of AYA enrolled with different AIDs			
• FMF	775	1363	587
• PFAPA	456	676	140
• SURF	312	429	83
• MKD	55	221	8
• CAPS	103	288	41
• TRAPS	56	287	47
• CNO	94	597	193
• Still's disease (soJIA)	393	6	262
• Behcet's	97	282	n/a

Reproduced/adapted with permissions from: Vyzhga et al.[3].

Legend. JIR Cohort Joint Inflammation Research Cohort, *Eurofever* European Registry for Autoinflammatory Disorders, *AID-Net* AutoInflammatory Diseases Network, *FMF* Familial Mediterranean Fever, *PFAPA* Periodic Fever, Aphthous Stomatitis, Pharyngitis, and Adenitis Syndrome, *SURF* Syndrome of Undifferentiated Recurrent Fever, *MKD* Mevalonate Kinase Deficiency, *CAPS* Cryopyrin-Associated Periodic Syndrome, *TRAPS* Tumor Necrosis Factor Receptor-Associated Periodic Syndrome, *CRMO* Chronic Recurrent Multifocal Osteomyelitis, *soJIA* Systemic Onset Juvenile Idiopathic Arthritis, recently renamed Still's Disease, *Behçet's* Behçet's Disease

participating centres from 46 countries. The project included mainly paediatric cases but also adults with newly diagnosed SAIDs. Although the mean age at diagnosis was before adolescence, individuals were diagnosed between 0.6 and 72 years (Table 14.1), highlighting that adolescents and young adults (AYA) with SAIDs are an important group to consider.

Presenting Features of SAIDs

Key features suggesting possible SAIDs are recurrent febrile episodes, sometimes with predictable timing, associated with stereotypical and repeated symptoms of multiorgan inflammation. SAIDs often present with rashes such as urticarial, maculopapular, erysipelas-like erythema, migratory erythematous patches, erythema nodosum, livedo racemosa, vasculitic, and granulomatous dermatitis. There can be periorbital or perioral swelling, inflammation of mucosal and serous membranes or serositis. Myalgia and arthralgia with intermittent muscle, joint and fascial inflammation may mimic other rheumatological conditions. Gastrointestinal symptoms, including vomiting and mouth ulcers, are common with hepatosplenomegaly with or without lymphadenopathy. Central nervous system, hearing, and eye features all vary in severity.

As the spectrum of recognised autoinflammatory disorders has expanded, other presenting features have been recognised, such as vasculitic rashes, enterocolitis, stroke, interstitial lung disease and basal ganglia calcifications [5, 6].

Acute phase reactants are raised, and neutrophilia is common with episodes, such that infections are rightly considered and ruled out with significant flares. Typically, autoantibodies are not present in SAIDs.

Genetics can lead to a definitive diagnosis, and given the relatively low cost of panels for multiple disorders, it should represent an early step in evaluating suspected autoinflammation. Where a specific diagnosis is strongly suspected, targeted single-gene sequencing is a cost-effective option. However, results require careful interpretation, especially for variants of uncertain significance [5]. Only 1/3 of cases receive a precise genetic diagnosis [7].

The Eurofever/Paediatric Rheumatology International Trials Organisation (PRINTO) group developed and validated evidence-based classification criteria for PFAPA (Periodic Fever, Aphthous Stomatitis, Pharyngitis, and Adenitis Syndrome), CAPS (Cryopyrin-Associated Periodic Syndrome), FMF (Familial Mediterranean Fever), TRAPS (Tumour Necrosis Factor Receptor-Associated Periodic Syndrome) and MKD (Mevalonate Kinase Deficiency) [8]. These are presented in a user-friendly chart that takes the presence and absence of clinical criteria into account. Performance was tested on 281 patients, and based on clinical criteria alone, the sensitivity ranged from 0.8 to 0.97 and the specificity from 0.82 to 0.93. Once a confirmatory or non-confirmatory genetic criteria was included, the sensitivity range increased to 0.94–1 and the specificity to 0.95–1.

Further classification criteria have been published for paediatric Behcet's [9].

A growing number of AYA with self-limiting episodes of systemic inflammation do not have a molecular diagnosis and do not fulfill the criteria of any known SAID or PFAPA. This is a heterogeneous group, often referred to as 'Syndrome of Undifferentiated Recurrent Fever' (SURF) [10].

Pathogenesis

Many SAIDs are caused by defined mutations affecting the function of the innate immune system. Some are clear monogenic autoinflammatory disorders, and others are considered polygenic, such as Still's disease, formerly known as systemic onset juvenile idiopathic arthritis, chronic non-bacterial osteomyelitis and Behcet's disease [2]. PFAPA syndrome, the most common autoinflammatory syndrome in children, is not considered a classic genetic disorder, but genetic factors may play a role in its development, contributing to the immune system dysregulation seen in affected individuals.

In contrast to autoimmune diseases, there is no autoantibody production and no antigen-specific T-lymphocyte responses. However, the emerging picture is that many disorders, generally regarded as autoimmune diseases, probably also include aspects that could be considered autoinflammatory.

SAIDs can be broadly divided into four main categories by the mechanism of pathogenesis [11]:

- Diseases of inflammasomes and related interleukin-1-family cytokines, e.g. FMF, MKD, PAPA (Pyogenic Arthritis, Pyoderma Gangrenosum, and Acne syndrome), CAPS, AIFEC (Autoinflammation with Infantile Enterocolitis), DIRA (Deficiency of the Interleukin-1 Receptor Antagonist)

- Diseases of interferon production and signalling, e.g. Aicardi-Gutieres syndrome, SAVI (STING-associated Vasculopathy with onset in Infancy), CANDLE (Chronic Atypical Neutrophilic Dermatosis with Lipodystrophy and Elevated temperature)
- Diseases of NFkB and/or tumour necrosis factor (TNF) activity, e.g. A20 haploinsufficiency, Blau syndrome, TRAPS, DADA2 (Deficiency of Adenosine Deaminase 2)
- Autoinflammation mediated by miscellaneous mechanisms, e.g. APLAID (Autoinflammation with PLA2G6-associated Dystrophy) and disorders of complement activation.

These impaired processes lead to recurrent infection-like symptoms with raised inflammatory cytokines without a specific infectious trigger. Flares can occur with stress, including psychological stress, menstruation, physical exercise, immunisations, minor trauma, surgery or viral infections, but more often without any specific trigger.

SAIDs have variable genetic penetrance and may only be diagnosed in adulthood [2, 4]. As relatively recently described conditions and considered incredibly rare, they may not appear in adolescent or adult differential diagnoses lists. Any late diagnosis does matter, however, as treatment is needed as early as possible to avoid complications such as life-threatening systemic secondary amyloidosis and to provide timely genetic counselling.

Labelling the genetically negative cases is difficult in practice. Teams need access to a diagnostic chart of classical features of SAIDs to acquire clinical skills from the experience of diagnosing these conditions. The Human Phenotype Ontology (available at http://www.human-phenotype-ontology.org is a diagnostic tool increasingly used to guide the diagnosis of these conditions and primary immunodeficiencies that may overlap with SAIDs. The Autoinflammatory Alliance (www.autoinflammatory.org) provides valuable information for young people and professionals alike regarding this aspect of care.

Types of Systemic Autoinflammatory Diseases

A summary of current knowledge of selected SAIDs is given in Table 14.2.

Table 14.2 Summary of selected, well-described systemic autoinflammatory conditions

Name	Inheritance and associated gene	Mutated protein	Clinical features and treatment	AYA specifics
FMF	AR Some cases are AD with low penetrance MEFV gene More than 380 variants have been reported.	Pyrin	Recurrent self-limited inflammatory episodes with fever, serositis (abdominal and chest pain), arthralgia or arthritis and erysipelas-like skin eruption on lower legs. Often raised acute phase reactants and SAA. Flares typically last 1–3 days and occur weekly or only a few times a year. The number of episodes is the key element of disease activity. Amyloidosis is a major complication and can be prevented and treated with colchicine. Aphthous stomatitis, urticarial and maculopapular rash and painful lymph nodes are typically absent [8]. Lifelong prophylaxis with colchicine is recommended. In colchicine intolerance or treatment resistance (5–10%), IL-1 blockade can be successful. Steroids are only indicated for protracted febrile myalgia [12].	Most common monogenic SAID. Most frequently reported SAID in adolescents and young adults. Fever can be the only presenting symptom in children. Periods of physical or emotional stress, e.g., cold exposure and menstrual cycle, can trigger attacks [12]. Colchicine may induce lactose intolerance, which can be corrected with a lactose-free diet. Adult-onset can occur. Individuals with FMF have higher fatigue levels, and adolescents' sleep quality is poorer [13].

CAPS including FCAS, MWS, NOMID/ CINCA	AD NLRP3 gene	Cryopyrin	Clinical spectrum from mild to severe: FCAS: Recurrent fever with cold-induced urticaria and constitutional symptoms. MWS, additional arthritis, sensorineural hearing loss and amyloidosis. NOMID, additional sub-continuous fever, chronic urticaria, uveitis, papilledema, deforming arthritis and chronic aseptic meningitis. Flares last 12 h to 3 days and may be continuous in NOMID. Often raised acute phase reactants and SAA. Treatment with IL-1 blockade can lead to complete symptom resolution and is considered standard of care [14]. Life-long treatment is recommended. Steroids may have a role in on-demand therapy.	Cold exposure and stress can trigger flares. Some cases of FCAS and MWS present in adolescence. Neurological involvement in CAPS is frequent, and most young people have difficulties with school performance, which has consequences for adult life chances [14, 15]. Sensorineural hearing loss starts in adolescence.
TRAPS	AD TNFRSF1A gene	Tumour necrosis factor 1	Recurrent fever, serositis (chest and abdominal pain), arthritis, conjunctivitis, periorbital swelling, muscle pain and painful migrating rash. Amyloidosis occurs in 10–20% if untreated. Flares typically last more than 7 days, on average, 3 weeks. Aphthous stomatitis and pharyngotonsillitis are typically absent [8]. Steroids may have a role in on-demand therapy. Treatment with IL-1 blockade has proven efficacy, while anti-TNF-α inhibition is no longer recommended [14].	Especially in adults, a sub-chronic disease course might be observed, with fatigue, diffuse limb pain and persistent elevation of acute phase reactants [14]. Individuals with low penetrance variants (e.g.R121Q) tend to have milder or atypical symptoms than those with more penetrant variants [16].

(continued)

Table 14.2 (continued)

Name	Inheritance and associated gene	Mutated protein	Clinical features and treatment	AYA specifics
MKD (HIDS)	AR MVK gene	Mevalonate kinase	Recurrent fever, polymorphous rash, arthralgias, abdominal pain, vomiting and diarrhoea, painful lymphadenopathy, hepatosplenomegaly, headache, oral and genital aphthosis, large joint arthritis. Severe forms show neurodevelopmental delay, muscular hypotonia, ataxia, cerebellar atrophy, and eye symptoms. Reduced levels of mevalonate kinase activity. Often elevated IgD. Amyloidosis in 5%. Flares typically occur every 2–12 weeks, lasting 3–7 days. Symptoms onset typically <6 months. Treatment with IL-1 blockade is recommended.	Attacks may decrease in frequency and severity in young adult life, and some resolve completely during adulthood. Menstruation and vaccines can trigger attacks.
Blau syndrome	AD NOD2 gene	NOD2	Intermittent fever, granulomatous dermatitis with ichthyosis-like changes, polyarthritis with boggy appearance due to tenosynovitis, recurrent panuveitis. Symptom onset typically <5 years. Treatment options include corticosteroids, DMARDs and anti-TNF-α blockade.	Usually, a diagnosis of young children. Monitor for eye disease with a high rate of ocular damage and sometimes blindness.
DIRA	AR IL1RN gene	Interleukin-1 receptor antagonist	Neonatal onset-multifocal osteomyelitis with severe bone pain, joint and rib swelling, aphthous ulcers and pustular-psoriasis rash. Dramatic response to anakinra in preventing disease flares and long-term complications.	

DADA2	AR ADA2/CECR1 gene	Adenosine deaminase 2	Intermittent, recurrent fevers, livedoid skin rash, early onset vasculopathy and high risk of stroke. Mild immunodeficiency is possible. Thrombosis is primarily inflammation-driven rather than due to classical hypercoagulability. Decrease in ADA2 enzyme activity. Anti-TNF-α treatment can lead to complete control of inflammation, reduced vasculitis disease activity and prevention of vascular events. Life-long treatment is recommended.	Genetic testing should be offered to healthy siblings, and prophylactic treatment with anti-TNF-α should be considered. Anti-drug antibodies are a major concern, especially in AYA, after several years of treatment. Strokes can cause blindness.
PFAPA	Likely multifactorial, involving both genetic predisposition and environmental triggers	No genetic mutation identified	Periodic episodes (every 21–28 days) with fever, aphthous stomatitis, pharyngitis, abdominal pains, diarrhoea, cervical lymphadenopathy, and arthralgia. Symptoms usually start at ages 2–5, with fever attacks lasting 3–6 days. Well in between episodes. Diarrhoea, chest pain, skin rash and arthritis are typically absent [8]. High rate of spontaneous resolution. Corticosteroids can abort attacks, and colchicine can prevent attacks. Adenotonsillectomy can cure the syndrome in many cases. Probiotics might be beneficial [17].	Most common recurrent fever disorder in children. Attacks are often outgrown within adolescence, but some may require transition of care. A few adult-onset cases have been reported. Corticosteroids may lead to an increased frequency of attacks.

(continued)

Table 14.2 (continued)

Name	Inheritance and associated gene	Mutated protein	Clinical features and treatment	AYA specifics
Behcet's	Strong genetic component with HLA-B51 and other genetic factors identified; also involves environmental triggers.	Likely polygenic	Flares with aphthous and genital ulcers, eye inflammation, acneiform or erythema nodosum type skin rashes and arthritis; 20–40% have neurological involvement, myocarditis, vasculitis, splenomegaly, lymphadenopathy. Association with HLA-B51. Flares last around 10 days. Treatment options include colchicine, azathioprine, topical and oral steroids, anti-TNF-α, IL-1 and IL-6 blockade.	Most show symptoms in early adulthood. Monitor for eye damage. See Chap. 10
CNO/ CRMO	Likely multifactorial, involving polygenic inheritance and environmental triggers	Likely polygenic	Chronic relapsing, often painful bone inflammation, sometimes with fevers, ¼ have associated inflammatory disorders such as palmar-plantar pustulosis, psoriasis, and inflammatory bowel disease. Treatment options include NSAIDs, bisphosphonates, and anti-TNF-α.	Many bone lesions heal completely. Some adult-onset cases. See Chap. 18

Legend. FMF Familial Mediterranean Fever, *AR* Autosomal Recessive, *AD* Autosomal Dominant, *SAA* Serum Amyloid A, *CAPS* Cryopyrin-Associated Periodic Syndrome, *FCAS* Familial Cold Autoinflammatory Syndrome, *MWS* Muckle-Wells Syndrome, *IL* interleukin, *NOMID* Neonatal-Onset Multisystem Inflammatory Disease, *CINCA* Chronic Infantile Neurologic, Cutaneous, and Articular Syndrome, *TRAPS* Tumour Necrosis Factor Receptor-Associated Periodic Syndrome, *MKD* Mevalonate Kinase Deficiency Syndrome, *HIDS* Hyper IgD Syndrome, *DMARDS* Disease-Modifying Antirheumatic Drugs, *DIRA* Deficiency of Interleukin-1 Receptor Antagonist, *DADA2* Deficiency of Adenosine Deaminase 2, *PFAPA* Periodic Fever, Aphthous Stomatitis, Pharyngitis and Cervical Adenitis, *CNO* Chronic Non-bacterial Osteomyelitis, *CRMO* Chronic Recurrent Multifocal Osteomyelitis, *NSAIDs* Nonsteroidal Anti-Inflammatory Drugs, *TNF* tumour necrosis factor

AYA-Specific Features of SAIDs

These rare conditions are usually diagnosed in childhood in specialist services, but late diagnoses still occur in AYAs due to a lack of awareness. Furthermore, milder or atypical forms can present de novo in adults [2, 4].

The implications of a late diagnosis in young adult life are significant, especially as some, for example, NOMID/CINCA, can cause developmental delay if untreated early in childhood [15].

A delay in diagnosis may contribute to significant psychological and emotional delay for the patient and the family and might be a risk factor for developing neurodevelopmental disorders [1]. It is also potentially devastating to face the fact of a lifelong genetic disorder being diagnosed for the first time as an AYA.

SAIDs differ in their clinical presentations, and the AYA needs to be monitored for specific aspects of their condition. For example, some diseases can lead to developmental delay, so learning assessment and support should be available. Growth delay is common and might be addressed before puberty. Hearing tests should be offered to some to avoid problems in school.

A crucial long-term outcome of SAIDs, if untreated, is amyloidosis; therefore, keeping AYA engaged with treatment for SAIDs is vital (see Chap. 21). Specific AYA considerations for selected SAIDs are summarised in Table 14.2.

Principles of Treatment in SAIDs

Treatment objectives are controlling symptoms, improving quality of life, and preventing long-term complications.

Treatment is focused on blocking the primary inflammatory pathway involved in each disease. While steroids can be used to manage acute symptoms in many autoinflammatory diseases, their long-term use is generally limited due to side effects. Colchicine is the mainstay of treatment in FMF. However, for many other conditions, interleukin-1 blockade has proven effective in bringing lasting control (e.g., inflammasome disorders and

TRAPS). TNF blockade is typically effective in DADA2 and CNO. Diseases mediated by interferon may respond to Janus kinase (JAK) inhibition.

Colchicine is usually a long-term and, for many, lifelong medication. It is a safe drug that has been used for a long time; however, it has a narrow therapeutic range, and its most common side effects may occur even at treatment dosages. These side effects are mainly gastrointestinal and tend to resolve after a period of treatment or dose reduction. Side effects can be reduced by splitting the dose, although adherence, especially in AYA may be better with once-daily dosing [12]. Colchicine adherence can be a problem during adolescence and needs to be considered in cases of increased attack frequency in FMF. Colchicine should not be discontinued during conception, pregnancy, or lactation, and in general, men do not need to stop colchicine before conception [12].

For pregnant women with interleukin-1-mediated SAIDs on biological therapies, it is essential to evaluate the benefits and potential hazards to both the mother and unborn child of continuing treatment versus leaving the condition untreated. Current guidelines and clinical observations endorse a preference for anakinra over other interleukin-1 inhibiting drugs during pregnancy [14].

It is important to monitor the AYA for inflammation during flares and periods of remission to avoid inadequate disease control. For many established autoinflammatory diseases, management recommendations have been published, and these can help the team treat and monitor the AYA:

- In 2016, the European Alliance of Associations for Rheumatology (EULAR) published guidelines for the management of FMF [12].
- The Childhood Arthritis and Rheumatology Research alliance (CARRA) group has published consensus treatment plans for PFAPA [18].
- In 2021, EULAR and the American College of Rheumatology (ACR) published points to consider for the diagnosis, management, and monitoring of the interleukin-1-mediated autoinflammatory diseases CAPS, TRAPS, MKD, and DIRA [14].

- The EULAR/ACR published points to consider for the diagnosis and management of autoinflammatory type I interferonopathies: CANDLE/PRAAS, SAVI, and AGS [19].

Transition and Practical Care Considerations

Effective transition from paediatric to adult services significantly improves adherence to treatment and long-term outcomes.

There are no specific publications prepared for transition in SAIDs and principles for supporting psychological wellbeing and coping strategies are therefore extrapolated from work on other genetic conditions that cause chronic health problems (see Chap. 23) [20]. A recent survey by the European Reference Networks (ERN) on current transition practices for AIDs in Europe was conducted as a first step towards creating global guidance for the transition of young people with these conditions [21].

Reproductive genetic counselling should be offered to all individuals, starting from adolescence and continuing throughout adulthood. Gynaecologic counselling during adolescence should be provided to prevent unplanned pregnancies.

Treatment with expensive biologic therapies such as canakinumab has led to the initiation of national schemes to facilitate access: e.g. the National Amyloidosis Centre in the UK. In this care pathway, there is the benefit of major expertise in rare conditions focused in one place, but with the drawback of the need to travel for medical care.

There is always the need to balance short-term wellbeing with known long-term risks of untreated conditions, such as neurological impairment in CAPS or the development of amyloidosis in later life. In young people, the concept of long-term preventive treatment versus screening for amyloidosis with treatment at a later date also needs to be discussed. There is the possibility of episodic flare-abortion treatment for acute flares versus long-term regular treatment to maintain symptom control. Counselling for each of these aspects of care is now assisted by data from disease registries and their potential to answer questions about long-term or lifelong treatment.

Psychological Well Being and Coping Strategies

Having a rare disease that no one knows much about during adolescence can prove a challenge for the AYA, especially during transition [21]. However, this is also an opportunity for them to become real experts in their own condition and to take self-advocacy to a new level, as in reality, they can know more about the condition than many of the health care professionals (HCPs) they will encounter. It is empowering to have clear links to good sources of up-to-date information that the AYA could refer the HCP to.

The Autoinflammatory Alliance (available at www.autoinflammatory.org) offers many online resources, including patient information guides, the Autoinflammatory Alliance blog, and a booklet on injection tips. Further information on many autoinflammatory conditions is available on the PReS/SHARE/PRINTO website (accessible at https://www.printo.it/pediatric-rheumatology/GB/info/sub/11/Autoinflammatory-Diseases).

Key Management Points

1. Care should be provided by inter-specialty teams with a special interest in the conditions, combining rheumatology, immunology and genetics.
2. The Autoinflammatory Alliance (www.autoinflammatory.org) offers a comprehensive comparison chart of currently known SAIDs.
3. Genetics is a mainstay of diagnosis and should be performed early, but it requires careful interpretation.
4. Recommendations for the management of many established autoinflammatory diseases have recently been published.
5. It is important to monitor the AYA for inflammation both during flares and in periods of remission to avoid inadequate disease control.
6. Support and information are available to the AYA on the autoinflammatory Alliance and PRINTO websites.

References

1. Hausmann JS, Lomax KG, Shapiro A, Durrant K. The patient journey to diagnosis and treatment of autoinflammatory diseases. Orphanet J Rare Dis. 2018;13(1):156. https://doi.org/10.1186/s13023-018-0902-7.
2. Borges T, Barbosa A, Silva S. Adult-onset systemic autoinflammatory disorders: a clinical approach. Reumatismo. 2020;71(4):177–88. https://doi.org/10.4081/reumatismo.2019.1192.
3. Vyzhga Y, Hentgen V, Caorsi R, et al. Breaking down the fences among registries on autoinflammatory diseases: the E-Merge project. Orphanet J Rare Dis. 2023;18(1):191. https://doi.org/10.1186/s13023-023-02812-4.
4. Papa R, Doglio M, Lachmann HJ, Ozen S, Frenkel J, Simon A, Neven B, Kuemmerle-Deschner J, Ozgodan H, Caorsi R, Federici S, Finetti M, Trachana M, Brunner J, Bezrodnik L, Pinedo Gago MC, Maggio MC, Tsitsami E, Al Suwairi W, Espada G, Shcherbina A, Aksu G, Ruperto N, Martini A, Ceccherini I, Gattorno M, Paediatric Rheumatology International Trials Organisation (PRINTO) and the Eurofever project. A web-based collection of genotype-phenotype associations in hereditary recurrent fevers from the Eurofever registry. Orphanet J Rare Dis. 2017;12(1):167. https://doi.org/10.1186/s13023-017-0720-3.
5. Kul Cinar O, Putland A, Wynne K, Eleftheriou D, Brogan PA. Hereditary systemic autoinflammatory diseases: therapeutic stratification. Front Pediatr. 2022;10:867679. https://doi.org/10.3389/fped.2022.867679.
6. Ashari KA, Hausmann JS, Dedeoglu F. Update on autoinflammatory diseases. Curr Opin Rheumatol. 2023;35(5):285–92. https://doi.org/10.1097/BOR.0000000000000953.
7. Similuk M, Yan J, PhD MS, et al. Clinical exome sequencing of 1000 families with complex immune phenotypes: toward comprehensive genomic evaluations. J Allergy Clin Immunol. 2022;150(4):947–54. https://doi.org/10.1016/j.jaci.2022.06.009.
8. Gattorno M, Hofer M, Federici S, et al. Classification criteria for autoinflammatory recurrent fevers. Ann Rheum Dis. 2019;78(8):1025–32. https://doi.org/10.1136/annrheumdis-2019-215048.
9. Kone-Paut I, Shahram F, Darce-Bello M, et al. Consensus classification criteria for paediatric Behcet's disease from a prospective observational cohort: PEDBD. Ann Rheum Dis. 2016;75(6):958–64. https://doi.org/10.1136/annrheumdis-2015-208491.
10. Papa R, Penco F, Volpi S, Sutera D, Caorsi R, Gattorno M. Syndrome of Undifferentiated Recurrent Fever (SURF): an emerging group of autoinflammatory recurrent fevers. J Clin Med. 2021;10(9):1963. https://doi.org/10.3390/jcm10091963.
11. Nigrovic PA, Lee PY, Hoffman HM. Monogenic autoinflammatory disorders: conceptual overview, phenotype, and clinical approach. J Allergy Clin Immunol. 2020;146(5):925–37. https://doi.org/10.1016/j.jaci.2020.08.01.
12. Ozen S, Demirkaya E, Erer B, et al. EULAR recommendations for the management of familial Mediterranean fever. Ann Rheum Dis. 2016;75(4):644–51. https://doi.org/10.1136/annrheumdis-2015-208690.

13. İncesu Ç, Kayaalp GK, Demirkan FG, et al. The assessment of fatigue and sleep quality among children and adolescents with familial Mediterranean fever: a case-control and correlation study. Eur J Pediatr. 2024;183(5):2223–9. https://doi.org/10.1007/s00431-024-05442-5.
14. Romano M, Arici ZS, Piskin D, et al. The 2021 EULAR/American College of Rheumatology points to consider for diagnosis, management and monitoring of the interleukin-1 mediated autoinflammatory diseases: cryopyrin-associated periodic syndromes, tumour necrosis factor receptor-associated periodic syndrome, mevalonate kinase deficiency, and deficiency of the interleukin-1 receptor antagonist. Arthritis Rheum. 2022;74(7):1102–21. https://doi.org/10.1002/art.42139.
15. Mamoudjy N, Maurey H, Marie I, Koné-Paut I, Deiva K. Neurological outcome of patients with cryopyrin-associated periodic syndrome(CAPS). Orphanet J Rare Dis. 2017;12:33. https://doi.org/10.1186/s13023-017-0589-1.
16. Ruiz-Ortiz E, Iglesias E, Soriano A, Buján-Rivas S, Español-Rego M, Castellanos-Moreira R, Tomé A, Yagüe J, Antón J, Hernández-Rodríguez J. Disease phenotype and outcome depending on the age at disease onset in patients carrying the r92Q low-penetrance variant in TNFRSF1A gene. Front Immunol. 2017;8:299. https://doi.org/10.3389/fimmu.2017.00299.
17. Batu ED, Kaya Akca U, Basaran O, Bilginer Y, Özen S. Probiotic use in the prophylaxis of periodic fever, aphthous stomatitis, pharyngitis, and adenitis (PFAPA) syndrome: a retrospective cohort study. Rheumatol Int. 2022;42(7):1207–11. https://doi.org/10.1007/s00296-021-05084-y.
18. Amarilyo G, Rothman D, Manthiram K, et al. Consensus treatment plans for periodic fever, aphthous stomatitis, pharyngitis and adenitis syndrome (PFAPA): a framework to evaluate treatment responses from the childhood arthritis and rheumatology research alliance (CARRA) PFAPA work group. Pediatr Rheumatol. 2020;18(1):31. https://doi.org/10.1186/s12969-020-00424-x.
19. Gedik KC, Lamot L, Romano M, et al. The 2021 European alliance of associations for rheumatology/American College of rheumatology points to consider for diagnosis and management of autoinflammatory type I interferonopathies: CANDLE/PRAAS, SAVI and AGS. Ann Rheum Dis. 2022;81(5):601–13. https://doi.org/10.1136/annrheumdis-2021-221814.
20. Foster HE, Minden K, Clemente D, Leon L, McDonagh JE, Kamphuis S, Berggren K, van Pelt P, Wouters C, Waite-Jones J, Tattersall R, Wyllie R, Stones SR, Martini A, Constantin T, Schalm S, Fidanci B, Erer B, Dermikaya E, Ozen S, Carmona L. EULAR/PReS standards and recommendations for the transitional care of young people with juvenile-onset rheumatic diseases. Ann Rheum Dis. 2017;76(4):639–46.
21. Israni M, Nicholson B, Mahlaoui N, et al. Current transition practice for primary immunodeficiencies and autoinflammatory diseases in Europe: a RITA-ERN survey. J Clin Immunol. 2023;43(1):206–16. https://doi.org/10.1007/s10875-022-01345-y.

Back Pain in Adolescence and Young Adulthood

15

Verna Cuthbert and Ellie Elliott

Introduction

Back pain in adolescence is common and presents a significant global health burden. Musculoskeletal (MSK) disorders have become the third most prevalent cause of global disability according to the World Health Organisation (WHO) and assessed using Disability-Adjusted Life Years (DALYs), of which back and neck pain are the most common [2]. It is estimated there is a 39% of lower back pain lifetime prevalence in adolescents [1].

There is broad acknowledgement of the major impact of low back pain (LBP) among adults on disability, quality of life, and healthcare consumption [3, 4]. However, the significance of LBP among adolescents and young adults (AYA) has received less attention, both in society and in the scientific literature. This lack of investigation is of concern not only due to the considerable

V. Cuthbert (✉)
Department of Paediatric and Adolescent Rheumatology, Royal Manchester Children's Hospital, Manchester University Hospitals NHS Trust, Manchester, UK
e-mail: Verna.cuthbert@mft.nhs.uk

E. Elliott
Adolescent and Young Adult Rheumatology Service, University College London Hospitals NHS Foundation Trust, London, UK
e-mail: Ellie.elliott1@nhs.net

C. Ciurtin, J. Hackett (eds.), *Adolescent and Young Adult Rheumatology In Clinical Practice*, In Clinical Practice, https://doi.org/10.1007/978-3-031-82102-8_15

impact of LBP on AYA's quality of life (e.g., school and work absenteeism, reduced physical activity and poor sleep) but also due to the relationship between adolescent LBP and the development of disabling LBP later in life [5]. Weiss & Stinson acknowledge the impact of adolescent back pain and suggest that the health burden is high economically, and negatively affects physical, social, academic and psychological function [6].

Studies have shown that adolescent back pain can be predictive of chronic pain in adults [7]. Similar to findings in adults, research has shown an association between multi-site MSK pain (of which back pain is a common site) and psychological problems in adolescents, specifically anxiety and low mood [8–10], and reduced quality of life [11]. There is evidence that central sensitisation and chronic LBP are related to pre-morbid trait anxiety sub-types and abnormal trait sensory processing profiles [12], but further research is required to better understand adolescent chronic back pain.

Additionally, there is a growing awareness of neurodiversity within adolescent clinics, specifically including young people who present with back pain. It is estimated that 1 in 36 young people have autistic spectrum disorder [13]; therefore, it is important to consider making reasonable adjustments to the subjective and objective examination of AYA with LBP. Young people with neurodiversity are likely to have a different clinical history and presentation and may not be able to articulate specific pain sensations due to atypical sensory modulation and intraception [14].

Adolescents are less likely to have a disc prolapse, suffer from spondylotic changes in the spine or be affected by spinal stenosis, compared with adults. Back pain in adolescents is less likely to be due to serious pathology compared to children below aged 12. Adolescents report both thoracic and lumbosacral back pain equally, whilst adults tend to report more lumbosacral back pain and younger children more thoracic pain. Adolescents are more likely to suffer back pain related to overuse and injury, particularly if they participate in sports.

It is important to note there is a lack of robust data detailing specific types of exercise, duration and frequency for management of back pain in AYA [15]. For young people to date, there is good evidence for benefits related to back care education, postural hygiene along with keeping physically active [2]. The advice from the National Institute for Health and Clinical Excellence (NICE) in the UK guidelines includes: "Take people's specific needs, preferences and capabilities into account when choosing the type of exercise" [15]. For someone who is unable to engage with this advice, a referral to physiotherapy should be considered for a more individualised management approach.

It is pivotal for Health Care Professionals (HCPs) to provide holistic developmentally appropriate care, including psychosocial assessment to ensure early and effective intervention and thus reduce disability and the likelihood of LBP symptoms becoming chronic into adulthood. Key factors to take into account when assessing AYA with LBP are detailed in Table 15.1.

Table 15.1 Potential Risk Factors for Back Pain in AYA

• **Gender**—Adolescent girls report spinal pain more frequently than boys [8, 16].
• **Age—**The prevalence of spinal pain increases from childhood to adolescence, from 10–12 years onwards.
• **Family history of back pain.**
• **Mechanical load** such as heavy bags and asymmetrical load may play a role, especially in taller young people though evidence is unclear [30].
• **Longer time spent using electronic devices/screen time** [17, 18].
• **Smoking, drugs and alcohol**— linked to an increase in the risk of back pain [19].
• **Physical activity and sports.**
• **Symptomatic hypermobility** [20].
• **Sedentary lifestyle, obesity** [17].
• **Psychosocial factors—**anxiety, emotional and behavioural problems, depressive symptoms and sleep difficulties [21]; social factors such as loneliness and lack of peer acceptance [9].
• **Adverse childhood experiences (ACE's)**—key contributor to chronic pain [22].
• **Co-occurrence of other somatic symptoms** e.g. headaches and abdominal pain.

Table 15.2

• **Nonspecific**—majority of cases.
• **Mechanical**—hypermobility (see Chap. 12), postural, mechanical load, increased BMI, Scheuermann's disease, spondylosis, spondylolisthesis, idiopathic scoliosis, disc related.
• **Inflammatory**—enthesitis related arthritis (ERA), ankylosing spondylitis (if onset >16 years) (see Chap. 7).
• **Metabolic**—osteoporosis both idiopathic or secondary e.g. eating disorders (see Chap. 17).
• **Vascular**—sickle cell, arteriovenous malformation, spinal infarct.
• **Infectious**—osteomyelitis, discitis, epidural abscess.
• **Tumour**—benign (osteoid osteoma), malignant (Ewing's sarcoma, osteosarcoma, and lymphoma), spinal cord involvement.
• **Referred Pain**—from hip or sacro-iliac joints or abdomen, pelvis, thorax (pneumonia, pleuritis), or due to gynaecological pathology (pelvic inflammatory disease or ovarian pathology).
• **Idiopathic pain syndromes** (as in hypermobility, see Chap. 12).

Causes of AYA Back Pain

The differential diagnosis of back pain in AYA are listed in Table 15.2.

National UK guidelines [23, 24] suggest the importance of risk stratification using assessment tools, such as the STarT Back Risk Assessment Tool, which help identification of young people over 16 years at risk of their back pain becoming chronic. A comprehensive history including relevant psychosocial assessment in young people, such as the HEADSSS assessment [25] (see Chaps. 4 and 23) and general and physical examination (see Chap. 6) should reveal more serious aetiologies and guide HCPs toward appropriate investigation and management.

Clinical Presentation of Back Pain in AYA

Symptom pattern recognition is the key to diagnosis in any age group and are no different. Key points will be highlighted here, as they are extensively reviewed elsewhere [26].

Symptom Pattern and Spinal Red Flags

Spinal red flags are listed in Table 15.3. These symptoms may be characteristic of serious conditions such as infection, tumours, inflammatory bowel disease (IBD) or rheumatic conditions. Bone-related pain tends to occur centrally in the spine, is usually exacerbated by extension and can be aggravated by percussing the spinous processes. Malignant tumours are more likely to present with neurological signs and symptoms. Scoliosis associated with severe pain, a very rigid scoliosis, rapid progression, and lack of compensatory curves above or below should be regarded as concerning and investigated as possible serious pathology. The most common benign tumour in adolescence is osteoid osteoma and may be reported to be relieved by non-steroidal anti-inflammatories (NSAIDS). Chronic recurrent multifocal osteomyelitis (CRMO or CNO) can rarely present as back pain (see Chap. 18). Common infectious causes include vertebral osteomyelitis (most common in the lumbosacral spine), discitis and epidural abscess (more common in adolescent males). Discitis is less common in adolescence compared with younger children and less severe than the adult-onset presentation. Discitis most frequently affects the thoracic and lumbar spine and usually only one disc space is affected. If more than one level is affected, tuberculosis (TB) should be excluded.

Table 15.3

Spinal Red Flags
– Constant, severe back pain
– Nocturnal pain or pain that wakes them up at night
– Systemic symptoms such as fever, weight loss, malaise, or night sweats
– Severe or rapidly progressing neurological deficit
– Cauda equina symptoms
– Limping, refusal to mobilise or significant gait changes
– Stiffness that is worse at rest or lasts for longer than 30 mins in the morning
– Localised spinal tenderness (including sacroiliac joints)
– Acute onset spinal deformity
– Pain spreading into the legs or buttocks

Reference: NICE guidelines, 2019—Scenario: Back pain in Children

Exposure to TB contacts and recent foreign travel should be elicited in the history taking. A history of intravenous drug use increases the risk in this age group. AYA with sickle cell anaemia may develop a vaso-occlusive crisis causing spinal pain, be more prone to osteomyelitis and may present acutely with red flag features. Fractures due to primary (idiopathic) or secondary causes for low bone density (see Chap. 17), may present with localised bony pain.

Investigations

Subjective and objective examination suggesting serious pathology warrants concern and further investigation. This is likely to include: routine blood tests, including blood cell counts, bone profile and inflammatory markers, and additional imaging, including magnetic resonance imaging (MRI), computed tomography (CT), dual-energy X-ray absorptiometry (DEXA) bone scan (if low bone density is suspected). If infection or systemic inflammatory diseases are presumed, in addition to routine blood tests, a sepsis screen including blood cultures, blood film, and autoantibody profiling, ferritin or HLA-B27 testing may be useful. MRI does not involve radiation exposure and provides better visualisation of soft tissue and spinal canal and thus is indicated when disc pathology or neural compromise are suspected. CT has superior depiction of cortical bone than MRI. Thus, when assessment of bone anatomy is critical, CT is preferable. Isotope bone scans and positron emission tomography (PET) scans are recommended in selected cases, and are used mainly to detect occult fractures, stress fractures, atypical infections or bone cancers and metastases. A drawback of ionising radiation imaging (including lumbar radiography, CT, PET and isotope bone scans) is the gonadal exposure, particularly relevant in young people and in the context of multiple exposures.

Adolescent Mechanical Back Pain

"Mechanical" back pain (see Table 15.2) is usually intermittent in nature. Symptoms are usually related to postures, positions, or movement. Pain is usually worse later in the day or after activity.

Scheuermann's Disease

Scheuermann's disease commonly affects males aged 12–18 years. Abnormal growth of different parts of the young person's vertebrae during the growth spurt, causes some of the vertebrae to become wedge shaped. Scheuermann's disease is associated with Schmorl's nodes: protrusions of the intervertebral disc into the cancellous bones of the vertebral body. The aetiology is unknown. Prevalence is between 0.4% and 8% of the general population. The condition is commonly associated with 20–45° kyphosis, and higher incidence of disc degeneration, while one third of AYA affected typically have a degree of scoliosis.

Young people may present with thoracic pain and a thoracic kyphotic deformity (about which they may feel very self-conscious) and complain of intermittent back aching and/or fatigue, particularly at the end of the day or after activity. Clinical features include altered posture—a forward head position, lumbar lordosis, rounded shoulders, possible contractures of the shoulder and hip joint, a protruded abdomen, and tight hamstrings. A structural kyphosis will still be present in prone lying; a postural kyphosis on sitting will disappear in a prone position. Adam's Forward Bend Test will reveal the presence of a scoliosis. The adolescent is asked to bend forward until their back is in an horizontal plane with arms hanging and knees in extension and the HCP then looks for an abnormality of the spinal curve and/or asymmetry of the trunk. In severe but rare cases, there may be cardio-pulmonary compromise or neurological symptoms associated with scoliosis. Further investigations, including lateral spinal X-ray and/or MR scans, if disc degeneration or neurological compromise are suspected, are warranted. The management of AYA with Scheuermann's disease includes physiotherapy, bracing and in the most severe cases, corrective surgery.

Spondylolysis or Pars Defect

Spondylolysis is a condition, affecting up to 6% of children and young people [28], associated with a unilateral or bilateral defect in the pars interarticularis of the vertebra, affecting the L5/S1 level in 71–95% cases [28]; the defect can also occur at L4/5 level, but rarely at a higher level. It has been proposed that pars defects are due to stress fractures and a genetic predisposition has been hypothesised. This condition commonly affects sporty teenagers participating in repetitive extension type activities: e.g. gymnastics, cricket (particularly bowling), basketball, football, dancing and swimming. If spondylolysis occurs bilaterally, this can give rise to a slip of the top vertebra on the one below, either anteriorly– *spondylolisthesis*, or less commonly, posteriorly (*retro spondylolisthesis*). Progression of a spondylolysis to a spondylolisthesis has been reported in approximately 15% of cases and this generally occurs during the teenage growth spurt, and rarely changes after age 16.

A high-grade spondylolisthesis (slip >50% of the anteroposterior vertebral body width) may present with symptoms commonly at the lumbosacral level, particularly worse after sport/activity and extension movements, and relieved by rest. Clinical signs may reveal a palpable step from the sacrum to the spinous process of L5, if a spondylolisthesis is present at this level. Back pain may be reproduced with spinal extension movement and pinpoint tenderness elicited by the palpation of the spinous process. Hamstrings may be restricted. More than 90% of AYA with spondylolysis respond to conservative treatment [29], including rest from repetitive activities/loading, bracing, physiotherapy but for some more severe cases, surgery, including laminectomy and spinal fusion, may be advised.

Postural Back Pain

Recent evidence suggests that perceived heavy backpack weight may be linked to postural back pain [27]. Asymmetrical forces acting through the spine related to carrying a heavy school bag over one shoulder, poor sustained posture/positions, e.g. “I-pad neck”, or heavy use of gaming consoles (current evidence suggests over 10 hours use per week), may all be risk factors [9]. Symptoms are often reported with a time delay. There is often little to find on clinical examination. There is recent evidence to suggest that posture education, physical activity and exercise, alongside back care knowledge can help prevent back pain [30]. Additionally, a pelvic tilt caused by a leg length discrepancy can contribute to mechanical back pain. Referral for consideration of leg length correction with a shoe raise may be indicated.

Disc/Nerve Root Related Pathology

Approximately 10% persistent adolescent back pain is thought to be due to a disc related problem and is much less common than in adults. The risk is higher in adolescent males, sporty adolescents—especially those involved in activities such as weight lifting, wrestling, gymnastics and impact sports, and those with a history of disc related back pain in the family. It may commonly occur following trauma. Symptomatic disc degeneration may start in adolescence and is best detected on MRI scans.

Back pain caused by a disc-related problem is usually exacerbated by forward flexion and may radiate and even change sides. Disc pathology can be accompanied by acute deformities of the spine.

Advice with regards to self-management, keeping active, continuing with daily tasks as possible and/or referral to a MSK adolescent physiotherapist for advice, pain management and treatment should be considered. Referrals to a wider multidisciplinary team (MDT) may be indicated if psychosocial factors present.

Adolescent Idiopathic Scoliosis

Scoliosis is common during adolescence. Studies suggest that 10% AYA have a detectable scoliosis. Scoliosis is defined as a lateral deviation from the vertical midline of the spine of at least 10° on a posterior-anterior radiograph associated with vertebral rotation, and most cases are idiopathic.

Scoliosis however, is a 3-dimensional change to the spine in the coronal, sagittal and axial planes. It causes the bones of the spine to twist or rotate so that the spine curves sideways [15].

Spinal deformity may cause an increased risk of chronic pain [11]. Mild to moderate scoliosis does not cause health problems but can be a source of cosmetic concern to the young person. Postural scoliosis may be due to leg length discrepancy, muscle weakness and/or unilateral tightness causing pelvic tilt, and management will need to be directed accordingly. If unsure whether a scoliosis is postural or structural, sit the young person on a plinth—postural scoliosis will disappear when sitting.

The time of peak progression of a spinal abnormal curvature is at the beginning of puberty. The older the adolescent becomes, the less likely a curve will progress. The greater the curve at presentation, the more likely it is to progress, and adolescent girls have a much greater chance of their scoliosis progressing to be clinically significant. A curve in the thoracic spine is more likely to progress than a lumbar curve.

The clinical examination for scoliosis requires that the young person is adequately undressed to provide visual access to the spine from the waist up. The examiner looks for specific signs, such as asymmetry of shoulder levels, asymmetry of scapulae, tilting of the hips or unequal waist creases and then asks the young person to bend forwards with knees extended (Adam's Forward Bend Test)) to examine for a rib cage hump and/or a lateral curve of the spine.

Knowledge of the factors likely to predict a worsening of a scoliosis will guide management. Adolescents who are early in puberty and who have an obvious scoliosis on presentation can be referred to a paediatric spinal surgeon for monitoring of Cobb angle (angle that measures in coronal plane the spinal deformity on a posterior-anterior projection radiography), or possible treatments including bracing or instrumented surgical correction.

In summary, a young person presenting with back pain needs a developmentally appropriate holistic assessment with reference to any red flags.

Key points for back pain management in AYA are highlighted below in Table 15.4.

Table 15.4

• Most back pain in adolescence is non- specific and non- serious with no demonstrable cause.
• Comprehensive developmentally appropriate history taking is important, asking about possible lifestyle, mechanical loading, family history, sporting, and leisure activities.
• Awareness of psychosocial factors linked with MSK symptoms and back pain presentations is important to offer early psychological intervention.
• Pre-pubertal children are more likely to have serious pathology. Recognition of spinal red flags and appropriate targeted investigation to rule out serious pathology are imperative.
• Physical exam should include postural and structural spinal examination.
• Pubertal assessment is important to stratify young people at risk for spinal structural abnormality progression during growth spurt.
• Early recognition of the need for holistic management and referral to wider MDT is important.

Useful Resources to Support Back Pain Management in AYA (Table 15.5)

Table 15.5

Mental Health:	https://www.youngminds.org.uk/
	https://www.themix.org.uk/
Sleep	https://teensleephub.org.uk
Ergonomics	https://www.ergonomics4kids.co.uk/
School Bag	apcp.csp.org.uk Parent Leaflet—Choosing the right school bag
Exercise	https://www.nhs.uk/live-well/exercise/physical-activity-guidelines-children-and-young-people/ Physical activity guidelines for children and young people
Spinal red flags:	https://versusarthritis.org/media/25276/red-whale-pearl-on-paediatric-red-flags-and-normal-variants.pdf
Although not adolescent specific, the CSP have some useful information on management of back pain:	https://www.csp.org.uk/conditions/back-pain
Adolescent back pain:	https://www.physio-pedia.com/Adolescent_Back_Pain#cite_note-Jones_et_al_2003-67

References

1. Garcia-Moreno JM, Calvo-Munoz I, Gomez-Conesa A, Lopez-Lopez JA. Effectiveness of physiotherapy interventions for back care and the prevention of non-specific low back pain in children and adolescents: a systematic review and meta-analysis. BMC Musculoskelet Disord. 2022;23(1):314.
2. Guan SY, Zheng JX, Sam NB, Xu S, Shuai Z, Pan F. Global burden and risk factors of musculoskeletal disorders among adolescents and young adults in 204 countries and territories, 1990–2019. Autoimmun Rev. 2023;22(8):103361.
3. Kamper SJ, Henschke N, Hestbaek L, Dunn KM, Williams CM. Musculoskeletal pain in children and adolescents. Braz J Phys Ther. 2016;20(3):275–84.
4. Kamper SJ, Yamato TP, Williams CM. The prevalence, risk factors, prognosis and treatment for back pain in children and adolescents: an overview of systematic reviews. Best Pract Res Clin Rheumatol. 2016;30(6):1021–36.
5. Goncalves TR, Mediano MF, Sichieri R, Cunha DB. Is health-related quality of life decreased in adolescents with back pain? Spine. 2018;43(14):E822–9.
6. Weiss JE, Stinson JN. Pediatric pain syndromes and noninflammatory musculoskeletal pain. Pediatr Clin N Am. 2018;65(4):801–26.
7. Minghelli B. Musculoskeletal spine pain in adolescents: epidemiology of non-specific neck and low back pain and risk factors. J Orthop Sci. 2020;25(5):776–80.
8. Bento TPF, Cornelio GP, Perrucini PO, Simeao SFAP, De Conti MHS, De Vitta A. Low back pain in adolescents and association with sociodemographic factors, electronic devices, physical activity and mental health. J Pediatr. 2020;96(6):717–24.
9. Batley S, Aartun E, Boyle E, Hartvigsen J, Stern PJ, Hestbaek L. The association between psychological and social factors and spinal pain in adolescents. Eur J Pediatr. 2019;178(3):275–86.
10. Beynon A, Hebert J, Hodgetts C, Boulos LM, Walker B. Chronic physical illnesses, mental health disorders, and psychological features as potential risk factors for back pain from childhood to young adulthood: a systematic review with meta-analysis. Eur Spine J. 2020;29:480–96.
11. Teles AR, Ocay DD, Bin Shebreen A, Tice A, Saran N, Ouellet JA, Ferland CE. Evidence of impaired pain modulation in adolescents with idiopathic scoliosis and chronic back pain. Spine J. 2019;19(4):677–86.
12. Clark JR, Nijs J, Yeowell G, Holmes P, Goodwin PC. Trait sensitivity, anxiety, and personality are predictive of central sensitization symptoms in patients with chronic low back pain. Pain Pract. 2019;19(8):800–10.

13. Han GT, Heavner HS, Rains TR, Hoang AH, Stone AL. Chronic pain in autistic youth: clinical prevalence and reflections on tailoring evidence-based interventions from an interdisciplinary treatment team. Children (Basel). 2024;11(3):312. https://doi.org/10.3390/children11030312.
14. Bogdanova O, Bogdanova V, et al. The current view on the paradox of pain in autism spectrum disorders. Front Psych. 2022;13:910824. https://doi.org/10.3389/fpsyt.2022.910824.
15. NICE.org.uk. Vertebral body tethering for idiopathic scoliosis in children and young people. Guidance published 29 June 2022—Overview | Vertebral body tethering for idiopathic scoliosis in children and young people | Guidance | NICE.
16. Masiero S, Sarto F, Cattelan M, Sarto D, Felice A, Agostini F, Scanu A. Lifetime prevalence of nonspecific low back pain in adolescents: a cross-sectional epidemiologic survey. Am J Phys Med Rehabil. 2021;100(12):1170–5.
17. Baradaran Mahdavi S, Riahi R, Vahdatpour B, Kelishadi R. Association between sedentary behavior and low back pain; a systematic review and meta-analysis. Health Promot Perspect. 2021;11(4):393–410. https://doi.org/10.34172/hpp.2021.50.
18. Joergensen AC, Strandberg-Larsen K, Andersen PK, Hestbaek L, Andersen AN. Spinal pain in pre-adolescence and the relation with screen time and physical activity behavior. BMC Musculoskelet Disord. 2021;22(1):393. https://doi.org/10.1186/s12891-021-04263-z.
19. Kamper SJ, Michaleff ZA, Campbell P, Dunn KM, Yamato TP, Hodder RK, Wiggers J, Williams CM. Back pain, mental health and substance use are associated in adolescents. J Public Health (Oxf). 2019;41(3):487–93. https://doi.org/10.1093/pubmed/fdy129.
20. Hershkovich O, Gordon B, Derazne E, Tzur D, Afek A, Lotan R. Symptomatic joint hypermobility is associated with low back pain: a national adolescents cohort study. J Clin Med. 2022;11(17):5105. https://doi.org/10.3390/jcm11175105.
21. Roman-Juan J, Jensen MP, Miró J. Increases in sleep difficulties and psychological symptoms are associated with the increase of chronic back pain in adolescents: the HBSC Study 2002 to 2018. J Pain. 2024;25(2):407–17. https://doi.org/10.1016/j.jpain.2023.09.004.
22. Groenewald CB, Murray CB, Palermo TM. Adverse childhood experiences and chronic pain among children and adolescents in the United States. Pain Rep. 2020;5(5):e839.
23. National Institute for Health and Care Excellence. Low back pain and sciatica in over 16s: assessment and management guideline NG 59 Nov 2016: Updated Dec 2020. https://www.nice.org.uk/guidance/ng59.
24. National Institute for Health and Care Excellence. Low back pain and sciatica in over 16s. Quality Standard QS155. July 2017 last review 2020. https://www.nice.org.uk/guidance/qs155.

25. Doukrou M, Segal TY. Fifteen-minute consultation: communicating with young people-how to use HEEADSSS, a psychosocial interview for adolescents. Arch Dis Child Educ Pract Ed. 2018;103(1):15–9.
26. MacDonald J, Stuart E, Rodenberg R. Musculoskeletal low back pain in school-aged children: a review. JAMA Pediatr. 2017;171(3):280–7.
27. Akbar F, AlBesharah M, Al-Baghli J, Bulbul F, Mohammad D, Qadoura B, Al-Taiar A. Prevalence of low back pain among adolescents in relation to the weight of school bags. BMC Musculoskelet Disord. 2019;20(1):37.
28. Achar S, Yamanaka J. Back pain in children and adolescents. Am Fam Physician. 2020;102(1):19–28.
29. Sato M, Mase Y, Sairyo K. Active stretching for lower extremity muscle tightness in pediatric patients with lumbar spondylosis. J Med Investig. 2017;64(1.2):136–9.
30. Rodríguez-Oviedo P, Santiago-Pérez MI, Pérez-Ríos M, Gómez-Fernández D, Fernández-Alonso A, Carreira-Núñez I, García-Pacios P, Ruano-Ravina A. Backpack weight and back pain reduction: effect of an intervention in adolescents. Pediatr Res. 2018;84(1):34–40. https://doi.org/10.1038/s41390-018-0013-0.

Sports Medicine in the Adolescent and Young Adult Athlete

16

Rebecca Robinson

Introduction

Physical activity (PA) in adolescence can optimise musculoskeletal development and help maintain healthy weight. Optimal physical health positively impacts neuromuscular, cardiovascular and cognitive development, as well as benefiting mood, sleep, academic attainment and social behaviour [1].

Body maturation during puberty and adolescence ultimately leads to increased musculoskeletal and aerobic capacity to undertake physical activity, however, many AYA stop sport during adolescence. Reasons are multifactorial, including competing social and educational pressures and changes in the AYA inhibitory control during puberty. Physical inactivity (PIA) during formative years is an increasing trend. This can influence higher adiposity and lower aerobic fitness in AYA that can map to higher risk of morbidity from non-communicable chronic diseases into adulthood [2]. Conversely, higher rates of aerobic fitness and muscular strength are linked to lower morbidity lifelong [3]. Every healthcare consultation represents an opportunity to promote physical activity for the health of AYA.

R. Robinson (✉)
Department of Sports and Exercise Medicine, UK Sports Institute, Manchester, UK

C. Ciurtin, J. Hackett (eds.), *Adolescent and Young Adult Rheumatology In Clinical Practice*, In Clinical Practice,
https://doi.org/10.1007/978-3-031-82102-8_16

Sports-Related Injury in Young People

Most musculoskeletal injuries in AYA are minor, relating to muscles, ligaments and tendons. Whilst the gender gap in physical activity is decreasing, boys are more active than girls at all ages and more likely to participate in high-impact and contact sport, sustaining higher-injury rates [4]. Contact and jumping sports have the highest injury rates, and early specialisation is linked to overuse injuries (see below).

Management of minor muscular injury (e.g. a contusion or muscle strain) should follow the principle of rest, ice, elevation and compression. Whilst recovery is usually straightforward, there may be a need to review training, technique or equipment errors.

Bony Sport-Related Injuries

Physeal Fracture

In the older child and adolescent, 30% of acute fractures involve the developing growth plate (*physis*). This is a common site after an impact injury, such as a fall following a rugby tackle. The growth plate is vulnerable to injury at the junction between calcified and noncalcified hypertrophying cells, where turnover is rapid.

Investigations

X-Rays taken in 2 planes oblique views with classification made according to the Salter Harris system.

Management

Cast immobilisation and reduction to reduce the risks of growth disturbance at the affected site.

Spondylolysis and Spondylolisthesis

Spondylosis and spondylolisthesis occur more frequently in the young sporting population repetitively loading into extension, with rotation of the spine (e.g. cricket, gymnastics).

Spondylolysis

Spondylolysis is a defect of the vertebral arch at the pars interarticularis. The pars elongates during growth and is susceptible to stress from excessive repetitive loading and torsion. An underlying dysplastic pars is often found, with a genetic link to the condition. In 90% of cases spondylolysis occurs at L5 level.

Presentation

Unilateral back pain can be pathognomonic, although symptoms of non-specific persistent back pain in the AYA should raise suspicion.

Investigations

X-Ray may demonstrate acute fracture, however sensitivity is limited and stress reactions will not usually be seen. Both computer tomography (CT) and magnetic resonance imaging (MRI) can identify indicative signs, including deviation of the spinous process and sclerosis of the contralateral pedicle. MRI and Single Photon Emission computed tomography (SPECT) scintigraphy can usefully elucidate bony oedema where a stress reaction, but no cortical breach, has occurred.

Management

Rest for 4–6 weeks with progression thereafter guided by pain resolution, to optimise the potential for osseous union and prevention of progression to spondylolisthesis. Repeat imaging and medically supervised return to sport are required alongside a graded return to play.

Spondylolisthesis

Spondylolisthesis refers to displacement of one vertebra in relation to the vertebra below. In the AYA population, this can occur secondary to bilateral pars fractures and usually presents with bilateral, localised back pain. There is potential for nerve root compromise and full neurological assessment should be performed. Imaging is as for spondylosis.

Management

Spondylolisthesis is graded according to the degree of slippage. Less than 50% displacement is usually managed conservatively with rest, analgesia and bracing in combination with rehabilitation. Once pain settles, a comprehensive approach to posture optimisation, strengthening and movement pattern retraining is required before specific return to sport. Less than 5% of AYA with spondylolisthesis have a more significant slippage that could require surgery (e.g. fusion, decompressive laminectomy).

Avulsion Fractures

Sudden muscular force upon immature bone can cause bony avulsion at the tendinous attachment. Presentation typically involves sudden pain, difficulty weight bearing and point-tenderness after explosive activity. Chronic microtrauma from repetitive overload may lead to avulsion injury. Common bony sites for avulsion fractures are listed in Table 16.1.

Investigations

Radiographs demonstrate the degree of bony injury. Ultrasound is increasingly available and can delineate the muscle insertion and MRI can evaluate bony oedema. CT is not recommended first-line in view of radiation exposure, however may be considered if the diagnosis is unclear or if a surgical approach is considered.

Management

Rest from aggravating activity with appropriate analgesia and rehabilitative physiotherapy.

Recovery can be prolonged. Surgical opinion should be sought for a significantly displaced fragment.

Table 16.1 Common sites of avulsion injury

Bony avulsion	Muscle origin/ insertion	Mechanism	Sporting
Ischial tuberosity	Hamstrings (origin)	Passive hamstring lengthening (gymnastics) Explosive passive lengthening of habitually contracted hamstrings	Gymnastics, running
Anterior inferior iliac spine	Rectus femoris (origin)	Forceful hip-flexion, knee extension	Football, athletics, tennis
Anterior superior iliac spine	Sartorius (origin)	Forceful hip-flexion, knee extension	Football, athletics, gymnastics
Pubic symphysis	Rectus abdominis (insertion)	High velocity forces through trunk	Football, fencing
Iliac crest	Abdominal muscles (insertion)	High velocity rotation through trunk; change of direction	Football, gymnastics, tennis
Lesser trochanter	Iliopsoas (insertion)	Excessive passive stretch of chronically shortened muscles	Athletics

Overload Injury

Chronic Growth Plate Injury

Overuse injury can be sustained in AYA who specialise early in a sport or overtrain, relative to the body's ability to grow and repair.

Presentation

Pain is initially confined to sports practice, becoming pervasive if aggravating activity is continued. On examination, decreased range of active and passive movement at the affected joint is typical. Pain persisting at rest and reduced range of movement may indicate a stress fracture.

Investigations

Early radiographs may be normal. Widening at the growth plate level indicates a failed healing response and repetitive microtrauma to the developing bone. A fracture at the growth plate requires orthopaedic review.

Management

Initial rest from sport is usually required for 3–6 months. Successful rehabilitation and return to sport should involve a graded programme, including modified/adjusted excessive training practices.

Traction Apophysitis

The cartilaginous apophysis contributes to circumferential growth. In repetitive sport, repetitive traction forces through tendon and ligament attachments can cause osteochondral stress. Presentations peak between ages 8 and 15, and this injury occurs more frequently in males.

Common sites are summarised in Table 16.2.

Presentation

Pain associated with impact, local tenderness over the apophyseal prominence.

Investigations

Apophysitis can be diagnosed clinically, however differentials include inflammation, epiphysitis or, rarely, soft-tissue tumour. A thorough history is required and radiological imaging may be justified to exclude underlying disease.

Management

Conservative management succeeds in 90% cases with rest from aggravating activity and local ice treatment. Topical or systemic non-steroidal anti-inflammatory (NSAIDs) medication may be useful although it lacks evidence for efficacy. Alternative exercise

Table 16.2 Common sites of traction apophysitis in AYA

Common traction apophysitis site		Name	Enthesis	Insertion
Upper limb	Elbow	Medial epicondylar apophysitis	Ulnar collateral ligament	Medial epicondyle
Lower limb	Hip region		Gluteus medius, minimus Sartorius Rectus femoris Hamstring	Greater trochanter Anterior Superior Iliac Spine (ASIS) Anterior Inferior Iliac Spine (AIIS) Ischial tuberosity
	Knee	Osgood-Schlatters	Patella tendon	Tibial tubercle
	Knee	Sindig-Larssen Johansson	Patella tendon	Distal pole patella
	Heel	Severs calcaneal apophysitis	Achilles tendon	Calcaneum
	Foot	Iselin's disease	Peroneus brevis and tertius	5th metatarsal

(e.g. cycling, swimming) should be encouraged, to maintain cardiorespiratory fitness. In some cases, symptoms persist for 2–3 years until the growth plates fusion.

Bone Stress Injury

High-impact, multidirectional loading of bone during adolescence leads to remodelling, strengthening the bone during skeletal maturation. However, excessive bone loading with suboptimal recovery can exceed the bone's capacity for adaptation. Microfractures in the cortex propagate with accelerated osteoclast remodelling. Periosteal oedema, local hypoxia and chemical stimuli can lead to progression of injury, resulting in stress fracture (Fig. 16.1). The tibia is the most frequent site of stress-fracture

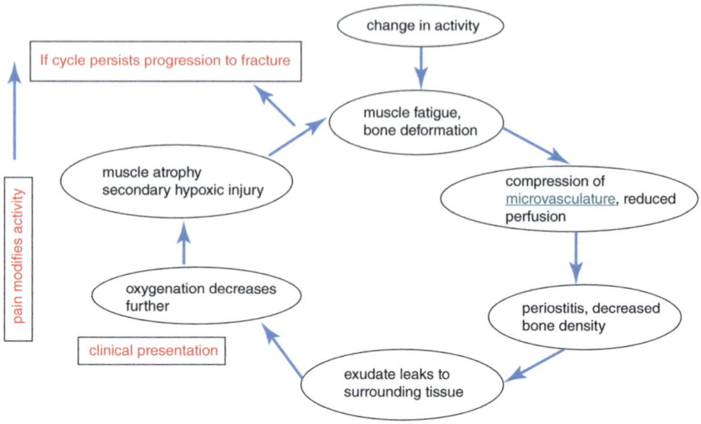

Fig. 16.1 Cyclical changes of stress fracture

(40%) followed by the metatarsal (25%). Sports-specific stress fracture patterns are seen, such as the rib in rowers and the lower back in cricketers (see above). The young athlete who continues to train through pain can develop a frank cortical fracture. Complete fracture at a high-risk site can be catastrophic, for example at the neck of the femur.

Presentation

Insidious pain during sporting activity becoming more persistent with continued training.

Acute presentation may be with inability to weigh bear with localised bony tenderness. There may be increased tone in surrounding musculature. A history of sudden increment in training load, change in footwear or training surface should raise concerns for bone stress injury.

Investigations

Plain radiographs are frequently negative in a stress reaction although delayed X-Ray may reveal callus formation on long bones. MRI is the gold standard in diagnosis. Classification systems have been developed according to the degree of oedema identified and whether a fracture line has formed [5]. Bone integrity should be assessed (see Chap. 17). All young athletes presenting with bone stress injuries should be assessed for extrinsic (e.g. training errors) and intrinsic risks (e.g. metabolic bone disease, hypothalamic causes of amenorrhoea in the female or the relative energy deficiency in sports (REDs) (see below), which should be addressed.

Management

Stress fracture at high-risk sites (see Table 16.3) benefit from added orthopaedic opinion. An isolated stress fracture in a young athlete can be treated with offloading, progressing from non-weight bearing to weight bearing once pain-free. Rehabilitation can include cross-training and a graded return to sport, usually at a minimum of 12 weeks.

Hip Pain in AYA

Femoroacetabular impingement (FAI) describes abnormal contact between the proximal femur and acetabulum and can be a source of pain in the young, non-arthritic hip. It may predispose to osteoarthritis. FAI subtypes are 'pincer' lesions; acetabular overcoverage and 'cam' deformity (aspherical change in the femoral head that can lead to chondrolabral damage). Aetiology is incompletely understood, with both genetic and acquired factors known. High-impact repetitive loading to the proximal femoral physis during adolescence may predispose to 'cam' lesion formation [6].

Table 16.3 High risk stress fracture sites

Neck of femur (superolateral-tension side)
5th metatarsal
Patella
Anterior tibia
Talus
Navicular
Sesamoids

Investigation

X-Rays can measure asphericity, femoral head coverage and the alpha angle (the degree to which the femoral head deviates from spherical).

MR arthrography is most sensitive to diagnose cartilage damage and labral tears closely associated with FAI.

Management

Non-operative management includes lumbopelvic strength and movement pattern training.

Surgical management may be arthroscopic or open hip surgery.

Adolescent Overtraining Syndrome and Relative Energy Deficiency in Sport

The relative energy deficiency in sports (REDs) syndrome describes low energy availability, calculated as energy intake minus the energetic cost of exercise relative to fat-free mass.

Excessive training and disordered eating are common but not universal causes of REDs [7].

Presentation

REDs may present as fatigue, overuse injury (particularly bone stress -see above), illness or unexplained underperformance. Training history enquiry can identify recent increases in volume or training type. The adolescent athlete should have lower training volumes than adult counterparts and coaching support is advised. Sensitive enquiry regarding history of disordered eating, pubertal development and female menstrual history should be made, as these may indicate differential diagnoses and should not be missed. REDs is now known to have multi-system negative effects upon bone health, metabolic health, fertility, cognitive and mental health, highlighting the need for early identification in the young athlete.

Mechanism

Low energy availability causes hormonal and metabolic abnormalities and may result in nutritional deficiencies. Suppression of insulin growth factor (IGF)-1, growth hormone and endogenous sex hormones occurs. Hypothalamic hypogonadism can arise in response to the body's attempts at energy conservation. Adolescent female athletes with primary or secondary hypothalamic amenorrhoea during the ages of peak bone mass attainment are at risk for low bone density/osteoporosis. Low testosterone in males also negatively impacts bone mineral density (see Chap. 17).

Initial Investigations

Screening is required to identify other causes of weight loss if present. A detailed history can provide direction for further investigations that may include blood tests and imaging. Inflammatory bowel disease, malabsorption and rarely malignancy can occur in the AYA as causes presenting similarly to REDs. For the female AYA, causes of amenorrhoea including hormonal disruption, metabolic bone disease or pregnancy should be considered.

Management

A multidisciplinary approach is recommended, including medicine, nutrition and psychology. First-line management for athletes with REDs is cessation or reduction of sports training until positive energy balance is attained; in young females, this is best demonstrated by resumption of menses. Consequences of impaired bone health should be managed with input from metabolic bone and gynaecology. In some cases, hormone replacement therapy may be instigated but expert guidance is advised. In female AYA, oral contraceptives may be detrimental to bone health and can mask the absence of periods. Concerns about disordered eating should prompt referral to specialist mental health and nutrition support. The REDs protocol (endorsed by the International Olympic Committee) recommends a return to training protocol [7].

Summary

This chapter covers the importance of physical activity in AYA and the common patterns of injury presentation and management.

It is recommended that discussing physical activity should be part of every consultation, from brief advice to signposting to specialist services. In this way, the healthcare professional can support the least active AYA and also the young sportsperson, to attain the optimal benefits from PA, which can be sustained into adulthood.

Key Management Points

1. Physical activity in adolescence is important for development of a healthy musculoskeletal system and has beneficial effects on physical, physiological, cognitive and social development.
2. Physical inactivity and obesity are increasing in adolescence and incur lifelong health-risks. The health care professionals (HCP) working with adolescents can offer support to promote sustained participation in physical activity.
3. Early specialisation in sport is linked to a higher risk of overuse injury, with particular vulnerability around the growth centres in bones and joints.
4. Whilst musculoskeletal injuries are relatively common in the active adolescent, a thorough work-up is required to recognise less common but serious conditions, such as tumours of bone or inflammatory conditions, which may present similarly.
5. Meeting the energy demands of sport can be challenging in the adolescent sporting population and an understanding of the principles of overtraining, overuse injury and the relative energy deficiency can help HCPs identify at-risk individuals.

References

1. Bidzan-Bluma I, Lipowska M. Physical activity and cognitive functioning of children: a systematic review. Int J Environ Res Public Health. 2018;15(4):800. https://doi.org/10.3390/ijerph15040800. PMID: 29671803; PMCID: PMC5923842.
2. Abarca-Gómez L, Abdeen ZA, Hamid ZA, et al. Worldwide trends in body-mass index, underweight, overweight, and obesity from 1975 to 2016: a pooled analysis of 2416 population-based measurement studies in 128.9 million children, adolescents, and adults. Lancet. 2017;390:2627–42.
3. Henriksson H, et al. Muscular weakness in adolescence is associated with disability 30 years later: a population-based cohort study of 1.2 million men. Br J Sports Med. 2018;53(19):1221–30. https://doi.org/10.1136/bjsports-2017-098723.
4. Costa E, Silva L, Teles J, Fragoso I. Sports injuries patterns in children and adolescents according to their sports participation level, age and maturation. BMC Sports Sci Med Rehabil. 2022;14(1):35. https://doi.org/10.1186/s13102-022-00431-3. PMID: 35264218; PMCID: PMC8908692.
5. Moreira CA, John P, Bilezikian JP. Stress fractures: concepts and therapeutics. J Clin Endocrinol Metabol. 2017;102(2):525–34. https://doi.org/10.1210/jc.2016-2720.
6. Siebenrock KA, Ferner F, Noble PC, et al. The cam-type deformity of the proximal femur arises in childhood in response to vigorous sporting activity. Clin Orthop Relat Res. 2011;469:3229–40.
7. Mountjoy M, Ackerman KE, Bailey DM, Burke LM, Constantini N, Hackney AC, Heikura IA, Melin A, Pensgaard AM, Stellingwerff T, Sundgot-Borgen JK, Torstveit MK, Jacobsen AU, Verhagen E, Budgett R, Engebretsen L, Erdener U. 2023 International Olympic Committee's (IOC) consensus statement on Relative Energy Deficiency in Sport (REDs). Br J Sports Med. 2023;57(17):1073–97. https://doi.org/10.1136/bjsports-2023-106994. Erratum in: Br J Sports Med. 2024 Feb 7;58(3):e4. doi: 10.1136/bjsports-2023-106994corr1. PMID: 37752011.

17 Adolescent and Young Adult Bone Health

Noor Alhamamy, Neil Gittoes,
Nicola Crabtree, and Zaki Hassan-Smith

Introduction

Childhood, adolescence and early adulthood are critical developmental stages for skeletal mineralisation. Optimal bone mass, defined as the maximum amount of bone mineral content present

N. Alhamamy · N. Gittoes
Department of Endocrinology, Queen Elizabeth Hospital Birmingham, Birmingham, UK

Centre for Endocrinology, Diabetes and Metabolism, Birmingham Health Partners, Birmingham, UK

N. Crabtree
Department of Nuclear Medicine, Birmingham Children's Hospital, Birmingham, UK

Z. Hassan-Smith (✉)
Department of Endocrinology, Queen Elizabeth Hospital Birmingham, Birmingham, UK

Centre for Endocrinology, Diabetes and Metabolism, Birmingham Health Partners, Birmingham, UK

Department of Endocrinology, Queen Elizabeth Hospital Birmingham, University Hospitals Birmingham NHS Foundation Trust, Birmingham, UK
e-mail: zaki.hassan-smith@uhb.nhs.uk; z.hassansmith@aston.ac.uk; z.hassansmith@bham.ac.uk

C. Ciurtin, J. Hackett (eds.), *Adolescent and Young Adult Rheumatology In Clinical Practice*, In Clinical Practice,
https://doi.org/10.1007/978-3-031-82102-8_17

at the end of skeletal maturation, is influenced by various factors, such as sex, ethnicity, genetics, as well as calcium and vitamin D intake, level of physical activity, weight, age at menarche, smoking and alcohol intake, and socio-economic factors, in addition to various medical conditions and medications [1]. As the vast majority of optimal bone mass is accrued in the first two decades of life, chronic diseases during this period can leave a life-long legacy. The effect can be further exacerbated by overexposure to glucocorticoids, a common treatment for a range of RMDs. Up to 50% of AYA with juvenile idiopathic arthritis (JIA) had decreased BMD, according to various studies [2].

The International Society for Clinical Densitometry (ISCD) consensus defines osteoporosis in young people in the context of clinically significant history of fractures rather than based on densitometric criteria alone [3]. The criteria for osteoporosis include the presence of a nontraumatic vertebral compression fracture (VF), irrespective of the BMD, to appropriately recognize the pathological nature of low-trauma VF in children. In the absence of a VF, the diagnosis requires the presence of both a clinically significant fracture history (≥2 long bone fractures by age 10 years, or ≥3 long bone fractures by 19 years), and a low age- and gender-matched BMD Z-score of ≤−2.0 (with appropriate corrections for bone size) [3, 4].

Despite being widely implemented, the ISCD criteria have also been criticised as they are potentially associated with a risk for underdiagnosis and undertreatment in children and young people with congenital forms of bone fragility, or with secondary osteoporosis (e.g. secondary to glucocorticoid toxicity or immobilisation) [5]. There are potential clinical scenarios in which the delay in treatment initiation following a single fracture can potentially lead to significant morbidity and even permanent disability: e.g. waiting for a second (or third) long bone fracture, or for a low BMD by dual-energy X-ray absorptiometry (DXA), following low-trauma fractures in a young person at high risk for osteoporosis.

As suboptimal bone mass increases the risk of osteoporosis earlier in life and as osteoporosis is a major cause of morbidity and mortality in adults, it is clear that prevention begins by optimising bone health at a young age.

Normal Bone Modelling

Bone structure is determined by bone modelling during childhood and remodelling throughout the life course. Modelling involves adaptation to mechanical loading and bone remodelling refers to the constant replacement of bone during life. This involves coordinated interaction of osteoclast-mediated bone resorption with osteoblast-mediated bone (re)formation. Bone remodelling occurs most often in areas high in trabecular (cancellous) bone such as the vertebrae, whilst cortical bone comprises the majority of the skeleton. In early adult life, endosteal apposition and trabecular thickening is crucial for optimum bone mass attainment, which is also influenced by various factors across the human evolution, from body composition, growth, sexual maturation, physical activity, nutritional status, as well as social context, and occupation, which all determine the development of skeletal strength [6].

Trabecular bone is susceptible to deleterious effects of supraphysiological glucocorticoids, particularly during adolescence [7]. Furthermore, during puberty, there are significant differences between males and females with regards to bone growth, especially in terms of bone size and mass. The development of adequate bone strength and the ability to respond to skeletal stress requires optimisation of numerous biochemical and physical factors at a young age. Genetic polymorphisms in the vitamin D, insulin growth factor (IGF)-1 and oestrogen receptor genes may influence bone phenotype [2]. Aside from these heritable influences, modifiable factors include diet, physical activity, lifestyle, body mass index (BMI) and hormonal status [5].

Assessment of Bone Health in Adolescence and Young Adulthood

Assessing the areal BMD (aBMD), defined as the bone mineral content divided by the bone area in square centimetres, and the fracture risk in clinical practice are both challenging in adolescence and young adulthood. In general, aBMD accelerates in puberty and peaks between the ages of 25–35 years [8]. The acceleration is associated with the period of rapid growth velocity and increased stature. The "gold standard" technique involves using DXA at skeletal sites, including the lumbar spine, hip or occasionally the forearm [9]. For children and adolescents, "posterior anterior" (PA) spine and "total body less head" (TBLH) are the preferred skeletal sites [10]. For children, adolescents, men under the age of 50 and premenopausal women, the Z-score is used to evaluate fracture risk, as expressed in the equation below. Manufacturer specific reference data is available to calculate gender and ethnicity specific aBMD Z-scores.

$$\text{Z score} = \frac{(\text{BMD}) - (\text{Age matched mean BMD})}{(\text{Standard deviation})}$$
$$*\text{BMD values expressed as g / cm}^2$$

Due to the technical limitation of DXA, which measures areal bone density (g/cm^2) rather than a true volumetric bone density (g/cm^3), anomalous results could be obtained when assessing children with reduced stature [11]. This may be of particular relevance in the context of chronic RMDs, such as JIA and childhood-onset systemic lupus erythematosus (cSLE) [12, 13]. When assessing a BMD in AYA, height, weight and pubertal stage should also be considered. The ISCD recommendations state that the term "low bone density or low bone mass" should be used "if the aBMD Z-score or BMC is ≤–2.0 S.D" [3]. A diagnosis of osteoporosis in younger men, premenopausal women and children should not be solely based on the BMD test result, as mentioned above. However, BMD is a useful predictor of fracture risk in an adult: each one standard deviation (SD) decrease below the reference population correlates to approximately double the fracture risk [14].

ISCD consensus is that the term 'osteoporosis' cannot be applied to AYA's without a clinically significant fracture history (see above); whilst the term 'osteopenia' should not be used in paediatric DXA reports at all [3, 10]. Additionally, due to the technical limitations of DXA, size adjustments should be made for young people with short stature or growth delay. Spine and

TBLH BMC and aBMD should be adjusted. With regards to the spine, either the bone mineral apparent density (BMAD) or the height for age Z-score should be calculated [15]. For the TBLH, the height for age Z-score should be used [9].

DXA reports should also include technical information on scanning hardware and software in addition to patient demographics, weight, height, medial history, bone age and Tanner stage. For AYA with an increased risk of clinically significant fractures, a DXA scan should be conducted as part of a comprehensive health assessment [9]. This is especially the case if the young person may benefit from intervention to decrease their fracture risk or if the results of the scan may affect the management plan [16].

General Approaches to Optimise Management and Promote Bone Health

Screening

Routine screening for osteoporosis in healthy AYA is not advised. However, those with RMDs or any other condition associated with decreased bone density and increased bone fragility should undergo baseline bone densitometry testing in addition to assessment of vitamin D status [16]. Recent consensus recommendations highlight BMD should be monitored at a minimum interval 1 year [2]. Screening criteria for osteoporosis in children and adolescents with chronic RMDs have been recommended [17], as outlined in Table 17.1. Vertebral fractures may be occult and represent a severe failure of bone strength. As many as 7% of young people had vertebral fractures at baseline (within 30 days) on commencing glucocorticoids for RMDs and 6% had incident fractures over 12 months follow up in the Steroid-associated Osteoporosis in the Paediatric Population (STOPP) study [18]. Thornton and colleagues advocate for measuring baseline BMD with surveillance every 2 years in adults with a background of JIA [19].

Table 17.1 Summary of key clinical points

History	Underlying diagnoses, including autoinflammatory and autoimmune conditions (e.g. RMDs), endocrine dysfunction, malabsorption, psychiatric diseases, cancer and cancer-treatment, gastric bypass surgery, thalassemia, human immunodeficiency virus, systemic mastocytosis, solid organ or bone marrow stem cell transplant, etc. Fractures (mechanism of injury, site, number, age; NB ≥2 long bone fractures by the age of 10; or ≥3 long bone fractures at any age up to 19 in presence of low BMD required for diagnosis of osteoporosis in young people). Glucocorticoid use (dose, duration). Bisphosphonate use.
Investigations	DXA (low BMD indicated by size adjusted BMD or BMC Z score ≤–2.0 S.D). Screening (suggested in the context of confirmed fractures, back pain; glucocorticoid therapy for more than 3 months, weight gain whilst on steroid treatment, active inflammation, and decreased Z-scores of the spine).
General advice and management	Glucocorticoids should be prescribed at the lowest effective treatment dose. Steroid sparing medications should be considered. Physical activity—weight bearing where possible, or low force activities if the RMD is active. Ensure optimal vitamin D status and calcium intake. Recommend stopping smoking and limiting alcohol intake. Address all additional risk factors for low BMD and fracture risk. Dietary recommendations in AYA with negative energy balance.
Assess potential for recovery from low BMD to decide need for additional pharmacological intervention	Re-assess and address persistent risk factors for low bone density. Annual spinal X-ray (earlier if back pain) and DXA scan. If >0.5 decline in BMD Z-score on two consecutive DXA scans or new fractures, escalate to bisphosphonate therapy (preferable IV).

Glucocorticoid Therapy

Adults have increased fracture risk with doses as low as 2.5–7.5 mg of oral prednisolone per day [20]. Effects on BMD are correlated with the cumulative glucocorticoid dose. Alternate-day rotations have been found to maintain growth in adolescents; however, the effects of glucocorticoid therapy on bone may not be reduced [21]. When long-term therapy is indicated or predicted, steroid-sparing medications, such as conventional or targeted disease modifying antirheumatic drugs (DMARDs) should be used where possible [22]. Exposure to glucocorticoids should be minimised with the use of lowest effective treatment dose and duration to prevent decreased bone accrual.

Physical Activity

Physical activity during child and adolescent development is a determinant of peak bone mass via effects on mechanical loading and osteocyte function. Exercise is deemed an essential component of long-term management for AYA with RMDs. Weight bearing physical activities such as walking, running, jumping and dancing are more effective at optimising bone health than swimming or cycling [23]. However during periods of inflammation of their underlying disease, low force activities are recommended, as they are better tolerated [24]. Furthermore, resistance training may be introduced, if tolerated, as it was found to be beneficial in increasing BMD in adolescents [25]. High impact activities of short duration with multiple rests are most effective in promoting bone metabolism. These maximal force activities enhance bone integrity [26]. Sedentary behaviour has negative impact on general health in adolescents; however, the impact of sedentary activities on the BMD of AYA is more nuanced, highlighting the distinct influence of BMI, as well as type of sedentary activity on bone health [27].

Vitamin D and Calcium Supplementation

Vitamin D deficiency is highly prevalent worldwide. Severe deficiency results in rickets and osteomalacia [28]. The most common risk factors in young people relate to reduced exposure to UVB light, low dietary intake and medication use (including glucocorticoids) [29]. There are also associations with chronic disease states. There is general agreement that calcium and vitamin D supplementation can improve skeletal outcomes as evidenced by epidemiological and a number of clinical trials, although there is no consensus over the vitamin D supplementation needs in adolescent population [30]. The Institute of Medicine (IOM) and UK National Osteoporosis Society advise deficiency as serum 25OHD <30 nmol/L, insufficiency between 30 and 50 nmol/L and sufficiency as >50 nmol/L [31]. The Endocrine Society recently published recommendations for general population supporting empiric vitamin D supplementation in children and adolescents younger than 18 years (equivalent of 1200 IU daily), and no empiric supplementation above the recommended daily allowance (RDA) established by the IOM (600 IU [15 μg] daily) for young adults and adults younger than 50 years [32].

The Endocrine Society suggested an induction dose of a vitamin D supplement (e.g. 300,000 IU total over 6–10 weeks) followed by maintenance dosing (e.g. 800 IU/day). The IOM endorses routine screening for vitamin D deficiency and higher recommended dietary allowances (RDA) for vitamin D supplements in AYA with chronic RMDs treated with glucocorticoids. Others have suggested an RDA for AYA with chronic inflammatory diseases should be at least twice the RDA of healthy controls [17]. It is clear that there is a need for high quality vitamin D supplementation studies in AYA to refine clinical protocols.

The management of bone health during pregnancy has been addressed in Chap. 19.

Diet and Nutrition

Clinicians are encouraged to promote healthy nutrition and enquire about the diet of their AYA with RMDs. During health maintenance visits, specifically ask about the use of calcium and vitamin D supplements, dairy intake, non-dairy sources of calcium or vitamin D and fizzy drinks consumption. Increased intake of foods and drinks that contain calcium and vitamin D should be encouraged. Dairy products are the major source of calcium in the diet, whilst cereals and beverages may be fortified [33]. Recent studies showed a positive impact of dairy product consumption on BMD of young people [34]. Reduced fat alternatives of dairy products such as reduced-fat milk and yoghurt also provide a good source of calcium. Misconceptions as to the caloric content of dairy products should be addressed and rectified in health maintenance visits. There is growing recognition that nutritional factors can act synergistically with exercise to impact on bone health [1].

Bisphosphonates and New Agents

Bisphosphonates are widely used in osteoporosis in older adults. Their mechanism of action involves inhibition of osteoclast-mediated bone resorption. They are recommended in children and adolescents with osteogenesis imperfecta (OI), an inherited skeletal dysplasia associated with bone fragility and skeletal deformities [35]. Outside of this context, the use of bisphosphonates in children and AYAs remains controversial due to safety concerns [36]. These agents are not licensed in pre-menopausal women and are contraindicated in pregnancy. Many specialists advocate that bisphosphonates should be limited to men with low-trauma fractures and post-menopausal women [36]. However, there is recent evidence that young people receiving steroids for RMDs may benefit from prophylactic treatment with bisphosphonates to increase lumbar spine BMD although the effect on fracture risk is uncertain [37]. At present their role is limited to use in OI and other diseases associated with frequent fractures, vertebral collapse or critical bone pain [38]. In RMDs, we recommend their use, if AYA experience decline in the BMD or new fractures despite adequate management (see Table 17.1). Denosumab, a monoclonal antibody anti-RANKL, is currently investigated in clinical trials in children and could become a potential alternative therapeutic option [37]. Additionally, sclerostin inhibitory antibodies and transforming growth factor (TGF)-beta inhibition are explored for the treatment of AYA with OI [35].

Conclusions

Careful consideration of bone health in AYA with RMDs is critical to ensure optimal long-term outcomes. AYA with RMDs may be exposed to a number of risk factors for low BMD including active inflammation, glucocorticoid use, and reduced activity. Osteoporosis in AYA is defined by clinically significant fracture history and confirmed low BMD. Young people with RMD should undergo baseline assessment of BMD by DXA. Principles of management as outlined in Table 17.1, include minimising glucocorticoid exposure to that which is required for disease control, encouraging weight bearing physical activity (where appropriate), and ensuring optimal vitamin D and calcium intake. Special attention should be given to the management of hypogonadism, anorexia nervosa, and detrimental lifestyle factors, as well as smoking, alcohol consumption and medication exposures with potential deleterious impact on bone health.

Acknowledgement Prof. Coziana Ciurtin, from the Centre for Adolescent Rheumatology, University College London, London, UK (email: c.ciurtin@ucl.ac.uk) reviewed and updated the previous version of the chapter published in 2018.

References

1. Zhu X, Zheng H. Factors influencing peak bone mass gain. Front Med. 2021;15(1):53–69.
2. Di Marcello F, Di Donato G, d'Angelo DM, Breda L, Chiarelli F. Bone health in children with rheumatic disorders: focus on molecular mechanisms, diagnosis, and management. Int J Mol Sci. 2022;23(10):5725. https://doi.org/10.3390/ijms23105725.
3. Bishop N, Arundel P, Clark E, Dimitri P, Farr J, Jones G, et al. Fracture prediction and the definition of osteoporosis in children and adolescents:

the ISCD 2013 Pediatric Official Positions. J Clin Densitom. 2014;17(2):275–80.

4. Weber DR, Boyce A, Gordon C, Hogler W, Kecskemethy HH, Misra M, et al. The utility of DXA assessment at the forearm, proximal femur, and lateral distal femur, and vertebral fracture assessment in the pediatric population: 2019 ISCD official position. J Clin Densitom. 2019;22(4):567–89.
5. Ward LM, Weber DR, Munns CF, Hogler W, Zemel BS. A contemporary view of the definition and diagnosis of osteoporosis in children and adolescents. J Clin Endocrinol Metab. 2020;105(5):e2088–97.
6. Kralick AE, Zemel BS. Evolutionary perspectives on the developing skeleton and implications for lifelong health. Front Endocrinol (Lausanne). 2020;11:99.
7. Ward LM. Glucocorticoid-induced osteoporosis: why kids are different. Front Endocrinol (Lausanne). 2020;11:576.
8. Karlsson MK, Rosengren BE. Exercise and peak bone mass. Curr Osteoporos Rep. 2020;18(3):285–90.
9. Guss CE, McAllister A, Gordon CM. DXA in children and adolescents. J Clin Densitom. 2021;24(1):28–35.
10. Crabtree NJ, Arabi A, Bachrach LK, Fewtrell M, El-Hajj Fuleihan G, Kecskemethy HH, et al. Dual-energy X-ray absorptiometry interpretation and reporting in children and adolescents: the revised 2013 ISCD Pediatric Official Positions. J Clin Densitom. 2014;17(2):225–42.
11. Messina C, Lastella G, Sorce S, Piodi LP, Rodari G, Giavoli C, et al. Pediatric dual-energy X-ray absorptiometry in clinical practice: what the clinicians need to know. Eur J Radiol. 2018;105:153–61.
12. d'Angelo DM, Di Donato G, Breda L, Chiarelli F. Growth and puberty in children with juvenile idiopathic arthritis. Pediatr Rheumatol Online J. 2021;19(1):28.
13. Ponin L, Poomthavorn P, Pirojsakul K, Lerkvaleekul B, Soponkanaporn S, Chitrapazt N, Vilaiyuk S. Long-term growth and final adult height outcome in childhood-onset systemic lupus erythematosus. Pediatr Rheumatol Online J. 2022;20(1):4.
14. Gregson CL, Armstrong DJ, Bowden J, Cooper C, Edwards J, Gittoes NJL, et al. UK clinical guideline for the prevention and treatment of osteoporosis. Arch Osteoporos. 2022;17(1):58.
15. Kocks J, Ward K, Mughal Z, Moncayo R, Adams J, Hogler W. Z-score comparability of bone mineral density reference databases for children. J Clin Endocrinol Metab. 2010;95(10):4652–9.
16. Ciancia S, van Rijn RR, Hogler W, Appelman-Dijkstra NM, Boot AM, Sas TCJ, Renes JS. Osteoporosis in children and adolescents: when to suspect and how to diagnose it. Eur J Pediatr. 2022;181(7):2549–61.
17. Cimaz R. In: Petty RE, Laxer RM, Lindsley CB, Wedderburn L, Mellins E, Fullbridgge R, editors. The impact of rheumatic diseases and their treatment on bone strength development in childhood. Textbook of pediatric rheumatology. 8th ed. Oxford: Elsevier Health Sciences; 2020. p. 644–57.

18. Rodd C, Lang B, Ramsay T, Alos N, Huber AM, Cabral DA, et al. Incident vertebral fractures among children with rheumatic disorders 12 months after glucocorticoid initiation: a national observational study. Arthritis Care Res (Hoboken). 2012;64(1):122–31.
19. Thornton J, Pye SR, O'Neill TW, Rawlings D, Francis RM, Symmons DP, et al. Bone health in adult men and women with a history of juvenile idiopathic arthritis. J Rheumatol. 2011;38(8):1689–93.
20. van Staa TP, Leufkens HG, Abenhaim L, Zhang B, Cooper C. Oral corticosteroids and fracture risk: relationship to daily and cumulative doses. Rheumatology (Oxford). 2000;39(12):1383–9.
21. Chaia-Semerena GM, Vargas-Camano ME, Alonso-Bello CD, Guillen-Toledo JJ, Guido-Bayardo RL, Lozano-Patino F, et al. The effects of alternate-day corticosteroids in autoimmune disease patients. Autoimmune Dis. 2020;2020:8719284.
22. Misra DP, Agarwal V. The perennial search for alternatives to corticosteroids in rheumatology: is there light at the end of the tunnel? Clin Rheumatol. 2020;39(10):2845–8.
23. Proia P, Amato A, Drid P, Korovljev D, Vasto S, Baldassano S. The impact of diet and physical activity on bone health in children and adolescents. Front Endocrinol (Lausanne). 2021;12:704647.
24. Iversen MD, Andre M, von Heideken J. Physical activity interventions in children with juvenile idiopathic arthritis: a systematic review of randomized controlled trials. Pediatric Health Med Ther. 2022;13:115–43.
25. Agostinete RR, Werneck AO, Narciso PH, Ubago-Guisado E, Coelho ESMJ, Bielemann RM, et al. Resistance training presents beneficial effects on bone development of adolescents engaged in swimming but not in impact sports: ABCD Growth Study. BMC Pediatr. 2024;24(1):247.
26. Simoes D, Craveiro V, Santos MP, Camoes M, Pires B, Ramos E. The effect of impact exercise on bone mineral density: a longitudinal study on non-athlete adolescents. Bone. 2021;153:116151.
27. Pelegrini A, Klen JA, Costa AM, Bim MA, Claumann GS, De Angelo HCC, de Araujo PA. Association between sedentary behavior and bone mass in adolescents. Osteoporos Int. 2020;31(9):1733–40.
28. Amrein K, Scherkl M, Hoffmann M, Neuwersch-Sommeregger S, Kostenberger M, Tmava Berisha A, et al. Vitamin D deficiency 2.0: an update on the current status worldwide. Eur J Clin Nutr. 2020;74(11):1498–513.
29. Corsello A, Spolidoro GCI, Milani GP, Agostoni C. Vitamin D in pediatric age: current evidence, recommendations, and misunderstandings. Front Med (Lausanne). 2023;10:1107855.
30. Patseadou M, Haller DM. Vitamin D in adolescents: a systematic review and narrative synthesis of available recommendations. J Adolesc Health. 2020;66(4):388–407.

31. Aspray TJ, Bowring C, Fraser W, Gittoes N, Javaid MK, Macdonald H, et al. National osteoporosis society vitamin D guideline summary. Age Ageing. 2014;43(5):592–5.
32. Demay MB, Pittas AG, Bikle DD, Diab DL, Kiely ME, Lazaretti-Castro M, et al. Vitamin D for the prevention of disease: an endocrine society clinical practice guideline. J Clin Endocrinol Metab. 2024;109(8):1907–47.
33. Ward LM. A practical guide to the diagnosis and management of osteoporosis in childhood and adolescence. Front Endocrinol (Lausanne). 2023;14:1266986.
34. Rizzoli R, Biver E, Brennan-Speranza TC. Nutritional intake and bone health. Lancet Diabetes Endocrinol. 2021;9(9):606–21.
35. Ying ZM, Hu B, Yan SG. Oral bisphosphonate therapy for osteogenesis imperfecta: a systematic review and meta-analysis of six randomized placebo-controlled trials. Orthop Surg. 2020;12(4):1293–303.
36. Herath M, Cohen A, Ebeling PR, Milat F. Dilemmas in the management of osteoporosis in younger adults. JBMR Plus. 2022;6(1):e10594.
37. Costi S, Giani T, Orsini F, Cimaz R. Drug treatment of low bone mass and other bone conditions in pediatric patients. Paediatr Drugs. 2022;24(2):103–19.
38. Sakka SD, Cheung MS. Management of primary and secondary osteoporosis in children. Ther Adv Musculoskelet Dis. 2020;12:1759720X20969262. https://doi.org/10.1177/1759720X20969262.

18 Chronic Non-bacterial Osteitis in Adolescence and Young Adulthood

Chandrika S. Bhat
and Athimalaipet V. Ramanan

Epidemiology

Chronic Non-bacterial Osteitis (CNO) can affect children and young people of all ethnicities, but the incidence varies between geographical regions due to differences in awareness amongst clinicians. The incidence of CNO in the United Kingdom and Republic of Ireland is estimated at 0.605 cases per 100,000 person years [1], and the prevalence is approximately between 1/160,000 and 1/2,000,000 [2]. The disease is predominantly seen in young girls between 9 and 12 years, with a median age of 10 years at diagnosis [3]. CNO in isolation is rarely seen in children below 3 years of age. The delay from symptom onset to diagnosis has been reported to be between 5 months and 2 years [4].

C. S. Bhat
Department of Pediatric Rheumatology, Rainbow Children's Hospital, Bangalore, India

A. V. Ramanan (✉)
Department of Pediatric Rheumatology, Bristol Royal Hospital for Children, Bristol, UK

C. Ciurtin, J. Hackett (eds.), *Adolescent and Young Adult Rheumatology In Clinical Practice*, In Clinical Practice,
https://doi.org/10.1007/978-3-031-82102-8_18

Nomenclature

The spectrum of CNO can range from mild, unifocal disease to a more severe, multifocal, and recurrent form also known as chronic recurrent multifocal osteomyelitis (CRMO) [5]. It has also been suggested that CNO could be the paediatric presentation of SAPHO syndrome (synovitis, acne, pustulosis, hyperostosis, osteitis). SAPHO is seldom seen in children and adolescents but is a well-recognized condition in adults. The axial skeleton, especially the costo-sterno-clavicular region, is more often involved in SAPHO compared to paediatric CNO [2, 4, 5].

Pathogenesis and Genetics

The precise pathophysiology of CNO is not clearly understood. Repeated attempts at isolating a causative organism have been unsuccessful. Whilst *Propionibacterium acnes*, *Bartonella* and other bacteria have been isolated, their role in pathogenesis is not clear [4, 5]. Studies published so far hypothesise that an imbalance between pro-inflammatory cytokines: e.g. tumour necrosis factor α (TNF-α), and interleukin (IL)-6 and anti-inflammatory (e.g. IL-10) cytokines is central to the pathogenesis of CNO. TNF-α and IL-6 support bone resorption through osteoclast differentiation and activation, whereas IL-10 has a potent inhibitory effect on osteoclastogenesis [2, 4, 5].

Evidence for a genetic predisposition in sporadic CNO stems from case reports of affected family members and monozygotic twins with CNO; however, a definite genetic locus continues to be elusive [2, 4]. A strong personal and family history of associated disorders, including psoriasis, inflammatory bowel disease and enthesitis-related arthritis, suggest a shared genetic and immunological pathogenesis [2, 4]. Mouse models with a homozygous mutation in the *pstpip2* gene manifested an autoinflammatory disease similar in phenotype to CNO. However, when a small cohort of 10 AYA with CNO was studied, no mutation in *pstipip1* or *pstpip2* was identified in any of the individuals affected [4]. Recently, a susceptibility gene (*FBLIM1*) has been demonstrated in two unrelated individuals from South Asia [6], and whole exome sequencing in a cohort of 99 individuals with CNO identified two cases with missense mutations in the *FGR* gene [7].

Clinical Features

Pain is the most common symptom at presentation with or without local swelling and increased warmth [3, 8]. Most children and young people appear well, but fatigue and delayed growth may be noted in a small proportion. The nature of pain may resemble 'growing pain' in children and may lead to a delay in diagnosis. The duration of symptoms can range from a few days to several years [4, 9]. Lesions can occur in any part of the skeleton but metaphyses of long bones such as the femur and tibia are more frequently affected [3, 8]. Localised swelling of the clavicle or mandible is the classic picture of CNO. A proportion of lesions can be asymptomatic in multifocal disease and are incidentally detected (usually after whole body imaging). Joint involvement with articular effusions or synovial hypertrophy has been reported in approximately 30% cases [3, 8]. Systemic symptoms may occur in up to 17% of children, adolescents and young adults (AYA), and are usually mild and include low grade fever, malaise or lethargy [4]. The presence of high-grade fever and overwhelming systemic symptoms should prompt investigations for an alternative, and potentially more severe, diagnoses.

Extraosseous manifestations include palmoplantar pustulosis, psoriasis, acneiform lesions and occasionally pyoderma gangrenosum [8, 10]. The term 'enteropathic CNO' is used when there is associated inflammatory bowel disease, most often Crohn's disease and less frequently ulcerative colitis [4, 5, 9]. There may be a history of inflammatory bowel or skin disease in first degree relatives of affected children and AYA [8].

Complications and sequelae are not uncommon in CNO). When a lesion involves the growth plate, growth abnormalities may result due to premature fusion resulting in limb length discrepancies. Other complications, including vertebral collapse, kyphosis, gibbus formation and growth arrests have been

Table 18.1 Differential diagnosis of CNO in children and AYA

Infections—Tuberculosis, Brucellosis, infection with *Kingella kingae*
Juvenile idiopathic arthritis—Enthesitis related arthritis, Psoriatic arthritis
Nutritional deficiency—Scurvy
Primary immune deficiency e.g. *Rag* deficiency
Benign bone tumours—Osteoid osteoma, Osteoblastoma
Malignant tumours—Osteosarcoma, Ewing's sarcoma, Neuroblastoma, Langerhans histiocytosis, Leukaemia, Lymphoma
Genetic disorders—Majeed syndrome, DIRA[a], Hypophosphatasia, Polyostotic fibrous dysplasia

[a] Deficiency of IL-1 receptor antagonist

described. A small subset of cases may evolve to a spondyloarthropathy [3, 8]. Conditions that can mimic CNO have been summarised in Table 18.1.

Diagnosis

Laboratory tests may show leukocytosis or elevated inflammatory markers (erythrocyte sedimentation rate—ESR or C-reactive protein—CRP). The elevation is not very significant and inflammatory markers tend to revert to normal when the disease is quiescent. Presence of very high inflammatory markers raises the probability of infection, and a bone biopsy is warranted in such situations [3, 8, 10]. Specific biomarkers or genomic markers are not yet available for diagnosis or measurement of disease activity [4, 5, 9]. A small proportion of children and AYA who present with or evolve to a spondyloarthropathy may test positive for the HLA-B27 gene [8].

Role of Biopsy

Although histopathology is typical for chronic inflammation, there are no features specific to CNO to help differentiate it from chronic infection. Nevertheless, affected areas are usually biopsied when the disease is unifocal, or occurs in unusual locations or/and in atypical age groups, and in the presence of systemic symptoms to exclude conditions like malignancy [4, 11–13]. The cellular infiltrate comprises predominantly of neutrophils in early lesions and monocytes, macrophages, lymphocytes, plasma cells during later stages. This parallels the immunological reaction characterised by activation of the innate immune system in early stages followed by the adaptive immune system in the chronic phases of the disease. Immunohistochemistry demonstrates the predominance of $CD3^{+}$, $CD45RO^{+}$ T-cells, which are mainly $CD4^{-}$ and $CD8^{+}$T cells. $CD20^{+}$ B-cell infiltrates are variable, but there is abundance of $CD68^{+}$ monocytes or macrophages [4, 9]. Osteoclastic bone resorption with secondary sclerosis, fibrosis and rarely, granulomatous foci can be seen in late phases [4, 9].

Imaging

Conventional radiographs may be normal in the early stages but as the disease progresses, AYA often develop features of osteolysis, sclerosis and new bone formation. Periosteal reactions or soft tissue swelling along with lytic areas that mimic bone tumours can also be seen [4, 5, 9, 14]. Where available, whole-body magnetic resonance imaging (WB-MRI) is now increasingly used, especially for multifocal disease, and has replaced other modalities of imaging. The advantages of a WB-MRI in the diagnosis of CNO cannot be overemphasised. It is particularly helpful in detecting asymptomatic lesions and, in early stages, to identify bone oedema before erosions or sclerosis become apparent. Short tau inversion recovery (STIR) or Turbo inversion recovery magnitude (TIRM) sequences are preferred, and typical lesions include bone marrow oedema, bone expansion, lytic areas and/or periosteal reaction. Andronikou et al. [14] reported two predominant phenotypes of radiological presentation of CNO: multifocal disease with mainly tibial involvement or pauci-focal clavicular and spinal disease [14]. Overall, the distal tibial metaphysis is the most involved site. Apart from diagnosis, WB-MRI is also used to monitor response to treatment [14–17]. Radionuclide bone scans and computed tomography scans are less preferred due to the risks associated with exposure to radiation. More recently, infrared thermal imaging was trialled in a small cohort to detect active lesions in the lower limbs, and significantly higher temperatures were detected for inflamed compared to uninflamed distal tibia/fibula segments [18].

Diagnostic Criteria

Diagnostic criteria can aid in early diagnosis and avoid unnecessary investigations. However, none of the proposed criteria has been evaluated in unrelated cohorts or are internationally accepted [4, 5, 8, 16, 19].

Treatment

Currently, there are no randomised control trials relating to treatment of CNO. The Childhood Arthritis and Rheumatology Research Alliance (CARRA) has recently proposed consensus treatment plans (CTP) with an intention to reduce variations in treatment practices [20]. A step-wise escalation pathway determined by the severity and location of disease has also been proposed (Fig. 18.1).

Non-steroidal Anti-inflammatory Drugs (NSAIDs)

Several studies have shown that NSAIDs are effective especially within 1–2 years of onset of disease and, generally, are the preferred first line drugs. Although any NSAID can be used, naproxen (15 mg/kg/day) is the only drug that has been studied prospectively. The mechanism of action probably involves inhibition of the cyclooxygenase pathway thereby decreasing prostaglandin synthesis. This helps with pain control and may also help prevent bone damage [4, 9, 19, 20]. NSAIDs have been used for primary lesions and to treat relapses. In one study involving 131 cases, 92 were commenced on naproxen and 57.6% of them attained clinical remission [8]. The effects of NSAIDs may take at least 4 weeks to be apparent.

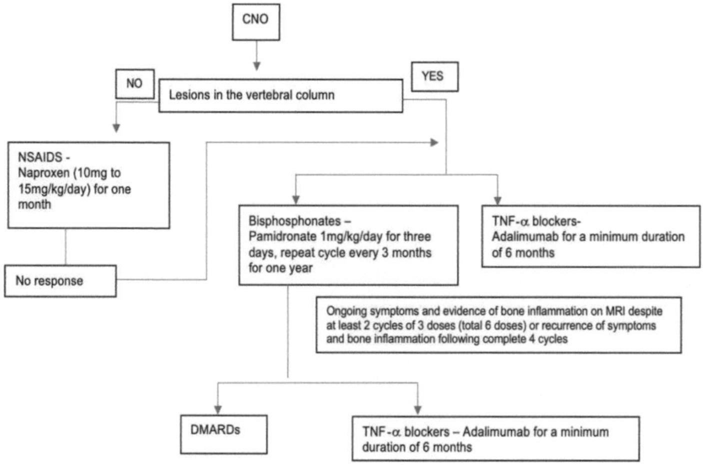

Fig. 18.1 Proposal of a treatment pathway (Bristol Children Hospital)

Bisphosphonates

There is increasing evidence to support the use of bisphosphonates when there is a failure to respond to NSAIDs. They are now used as the first line for spinal and mandibular disease [3, 8, 15, 16, 19]. Bisphosphonates reduce bone resorption by limiting osteoclastic apoptosis and also increase secondary mineralisation of bone. They have preferential affinity for sites of active bone remodelling such as areas of bone inflammation seen in CNO. Pamidronate was the first and most-commonly used bisphosphonate, but neridronate and zoledronate have also been used in CNO and appear to have similar effects to pamidronate [19, 20]. The protocol for pamidronate can vary between centres depending on clinical expertise, but is usually administered as 3-monthly cycles for a period of 12 months. Each cycle consists of 3 days of pamidronate at a dose of 1 mg/kg/day and a maximum of 60 mg/day. Vitamin D and calcium levels should be checked and corrected prior to treatment initiation [15, 16, 19]. Suppression of bone resorption is maximum within 3 months of initiation of therapy and is more rapid with intravenous than oral therapy. In a study by

Bhat et al. 70% of the radiologically-apparent lesions disappeared after treatment with pamidronate. Importantly, 82.3% of vertebral lesions resolved completely, demonstrating the benefit of bisphosphonates in treating spinal disease [15].

Biologics

TNF-α blockers: As per the CTP proposed by CARRA, TNF-α blockers (with or without methotrexate) can be used in the subset of AYA who are refractory to treatment with NSAIDs and/or in AYA with CNO and active spinal lesions [9, 20]. Access to TNF-α blockers has been variable worldwide, and this is reflected in treatment practices with some centres opting to use TNF-α blockers prior to bisphosphonates. Etanercept, adalimumab and infliximab have all been used with promising results [9, 20]. It is mandatory to test for and treat tuberculosis prior to initiation of treatment. More recently, fully humanised TNF-α inhibitor golimumab was used in 18 children and AYA with CNO with good outcomes [21].

IL-1 blockade: Anakinra has reportedly been used in one patient with some benefit. Currently the use of IL-1 blockade is restricted to autoinflammatory syndromes with inflammatory osteitis [2, 4].

Corticosteroids

In earlier studies, there was a tendency to use corticosteroids as second line therapy after NSAIDs [22]. It is now recognised that the effect of corticosteroids is transient and that there is a high likelihood of recurrence of disease when they are discontinued. Additionally, the toxicity profile of corticosteroids is unfavourable for long term use [3, 8, 10].

Other DMARDs

Methotrexate: Has been used in CNO with limited efficacy. It probably has a role as an adjunct therapy, but is less effective when used as a standalone drug [3, 8, 10, 23].

Sulfasalazine and Mesalazine: Their use is restricted to cases with associated inflammatory bowel disease. Sulfasalazine also reportedly has a higher efficacy in HLA-B27 positive individuals with CNO [8, 9, 20].

Long Term Outcome

Consensus guidelines for monitoring of disease activity are currently lacking. The disease course can be variable with intermittent flares and subsequent remission [3, 8]. In a recently published case series where 81 adolescents with a median age of onset at 11 years were followed for 4 years, an improvement in the physician global disease activity (PGDA), patient reported overall well-being and imaging-defined disease activity measures was documented, suggesting that good disease control in CNO can be reached. Sixty percent achieved inactive disease with zero lesions on WB-MRI after 4 years. Of note, only 5–7% of AYA had a severe disease course [24]. However, a large number of AYA can experience flares of pain despite radiological remission of disease. It is therefore important to monitor disease activity with a WB-MRI on follow-up [3, 8, 10, 12]. The impact of CNO on the growth of children and AYA is unclear. Height or weight at diagnosis were not associated with disease outcomes, but despite effective treatment, no significant increase in height or weight was documented [24].

Key Management Points

1. NSAIDs, particularly naproxen, are the preferred first-line treatment for CNO. Approximately 57.6% of AYA with CNO on naproxen achieve clinical remission, though courses of minimum 4 weeks are recommended.
2. Bisphosphonates are used when response to NSAIDs is suboptimal, and as first-line therapy for spinal and mandibular disease.
3. TNF-α blockers, such as adalimumab, are recommended for NSAID-refractory cases or for active spinal disease.
4. Corticosteroids are not recommended for CNO treatment due to their transient effects and high likelihood of disease recurrence after discontinuation.

References

1. Suo C, Chia D, Toms A, Sanghrajka A, Ramanan A, Killeen O, Jacobs B, Ilea C, Mahmood K, Compeyrot-Lacassagne S, Armon K. OA33 incidence of chronic recurrent multifocal osteomyelitis in the UK and Republic of Ireland: initial results from 13 months of surveillance study. Rheumatol Adv Pract. 2022;6(Suppl 1):rkac066.033.
2. Taddio A, Zennaro F, Pastore S, Cimaz R. An update on the pathogenesis and treatment of chronic recurrent multifocal osteomyelitis in children. Paediatr Drugs. 2017;19(3):165–72.
3. Wipff J, Costantino F, Lemelle I, Pajot C, Duquesne A, Lorrot M, et al. A large national cohort of French patients with chronic recurrent multifocal osteitis. Arthritis Rheumatol. 2015;67(4):1128–37.
4. Zhao DY, McCann L, Hahn G, Hedrich CM. Chronic nonbacterial osteomyelitis (CNO) and chronic recurrent multifocal osteomyelitis (CRMO). J Transl Autoimmun. 2021;4:100095.
5. Hofmann SR, Kapplusch F, Girschick HJ, Morbach H, Pablik J, Ferguson PJ, Hedrich CM. Chronic Recurrent Multifocal Osteomyelitis (CRMO): presentation, pathogenesis, and treatment. Curr Osteoporos Rep. 2017;15(6):542–54.
6. Cox AJ, Darbro BW, Laxer RM, Velez G, Bing X, Finer AL, et al. Recessive coding and regulatory mutations in FBLIM1 underlie the pathogenesis of chronic recurrent multifocal osteomyelitis (CRMO). PLoS One. 2017;12(3):e0169687.

7. Abe K, Cox A, Takamatsu N, Velez G, Laxer RM, Tse SML, et al. Gain-of-function mutations in a member of the Src family kinases cause auto-inflammatory bone disease in mice and humans. Proc Natl Acad Sci USA. 2019;116(24):11872–7.
8. Bhat CS, Anderson C, Harbinson A, McCann LJ, Roderick M, Finn A, et al. Chronic non bacterial osteitis- a multicentre study. Pediatr Rheumatol Online J. 2018;16(1):74.
9. Singhal S, Landes C, Shukla R, McCann LJ, Hedrich CM. Classification and management strategies for paediatric chronic nonbacterial osteomyelitis and chronic recurrent multifocal osteomyelitis. Expert Rev Clin Immunol. 2023;19(9):1101–16.
10. Girschick H, Finetti M, Orlando F, Schalm S, Insalaco A, Ganser G, et al. The multifaceted presentation of chronic recurrent multifocal osteomyelitis: a series of 486 cases from the Eurofever international registry. Rheumatology (Oxford). 2018;57(7):1203–11. https://doi.org/10.1093/rheumatology/key058.
11. Schnabel A, Range U, Hahn G, Siepmann T, Berner R, Hedrich CM. Unexpectedly high incidences of chronic non-bacterial as compared to bacterial osteomyelitis in children. Rheumatol Int. 2016;36(12):1737–45.
12. Walsh P, Manners PJ, Vercoe J, Burgner D, Murray KJ. Chronic recurrent multifocal osteomyelitis in children: nine years' experience at a statewide tertiary paediatric rheumatology referral centre. Rheumatology (Oxford). 2015;54(9):1688–91.
13. Girschick H, Finetti M, Orlando F, Schalm S, Insalaco A, Ganser G, et al. The multifaceted presentation of chronic recurrent multifocal osteomyelitis: a series of 486 cases from the Eurofever international registry. Rheumatology (Oxford). 2018;57(8):1504.
14. Andronikou S, Mendes da Costa T, Hussien M, Ramanan AV. Radiological diagnosis of chronic recurrent multifocal osteomyelitis using whole-body MRI-based lesion distribution patterns. Clin Radiol. 2019;74(9):737.e3–737.e15.
15. Bhat CS, Roderick M, Sen ES, Finn A, Ramanan AV. Efficacy of pamidronate in children with chronic non-bacterial osteitis using whole body MRI as a marker of disease activity. Pediatr Rheumatol Online J. 2019;17(1):35.
16. Roderick MR, Shah R, Rogers V, Finn A, Ramanan AV. Chronic recurrent multifocal osteomyelitis (CRMO)—advancing the diagnosis. Pediatr Rheumatol Online J. 2016;14(1):47.
17. Arnoldi AP, Schlett CL, Douis H, Geyer LL, Voit AM, Bleisteiner F, et al. Whole-body MRI in patients with non-bacterial osteitis: radiological findings and correlation with clinical data. Eur Radiol. 2017;27(6):2391–9.
18. Zhao Y, Iyer RS, Reichley L, Oron AP, Gove NE, Kitsch AE, et al. A pilot study of infrared thermal imaging to detect active bone lesions in children

with chronic nonbacterial osteomyelitis. Arthritis Care Res (Hoboken). 2019;71(11):1430–5.

19. Roderick MR, Sen ES, Ramanan AV. Chronic recurrent multifocal osteomyelitis in children and adults: current understanding and areas for development. Rheumatology (Oxford). 2017;57(1):41–8. https://doi.org/10.1093/rheumatology/kex066.
20. Zhao Y, Wu EY, Oliver MS, Cooper AM, Basiaga ML, Vora SS, et al. Consensus treatment plans for chronic nonbacterial osteomyelitis refractory to nonsteroidal antiinflammatory drugs and/or with active spinal lesions. Arthritis Care Res (Hoboken). 2017;70(8):1228–37. https://doi.org/10.1002/acr.23462.
21. Yang C, Rosenwasser N, Wang X, Xu Z, Scheck J, Boos MD, Gupta D, Brandling-Bennet HA, Sidbury R, Iyer RS, Zhao Y. Golimumab in children with chronic recurrent multifocal osteomyelitis: a case series and review of the literature. Paediatr Drugs. 2023;25(5):603–11.
22. Ishikawa-Nakayama K, Sugiyama E, Sawazaki S, Taki H, Kobayashi M, Koizumi F, et al. Chronic recurrent multifocal osteomyelitis showing marked improvement with corticosteroid treatment. J Rheumatol. 2000;27(5):1318–9.
23. Kaiser D, Bolt I, Hofer M, Relly C, Berthet G, Bolz D, et al. Chronic nonbacterial osteomyelitis in children: a retrospective multicenter study. Pediatr Rheumatol Online J. 2015;13:25.
24. Reiser C, Klotsche J, Hospach T, Heubner G, Windschall D, Trauzeddel R, Groesch N, Niewerth M, Minden K, Girschick H. Long-term follow-up of children with chronic non-bacterial osteomyelitis-assessment of disease activity, risk factors, and outcome. Arthritis Res Ther. 2023;25(1):228.

Part III

General Principles of Management of AYA with Rheumatic and Musculoskeletal Conditions

19 Managing Pregnancy in AYA with Paediatric Onset Rheumatic Diseases

Bethan Goulden, Sonji Clarke,
and Ian Giles

Pregnancy in Adolescence

Pregnant teenagers have an increased risk of pre-eclampsia, anaemia, and perinatal loss (e.g., miscarriage, stillbirth, neonatal death) (Box 19.1) [1]. Their infants are more likely to be born prematurely and with low birth weight, and may go on to have poor educational attainment and behavioural issues [2]. Post-partum depression and intimate partner violence are more common, and pregnancies are more likely to be complicated by smoking, substance misuse, and sexually transmitted infections (STIs) [2, 3]. Those at highest risk of teenage pregnancy include those living in poverty, not in education, and those with adverse childhood experiences [4, 5].

B. Goulden (✉) · I. Giles (✉)
Department of Ageing, Rheumatology and Regenerative Medicine, University College London, London, UK
e-mail: bethan.goulden@ucl.ac.uk; i.giles@ucl.ac.uk

S. Clarke
Department of Obstetrics, Guys and St Thomas' NHS Foundation Trust, London, UK
e-mail: Sonji.Clarke@gstt.nhs.uk

C. Ciurtin, J. Hackett (eds.), *Adolescent and Young Adult Rheumatology In Clinical Practice*, In Clinical Practice,
https://doi.org/10.1007/978-3-031-82102-8_19

Box 19.1 Glossary of Obstetric Terminology

Anaemia (in pregnancy): <110 g/L (first trimester), <105 g/L (second & third trimester), <100 g/L postpartum.

Instrumental delivery: Vaginal delivery with assistance from forceps or ventouse suction cup.

Intrahepatic cholestasis of pregnancy (ICP): Pruritus and elevated random total bile acid concentration (mild: ≥19–39 µmol/L; moderate 40–99 µmol/L, severe ≥100 µmol/L).

Miscarriage: Spontaneous pregnancy loss before 21 weeks and 6 days gestation.

Pre-eclampsia: New onset hypertension (≥140/90 mmHg) after 20 weeks of pregnancy associated with end-organ damage which can be maternal (e.g., proteinuria, seizures, haemolysis, elevated transaminases) or uteroplacental (e.g., foetal growth restriction, placental abruption).

Preterm birth: Liveborn infant delivered before 37 weeks of pregnancy.

Small for gestational age: Infant birth weight < tenth centile.

Stillbirth: Spontaneous pregnancy loss after 22 weeks gestation.

AYA with chronic health conditions are as sexually active as their peers and therefore regular, pre-emptive discussions are recommended [6, 7]. These discussions, however, are not routinely taking place in clinical practice. A survey of people with paediatric onset RMDs identified a lack of meaningful reproductive health counselling—AYA were being advised to avoid pregnancy but did not receive a clear explanation as to how or why [8]. Numerous resources exist to support prescribing and counselling discussions (Table 19.1).

Table 19.1 Resources for RMD pre-pregnancy counselling and prescribing

Resource	Weblink
United Kingdom Teratology Information Service (UKTIS)—for prescribing in pregnancy	https://uktis.org; UKTIS monographs also available on the Toxbase app
Drugs and Lactation Database (LactMed)—for prescribing in breastfeeding	https://www.ncbi.nlm.nih.gov/books/NBK501922; LactMed monographs also available on the LactRx app
Best Use of Medicines in Pregnancy (BUMPS)—for patient information on medications in pregnancy	https://www.medicinesinpregnancy.org
The Breastfeeding Network (BfN)—for patient information on medications in lactation	https://www.breastfeedingnetwork.org.uk
American College of Rheumatology Reproductive Health Guideline—for RMDs specific advice on contraception and assisted reproduction	https://acrjournals.onlinelibrary.wiley.com/doi/10.1002/art.41191
UK Medical Eligibility for Contraception Calculator	UKMEC Calculator
British Society for Rheumatology Prescribing in Pregnancy and Lactation guidelines—for RMDs specific prescribing recommendations	Part 1: Immunosuppressive medications: https://academic.oup.com/rheumatology/article/62/4/e48/6783012 Part 2: Co-morbidity medications: https://academic.oup.com/rheumatology/article/62/4/e89/6783013

Contraception

Male and female condoms protect against STIs but do not individually offer sufficiently reliable contraception for pregnancy prevention with typical use (Table 19.2).

All female AYA with RMDs should be recommended to consider long acting reversible contraception (LARC) including the progesterone intrauterine system (IUS), progesterone contraceptive implant and copper intrauterine device [10–12]. LARCs are as effective as surgical sterilisation, rapidly reversible on removal, and can be used in those with thrombotic risk factors, such as a high risk anti-phospholipid antibody profile (i.e., persistently positive lupus anticoagulant and/or medium/high anticardiolipin or anti-β2Glycoprotein I antibodies) or a previous thrombosis [9, 13]. The progesterone based methods, in particular the IUS, offer additional benefits including infrequent, light (or absent) men-

Table 19.2 Contraception and RMDs: Percentage efficacy at preventing pregnancy in first year of use

Method of contraception	Hormone content	Perfect use	Typical use
IUD	Nil	>99%	>99%
IUS	Progesterone	>99%	>99%
Implant	Progesterone	>99%	>99%
Injection	Progesterone	>99%	94%
POP	Progesterone	>99%	91%
COCP	Progesterone & oestrogen	>99%	91%
Patch	Progesterone & oestrogen	>99%	91%
Ring	Progesterone & oestrogen	>99%	91%
Male condoms	Nil	98%	82%
Female diaphragm	Nil	94%	88%

Adapted from Ref. [9]

COCP combined oral contraceptive pill, *IUD* Intra-uterine device (copper coil), *IUS* intra-uterine system (progesterone coil), *POP* progesterone only pill

struation—thereby reducing the risk of iron deficiency anaemia and the distress and disruption of heavy and/or painful periods [10]. All LARCs can be inserted in those who are immunosuppressed, anticoagulated and/or nulliparous, and a systematic review of contraceptive use in the general population confirmed LARC continuation rates were significantly higher than other contraceptive methods [14].

Whilst highly user dependent in terms of efficacy, oral contraceptive pills remain a popular option—they are non-invasive and often easier to access than LARCs. Efficacy may be reduced by missed pills (more likely to occur with AYA), taking enzyme inducing medications, and diarrhoea and vomiting. The combined oral contraceptive pill (COCP) typically comes as a pack with 21 days of active tablets followed by a 7 day break which triggers a withdrawal bleed. There is no health benefit conferred from this regimen; it may reduce contraceptive efficacy and cause side-effects (e.g., headache, mood disturbance) [12, 15]. Users increasingly take the COCP continuously or for extended periods. Non-contraceptive benefits of COCP include improvements in menorrhagia and acne, and a reduced risk of endometrial, ovarian and colorectal cancer. COCPs are associated with small increases in the risk of cervical and breast cancer, as well as thrombotic arterial and venous events with magnitude of risk dependent on the progesterone type and oestrogen dose [15]. COCPs are contraindicated in those with significant risk factors for thromboembolic disease (e.g., high-risk anti-phospholipid antibody profile) and should be used with caution in smokers or the significantly overweight. The progesterone only pill (POP)—often referred to as the mini-pill—is an alternative to the COCP. It can be safely taken by those with thrombotic risk factors but can cause an irregular bleeding pattern, especially during initial use, and needs to be taken daily within a narrow timeframe (3 or 12 h interval depending on the POP type) [16].

Less common alternatives include the progesterone contraceptive injection, and other combined oestrogen-progesterone methods (e.g., contraceptive patch, vaginal ring) [15]. The ring and patch have similar cautions and contraindications to the COCP, and alternatives should be offered to those at significant risk of thrombosis. Historically, the contraceptive injection was administered intramuscularly by a healthcare professional every 8–13 weeks but a newer product called the Sayana-Press can be self-administered subcutaneously at home [17]. All progesterone injections can cause an irregular and occasionally heavier bleeding pattern as well as a delayed return of fertility and reversible loss of bone density [17]. Other methods are preferable in those at high-risk of osteoporosis [12].

Emergency contraception can be used in AYA with RMDs, including those with active disease, a history of thrombosis, or antiphospholipid antibodies. The most effective emergency contraceptive is the copper IUD—it can be efficacious up to 5-days following unprotected sex and provides long-lasting contraception. Oral progesterone-only based alternatives exist though they are only effective if taken prior to ovulation and efficacy may be reduced if the individual is of higher weight or concurrently taking enzyme inducing medications.

Pre-pregnancy Counselling

Proactive referral for specialist pre-pregnancy counselling (PPC) is particularly important in those with conditions or complications which carry high maternal mortality, where alternative routes to motherhood such as adoption or surrogacy should be discussed (e.g., pulmonary arterial hypertension, ventricular ejection fraction <30%, vascular Ehlers Danlos syndrome) [18]. For others, meaningful discussions on how to avoid unplanned pregnancy and education regarding future reproductive health are welcomed by AYA and their parents regardless of whether they are actively planning pregnancy [8, 19].

Many RMDs-related factors can reduce fertility including active inflammation and established end-organ damage (e.g., chronic kidney disease; CKD). In females, cyclophosphamide may reduce ovarian reserve but risk of ovarian failure is low in those treated in adolescence, and co-administration with gonadotropin releasing hormone (GnRH) analogues may further mitigate risk [20].

For those actively planning pregnancy, 400 mcg/day folic acid and at least 400 IU/day vitamin D should be started 3 months prior to conception [21, 22]. Those on sulphasalazine, anti-epileptics, with diabetes or a body mass index >30 should take 5 mg/day of folic acid, until at least 12 weeks gestation, although evidence for this increased dose in pregnancy is lacking [23]. Those with high-risk anti-phospholipid antibody profiles should be offered low dose aspirin (LDA), 75–150 mg daily, from pre-conception or positive pregnancy test, and prophylactic low molecular weight heparin (LMWH) should be co-administered in those with obstetric antiphospholipid antibody syndrome (APS). If there is a history of thrombotic APS—then high-dose LMWH should be commenced with a positive pregnancy test (either started de novo or as a switch from existing oral anticoagulation) [24].

Achieving low disease activity or remission on pregnancy compatible therapies for 3–6 months before pregnancy (up to 12 months if organ dysfunction) is vital to optimise fertility, reduce early pregnancy loss and minimise antepartum flares [12]. Evidence based guidance advises on pregnancy compatible medication [12, 23] and increasingly, biologic therapy is considered to control disease activity in pregnancy [25]. Potentially teratogenic therapies should be discontinued in females before pregnancy in-line with guidance (Table 19.1 and Fig. 19.1); particularly, methotrexate, leflunomide, mycophenolate, cyclophosphamide and Janus kinase inhibitors. Renoprotective therapies such as ACE-inhibitors should also be stopped at a positive pregnancy test, and sodium-glucose co-transporter-2 (SGLT-2) inhibitors should be discontinued pre-conception. All biologic and conventional synthetic disease modifying anti-rheumatic drugs (DMARDs) can be continued in young men, with semen cryopreservation recommended prior to use of cyclophosphamide [23].

Finally, smoking, drug, and alcohol use should be addressed and screening for STIs instigated. Smoking contributes to 1 in 12 preterm births, 1 in 5 low birth weight infants, and 1 in 3 sudden unexplained deaths in infancy [26], and cessation is one of the most impactful steps an individual can take to improve future pregnancy outcomes. Recreational drug use may increase these risks further and, in some instances (e.g., opioid use), lead to neonatal abstinence syndrome postnatally as the infant withdraws.

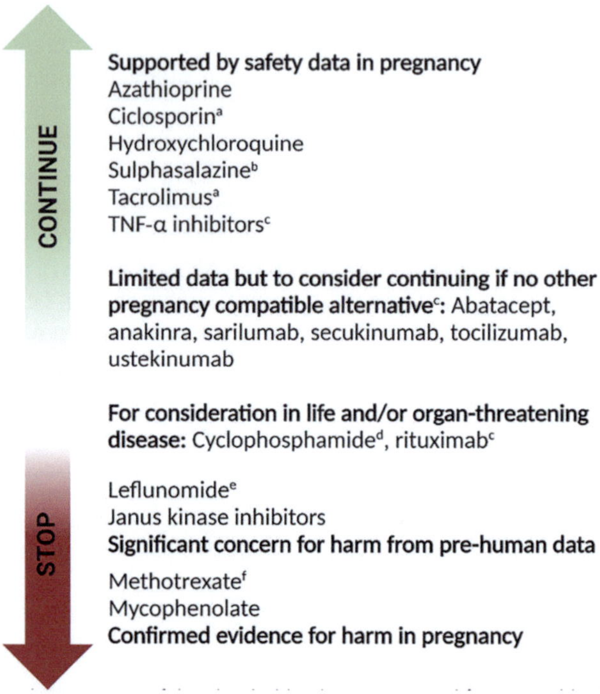

Fig. 19.1 Prescribing in pregnancy. (Created with BioRender.com). [a]With monitoring of drug levels, blood pressure, renal function & blood glucose. [b]Co-administer folic acid 5 mg/day 3 months pre-conception to 14 weeks pregnancy. [c]Use in later pregnancy necessitates adjustment of live vaccine schedule in infant. [d]Severe and/or life threatening disease in second/third trimester. [e]Increasing body of human data do not suggest harm, advice may change, but for now, recommendation is to avoid. [f]Data too limited for low dose (≤25 mg/week) to make evidence-based risk assessment, recommendation remains to avoid

Pregnancy Care

On being notified of pregnancy, rheumatology teams should review medications and disease activity, and if available, refer for specialist obstetrics and maternal medicine care (Fig. 19.2).

Risk stratification for pre-eclampsia is usually performed by 11–14 weeks using clinical factors alone or ideally, composite

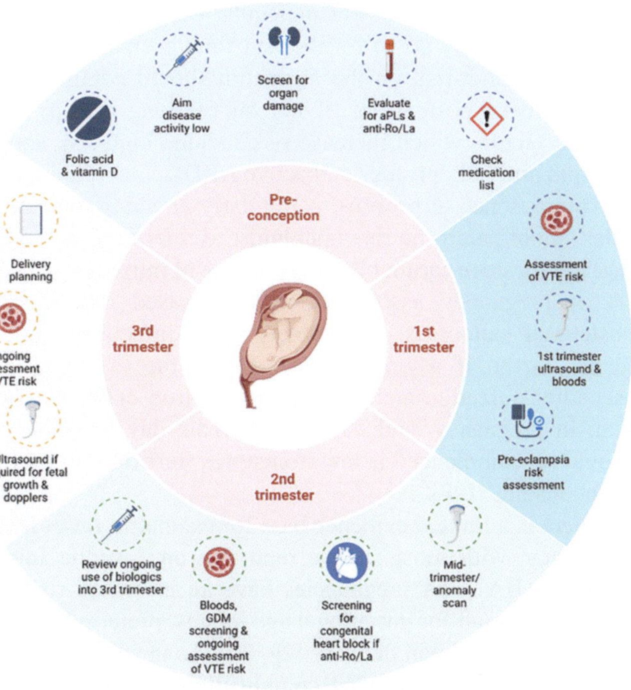

Fig. 19.2 Summary of pre-pregnancy and pregnancy care for AYA with RMDs. (Created with BioRender.com). *aPLs* antiphospholipid antibodies, *GDM* gestational diabetes, *VTE* venous thromboembolism

scores, including ultrasound and biochemistry. When reliant on clinical parameters alone, conditions such as systemic lupus erythematosus (SLE), APS, vasculitis, scleroderma, and active inflammatory arthritis may all influence risk. When these RMD-related factors are present, the pregnant person should be discussed with the obstetrician or obstetric physician regardless of risk score, to consider initiating LDA if <16 weeks gestation.

Thromboembolic risk should also be assessed on pregnancy notification and subsequent reviews using published algorithms such as that from the Royal College Of Obstetricians and Gynaecologists [27]. Risk varies throughout pregnancy and remains elevated in the postpartum period. Individuals who have not met the threshold for low molecular weight heparin (LMWH) in pregnancy may do so for the first time postpartum, and those considered high-risk on the algorithm should continue LMWH until 6-weeks postpartum (if not on life-long therapy). RMD-specific factors which increase risk include high-risk anti-phospholipid antibody profiles and active ARDs.

The presence of pruritus, particularly affecting the palms and soles, should alert the rheumatologist to refer urgently to obstetrics and measure serum bile acids in case of intrahepatic cholestasis of pregnancy associated with increased risk of adverse obstetrical outcomes. All urinary tract infections should be treated—even if asymptomatic—due to the increased risk of ascending infection and preterm labour. Iron deficiency is common in pregnancy, and daily or alternate day supplementation should be commenced if low iron stores (ferritin <30 μg/l), even if not anaemic [28].

There is a limited evidence base for paediatric-onset RMDs in pregnancy, with most studies reporting on Juvenile Idiopathic Arthritis (JIA). JIA pregnancies have an increased risk of pre-eclampsia, small for gestational age infants, preterm birth, instrumental and caesarean delivery [29, 30]. As in adult onset RMDs, the risk of these pregnancy complications is related to disease activity [31]. The highest-risk period for flare is postpartum [32, 33]. Discontinuation of DMARDs contributes to progressive articular damage over the course of pregnancy [34], increases risk of pregnancy complications and increases postpartum flare incidence [35]. We therefore recommend that pregnancy compatible therapies are continued throughout to suppress active RMDs for both maternal and infant benefit.

The limited data available for juvenile dermatomyositis (JDM) and juvenile SLE (JSLE) support a similar approach, although individuals with JDM and JSLE have a higher prevalence of end-organ damage (e.g., chronic kidney disease – CKD) and co-morbidities (e.g., hypertension) which may influence pregnancy outcomes independent of disease activity [36, 37]. The consequences of severe flare necessitate vigilant observation of maternal health—clinically, serologically, and with an awareness of normal gestational changes (e.g., complement should rise in healthy pregnancy and thus static as well as falling levels may indicate disease activity). In the event of a severe flare, cyclophosphamide may be used in the second/third trimester, and rituximab throughout pregnancy—though second/third trimester use will result in transplacental transfer and a risk of neonatal cytopenias. Anti-Ro/La antibodies confer a 1/75 risk of congenital heart block (CHB) in the foetus which typically becomes apparent between 20 and 30 weeks gestation. Enhanced surveillance is recommended with auscultation of foetal heart rate and urgent foetal echocardiogram if foetal bradycardia is detected. Evidence-based therapies to treat CHB are lacking but hydroxychloroquine halved the risk of recurrence in those with previously affected infants [38].

In all cases the priority is to ensure disease quiescence with adjustment to the most suitable pregnancy compatible medications several months before conception and continuation of these medications throughout pregnancy to maintain disease control (Fig. 19.1) [39]. Increasingly, biologic DMARDs are being continued throughout pregnancy and although the largest body of experience and safety exists for drugs that inhibit tumour necrosis factor (TNF)-α, many non-TNF-α inhibiting biologic DMARDs may be continued if they are the only drugs considered suitable to maintain disease control, given their emerging safety profile and benefits of disease suppression [25].

Late pregnancy use of biologics does mean that, if eligible, the Bacillus Calmette-Guérin (BCG) vaccine should be deferred until the infant is 6 months old [23]. The rotavirus vaccine is also live, but cannot be delayed beyond 6 months and as such should be missed if a non-TNF-α inhibiting biologic is used in late pregnancy [40]. This advice may change as the evidence base for these biologics expands.

Unplanned Pregnancy

Around 55% of pregnancies are unplanned, many of which will end in abortion [41]. The safety and availability of abortion varies worldwide and accidental conception should act as a prompt for rheumatologists to review STI risk, medication safety, contraception and, if applicable, address any safeguarding concerns. If AYA with RMDs decide to continue the pregnancy it is important to refer them early to maternity services, ensure disease activity is optimised on pregnancy-compatible therapies, initiate folic acid (5 mg/day if exposed to methotrexate or taking sulphasalazine) and vitamin D supplementation.

Accurate pregnancy risk prediction following teratogen exposure can be complex. Risk is determined by preconception compliance, length of pregnancy exposure, use of co-administered medications (e.g., other teratogens), and the specific exposure drug and dose. Some agents are avoided in pre-conception/early pregnancy due to well documented human teratogenicity (e.g., cyclophosphamide, mycophenolate) whilst others are avoided due to limited human data confirming safety and/or concerns from animal testing (e.g., leflunomide, janus kinase inhibitors, methotrexate).

Even for exposure to known teratogens there is a spectrum of possible outcomes. Mycophenolate more than doubles the risk of miscarriage, and causes a defined embryopathy with congenital defects in up to 1 in 4 subsequent live births, but healthy live births have also been reported [23]. Navigating this uncertainty can be difficult and even with enhanced foetal medicine surveillance, it is not always possible to identify congenital anomalies antenatally.

Safeguarding

Conversations with AYA about sex, contraception and pregnancy should include time without parents present, and if there is a language barrier, using independent translators. Interconnected issues include female genital mutilation, rape and sexual abuse, intimate partner physical and sexual violence, drug and alcohol use, and mental health issues. If the teenager is already pregnant then considering the needs of, and risks to, the unborn child is also required.

Liaison with safeguarding services and skilled paediatricians and obstetricians is essential in navigating teenage pregnancy, and when relevant, including outside agencies such as children's social care and learning disability services. Conversations must include an assessment of capacity during pregnancy and provide clarity regarding parental responsibility (particularly if the pregnant teenager is under 16).

These discussions require sensitivity and a clear understanding of relevant legal statutes. Region-specific guidance may dictate a minimum age to consent to sexual activity with associated safeguarding and legal consequences (e.g., the age at which any sexual activity would be considered statutory rape). Separate laws may also govern the ability of a child to consent to or decline medical treatment, and more specifically related to contraception, without parental consent—this once again varies worldwide. Countries such as the UK have specific legal rulings governing these aspects of paediatric care (e.g., Gillick competence, Fraser guidelines) but many countries worldwide do not have specific age cut-offs, and in these scenarios adhering to World Health Organisation advice is recommended [42].

Summary

Delivering regular, pre-emptive discussions addressing reproductive health should be a core component of holistic adolescent care. By ensuring that AYA with RMDs are on highly effective contraception (preferably a LARC), pregnancy can be planned for a time when disease is well-controlled on pregnancy-compatible therapies, and the individual is mentally, financially and emotionally prepared—thereby optimising outcomes for mother and infant.

Learning Points

1. Rheumatologists should have the skills to engage in meaningful discussions on contraception and reproductive health in the context of RMDs through adolescence and young adulthood.
2. Pregnancy should be planned when RMDs are well controlled on pregnancy-compatible therapies.
3. Unplanned and adolescent pregnancy come with unique challenges and an increased risk of adverse pregnancy outcomes including maternal and perinatal mortality.
4. Region specific laws should be considered when engaging in discussions around contraception, pregnancy and abortion with teenagers.
5. Integrated care with specialist obstetricians, obstetric physicians (where available) and midwives is essential in pregnancies complicated by RMDs.

References

1. Akseer N, Keats EC, Thurairajah P, Cousens S, Bétran AP, Oaks BM, Osrin D, Piwoz E, Gomo E, Ahmed F, Friis H, Belizán J, Dewey K, West K, Huybregts L, Zeng L, Dibley MJ, Zagre N, Christian P, Kolsteren PW, Kaestel P, Black RE, Arifeen SE, Ashorn U, Fawzi W, Bhutta ZA. Characteristics and birth outcomes of pregnant adolescents compared to older women: an analysis of individual level data from 140,000 mothers from 20 RCTs. EClinicalMedicine. 2022;45:101309. https://doi.org/10.1016/j.eclinm.2022.101309.
2. Paranjothy S, Broughton H, Adappa R, Fone D. Teenage pregnancy: who suffers? Arch Dis Child. 2009;94:239–45. https://doi.org/10.1136/adc.2007.115915.
3. Niccolai LM, Ethier KA, Kershaw TS, Lewis JB, Ickovics JR. Pregnant adolescents at risk: sexual behaviors and sexually transmitted disease prevalence. Am J Obstet Gynecol. 2003;188:63–70. https://doi.org/10.1067/mob.2003.119.
4. Bellis MA, Hughes K, Leckenby N, Perkins C, Lowey H. National household survey of adverse childhood experiences and their relationship with resilience to health-harming behaviors in England. BMC Med. 2014;12:1–10. https://doi.org/10.1186/1741-7015-12-72.

5. Ford K, Butler N, Hughes K, Quigg Z, Bellis MA, Barker P, Conrad D, O'Neill K, Bhattacharya C, Paterson B. Adverse childhood experiences (ACEs) in Hertfordshire. Luton and Northamptonshire: Centre for Public Health; 2016.
6. Hunt JA, Randell KA, Mermelstein S, Miller MK, Sherman AK, Philipose S, Masonbrink AR. Sexual health behaviors and pregnancy risk among hospitalized female adolescents. Hosp Pediatr. 2021;11:1129–36. https://doi.org/10.1542/hpeds.2021-005810.
7. Surís JC, Resnick MD, Cassuto N, Blum RW. Sexual behavior of adolescents with chronic disease and disability. J Adolesc Health. 1996;19(2):124–31. https://doi.org/10.1016/1054-139X(95)00282-W.
8. Carandang K, Mruk V, Ardoin SP, Huynh B, Clowse MEB, Berlan ED, Edens C. Reproductive health needs of adolescent and young adult women with pediatric rheumatic diseases. Pediatr Rheumatol Online J. 2020;18:66. https://doi.org/10.1186/s12969-020-00460-7.
9. FSRH. FSRH guideline (2016, amended September 2019) UK medical eligibility for contraceptive use. 2019.
10. FSRH. FSRH guideline (March 2023) intrauterine contraception. BMJ Sex Reprod Health. 2023;49:1–142. https://doi.org/10.1136/bmjsrh-2023-IUC.
11. FSRH. FSRH guideline (February 2021) progestogen-only implant. BMJ Sex Reprod Health. 2021;47:1–62. https://doi.org/10.1136/bmjsrh-2021-CHC.
12. Sammaritano LR, Bermas BL, Chakravarty EE, Chambers C, Clowse MEB, Lockshin MD, Marder W, Guyatt G, Branch DW, Buyon J, Christopher-Stine L, Crow-Hercher R, Cush J, Druzin M, Kavanaugh A, Laskin CA, Plante L, Salmon J, Simard J, Somers EC, Steen V, Tedeschi SK, Vinet E, White CW, Yazdany J, Barbhaiya M, Bettendorf B, Eudy A, Jayatilleke A, Shah AA, Sullivan N, Tarter LL, Birru Talabi M, Turgunbaev M, Turner A, D'Anci KE. 2020 American College of rheumatology guideline for the management of reproductive health in rheumatic and musculoskeletal diseases. Arthritis Rheumatol. 2020;72:529–56. https://doi.org/10.1002/art.41191.
13. Barbhaiya M, Zuily S, Naden R, Hendry A, Manneville F, Amigo M-C, Amoura Z, Andrade D, Andreoli L, Artim-Esen B, Atsumi T, Avcin T, Belmont HM, Bertolaccini ML, Branch DW, Carvalheiras G, Casini A, Cervera R, Cohen H, Costedoat-Chalumeau N, Crowther M, de Jesus G, Delluc A, Desai S, De Sancho M, Devreese KM, Diz-Kucukk R, Duarte-Garcia A, Frances C, Garcia D, Gris J-C, Jordan N, Leaf RK, Kello N, Knight JS, Laskin C, Lee AI, Legault K, Levine SR, Levy RA, Limper M, Lockshin MD, Mayer-Pickel K, Musial J, Meroni PL, Orsolini G, Ortel TL, Pengo V, Petri M, Pons-Estel G, Gomez-Puerta JA, Raimboug Q, Roubey R, Sanna G, Seshan SV, Sciascia S, Tektonidou MG, Tincani A, Wahl D, Willis R, Yelnik C, Zuily C, Guillemin F, Costenbader K, Erkan D, ACR/EULAR APS Classification Criteria Collaborators. The 2023

ACR/EULAR antiphospholipid syndrome classification criteria. Arthritis Rheumatol. 2023;75:1687–702. https://doi.org/10.1002/art.42624.

14. Usinger KM, Gola SB, Weis M, Smaldone A. Intrauterine contraception continuation in adolescents and young women: a systematic review. J Pediatr Adolesc Gynecol. 2016;29:659–67. https://doi.org/10.1016/j.jpag.2016.06.007.
15. FSRH. FSRH guideline (January 2019, amended October 2023) combined hormonal contraception. BMJ Sex Reprod Health. 2019;45:1–93. https://doi.org/10.1136/bmjsrh-2018-CHC.
16. FSRH. FSRH guideline (August 2022) progestogen-only pills. BMJ Sex Reprod Health. 2022;48:1–75. https://doi.org/10.1136/bmjsrh-2022-PoP.
17. FSRH. FSRH guideline (December 2014, amended July 2023) Progesterone-only Injectable Contraception (No. 02/FSRH/Injectable/2014). Faculty of Sexual and Reproductive Health. 2023.
18. Regitz-Zagrosek V, Roos-Hesselink JW, Bauersachs J, Blomström-Lundqvist C, Cífková R, De Bonis M, Iung B, Johnson MR, Kintscher U, Kranke P, Lang IM, Morais J, Pieper PG, Presbitero P, Price S, Rosano GMC, Seeland U, Simoncini T, Swan L, Warnes CA, ESC Scientific Document Group. 2018 ESC Guidelines for the management of cardiovascular diseases during pregnancy: the task force for the management of cardiovascular diseases during pregnancy of the European Society of Cardiology (ESC). Eur Heart J. 2018;39:3165–241. https://doi.org/10.1093/eurheartj/ehy340.
19. Matsumoto T, Mori M. Questionnaire survey on transitional care for patients with juvenile idiopathic arthritis (JIA) and families. Mod Rheumatol. 2021;31:691–6. https://doi.org/10.1080/14397595.2020.1813369.
20. Luong SN, Isaacs A, Liu Z, Sin FE, Giles I. A systematic review and meta-analysis of the gonadotoxic effects of cyclophosphamide and benefits of gonadotropin releasing hormone agonists (GnRHa) in women of child-bearing age with autoimmune rheumatic disease. Expert Rev Clin Immunol. 2020;16(3):321–33. https://doi.org/10.1080/1744666X.2020.1724091.
21. NICE. Recommendations | Vitamin D: supplement use in specific population groups | Guidance | NICE [WWW Document]. 2014. https://www.nice.org.uk/guidance/ph56/chapter/Recommendations. Accessed 30 July 2024.
22. NICE. Recommendations | Maternal and child nutrition | Guidance | NICE [WWW Document]. 2008. https://www.nice.org.uk/guidance/ph11/chapter/Recommendations. Accessed 30 July 2024.
23. Russell MD, Dey M, Flint J, Davie P, Allen A, Crossley A, Frishman M, Gayed M, Hodson K, Khamashta M, Moore L, Panchal S, Piper M, Reid C, Saxby K, Schreiber K, Senvar N, Tosounidou S, van de Venne M, Warburton L, Williams D, Yee C-S, Gordon C, Giles I, BSR Standards, Audit and Guidelines Working Group. British society for rheumatology

guideline on prescribing drugs in pregnancy and breastfeeding: immunomodulatory anti-rheumatic drugs and corticosteroids. Rheumatology. 2023;62:e48–88. https://doi.org/10.1093/rheumatology/keac551.

24. Tektonidou MG, Andreoli L, Limper M, Amoura Z, Cervera R, Costedoat-Chalumeau N, Cuadrado MJ, Dörner T, Ferrer-Oliveras R, Hambly K, Khamashta MA, King J, Marchiori F, Meroni PL, Mosca M, Pengo V, Raio L, Ruiz-Irastorza G, Shoenfeld Y, Stojanovich L, Svenungsson E, Wahl D, Tincani A, Ward MM. EULAR recommendations for the management of antiphospholipid syndrome in adults. Ann Rheum Dis. 2019;78:1296–304. https://doi.org/10.1136/annrheumdis-2019-215213.
25. Giles I, Thorne I, Schmidt NS, Reid C, Crossley A, Panca M, Freemantle N, Tower C, Dass S, Sharma SK, Williams D, O'Neill S, Dolhain RJEM, Toplak N, Hodson K, Nelson-Piercy C, Clowse MEB. The time of equipoise on the use of biological DMARDs in for inflammatory arthritis during pregnancy is finally over: a reappraisal of evidence to optimise pregnancy management. Lancet Rheumatol. 2024;6:e546–59. https://doi.org/10.1016/S2665-9913(24)00097-3.
26. Public Health England. Teenage mothers and young fathers: support framework—GOV.UK [WWW Document]. GOV.UK. 2019. https://www.gov.uk/government/publications/teenage-mothers-and-young-fathers-support-framework. Accessed 5 July 2024.
27. RCOG. Reducing the risk of thrombosis and embolism during pregnancy and the puerperium (Green-top Guideline No. 37a). Royal College of Obstetricians and Gynaecologists; 2015.
28. Pavord S, Daru J, Prasannan N, Robinson S, Stanworth S, Girling J. UK guidelines on the management of iron deficiency in pregnancy. Br J Haematol. 2020;188:819–30. https://doi.org/10.1111/bjh.16221.
29. Chen JS, Ford JB, Roberts CL, Simpson JM, March LM. Pregnancy outcomes in women with juvenile idiopathic arthritis: a population-based study. Rheumatology. 2013;52:1119–25. https://doi.org/10.1093/rheumatology/kes428.
30. Remaeus K, Johansson K, Askling J, Stephansson O. Juvenile onset arthritis and pregnancy outcome: a population-based cohort study. Ann Rheum Dis. 2017;76:1809–14. https://doi.org/10.1136/annrheumdis-2016-210879.
31. Götestam Skorpen C, Lydersen S, Salvesen KÅ, Wallenius M. A population-based study of caesarean section in women with juvenile idiopathic arthritis. Rheumatol Adv Pract. 2023;7:rkad062. https://doi.org/10.1093/rap/rkad062.
32. Gerosa M, Chighizola CB, Pregnolato F, Pontikaki I, Luppino AF, Argolini LM, Trespidi L, Ossola MW, Ferrazzi EM, Caporali R, Cimaz R. Pregnancy in juvenile idiopathic arthritis: maternal and foetal outcome, and impact on disease activity. Ther Adv Musculoskelet Dis. 2022;14:1759720X221080375. https://doi.org/10.1177/1759720X221080375.

33. Ursin K, Lydersen S, Skomsvoll JF, Wallenius M. Disease activity of juvenile idiopathic arthritis during and after pregnancy: a prospective multicenter study. J Rheumatol. 2018;45:257–65. https://doi.org/10.3899/jrheum.161410.
34. Nagase T, Takakubo Y, Yokoyama Y, Nagase S, Yang S, Honma R, Oki H, Ito J, Sasaki A, Takagi M. Progression of bone and joint destruction during the perinatal period in patients with rheumatoid arthritis and juvenile idiopathic arthritis in the last decade. Cureus. 2022;14:e25396. https://doi.org/10.7759/cureus.25396.
35. García-Fernández A, Gerardi MC, Crisafulli F, Filippini M, Fredi M, Gorla R, Lazzaroni MG, Lojacono A, Nalli C, Ramazzotto F, Taglietti M, Zanardini C, Zatti S, Franceschini F, Tincani A, Andreoli L. Disease course and obstetric outcomes of pregnancies in juvenile idiopathic arthritis: are there any differences among disease subtypes? A single-centre retrospective study of prospectively followed pregnancies in a dedicated pregnancy clinic. Clin Rheumatol. 2021;40:239–44. https://doi.org/10.1007/s10067-020-05404-w.
36. Ling N, Lawson E, von Scheven E. Adverse pregnancy outcomes in adolescents and young women with systemic lupus erythematosus: a national estimate. Pediatr Rheumatol Online J. 2018;16:26. https://doi.org/10.1186/s12969-018-0242-0.
37. Madu AE, Omih E, Baguley E, Lindow SW. Juvenile dermatomyositis in pregnancy. Case Rep Obstet Gynecol. 2013;2013:890107. https://doi.org/10.1155/2013/890107.
38. Izmirly P, Kim M, Friedman DM, Costedoat-Chalumeau N, Clancy R, Copel JA, Phoon CKL, Cuneo BF, Cohen RE, Robins K, Masson M, Wainwright BJ, Zahr N, Saxena A, Buyon JP. Hydroxychloroquine to prevent recurrent congenital heart block in fetuses of anti-SSA/Ro-positive mothers. J Am Coll Cardiol. 2020;76:292–302. https://doi.org/10.1016/j.jacc.2020.05.045.
39. Giles I, Yee C-S, Gordon C. Stratifying management of rheumatic disease for pregnancy and breastfeeding. Nat Rev Rheumatol. 2019;15:391–402. https://doi.org/10.1038/s41584-019-0240-8.
40. Bass AR, Chakravarty E, Akl EA, Bingham CO, Calabrese L, Cappelli LC, Johnson SR, Imundo LF, Winthrop KL, Arasaratnam RJ, Baden LR, Berard R, Bridges SL, Cheah JTL, Curtis JR, Ferguson PJ, Hakkarinen I, Onel KB, Schultz G, Sivaraman V, Smith BJ, Sparks JA, Vogel TP, Williams EA, Calabrese C, Cunha JS, Fontanarosa J, Gillispie-Taylor MC, Gkrouzman E, Iyer P, Lakin KS, Legge A, Lo MS, Lockwood MM, Sadun RE, Singh N, Sullivan N, Tam H, Turgunbaev M, Turner AS, Reston J. 2022 American College of Rheumatology guideline for vaccinations in patients with rheumatic and musculoskeletal diseases. Arthritis Care Res (Hoboken). 2023;75:449–64. https://doi.org/10.1002/acr.25045.

41. Wellings K, Jones KG, Mercer CH, Tanton C, Clifton S, Datta J, Copas AJ, Erens B, Gibson LJ, Macdowall W, Sonnenberg P, Phelps A, Johnson AM. The prevalence of unplanned pregnancy and associated factors in Britain: findings from the third national survey of sexual attitudes and lifestyles (Natsal-3). Lancet. 2013;382:1807–16. https://doi.org/10.1016/S0140-6736(13)62071-1.
42. WHO. Assessing and supporting adolescents' capacity for autonomous decision-making in health care settings: a tool for health-care providers. Geneva: World Health Organisation; 2021.

Supporting Self-Management Skill Development Among Adolescents and Young Adults with Rheumatic Musculoskeletal Disease

20

Chitra Lalloo, Jennifer Stinson, and Lawrence S. Bloomberg

C. Lalloo (✉)
Child Health Evaluative Sciences, The Peter Gilgan Centre for Research and Learning, The Hospital for Sick Children, Toronto, ON, Canada

Institute for Health Policy, Management and Evaluation, The University of Toronto, Toronto, ON, Canada
e-mail: chitra.lalloo@sickkids.ca

J. Stinson
Child Health Evaluative Sciences, The Peter Gilgan Centre for Research and Learning, The Hospital for Sick Children, Toronto, ON, Canada

Institute for Health Policy, Management and Evaluation, The University of Toronto, Toronto, ON, Canada

Department of Anesthesia and Pain Medicine, The Hospital for Sick Children, Toronto, ON, Canada
e-mail: jennifer.stinson@sickkids.ca

L. S. Bloomberg
Faculty of Nursing, University of Toronto, Toronto, ON, Canada

C. Ciurtin, J. Hackett (eds.), *Adolescent and Young Adult Rheumatology In Clinical Practice*, In Clinical Practice,
https://doi.org/10.1007/978-3-031-82102-8_20

Disease self-management has been defined as "the interaction of health behaviors and related processes that patients and families engage in to care for a chronic condition" [1]. This conceptualization of self-management acknowledges that strictly adult-focused self-management models are not designed to account for influences of the larger family system (e.g., caregivers, siblings) on self-management behaviors. Specifically, in their young person model, Modi and colleagues define three interdependent components of self-management: (1) self-management behaviors, (2), the contextual variables across four domains (i.e., influences of individual, family, healthcare system, and community) that impact the execution of those behaviors, and (3) the processes that link influences with behaviors [1]. Self-management behaviors are performed in the context of attempting to care for a chronic condition (e.g., an adolescent with arthritis who swims regularly to improve their aerobic fitness). However, it is important to note that self-management itself is a neutral concept and specific efforts to manage a condition may ultimately positively or negatively affect health outcomes.

The management of rheumatic musculoskeletal diseases (RMD) during adolescence and young adulthood is often complex, requiring diverse multifaceted therapies over long periods of time that necessitate frequent monitoring. As they grow older, adolescents and young adults (AYA) are expected to become more self-sufficient and independent in the management of their condition. In developmental terms, AYA are characterized by identity explorations, instability, self-focus, and continued development of executive cognitive functioning [2]. It is known that executive functioning is critical for the development of self-management skills [1, 3] (see Chap. 1).

Many AYA with RMD have ongoing disease into adulthood [4]. The self-management decisions made during adolescence and young adulthood can have lasting impacts later in the disease trajectory [5]. Overall, poor mastery of self-management skills by AYA is associated with an increased risk of treatment nonadherence and lack of follow-up, with subsequent negative consequences in terms of morbidity and mortality as well as in social, educational, and vocational outcomes [6–8]. Therefore, the provision and practice of positive self-management skills by young people with RMD is critically important.

The period of adolescence and young adulthood represents a window of opportunity to optimize and solidify positive health behaviors in order to minimize future disease-related disability [1, 9]. Unfortunately, evidence shows that many young people with RMD do not successfully transfer to adult care (i.e., they are not followed by an adult rheumatologist) and/or develop the self-management skills that are necessary to thrive in the adult setting [7, 10]. Notably, there is evidence that young people who choose to attend pediatric appointments alone may be more likely to be followed appropriately in adult centers [11]. By demonstrating independence and self-advocacy during clinic appointments, these young people may be described as "activated patients" (see Box 20.1).

Box 20.1. Patient Activation

What Is Patient Activation?

- Defined as "the degree to which the individual understands they must play an active role in managing their own health and health care, and the extent to which they feel able to fulfill that role" [12].
- Concept first operationalized through a rigorous process involving literature review, expert consensus, and patient focus groups [12].

How Can I Measure Patient Activation?

- Patient Activation Measure (PAM-13) is a widely used 13-item self-report tool to assess level of empowerment and self-management in individuals living with chronic illness [13].
- Extensively validated for use across diverse adult populations [14] and used in children as young as age 12 with chronic health conditions [15], although no studies specific for youth with RMD.
- Parent-Patient Activation Measure (P-PAM), a disease-agnostic version of PAM, is available to measure activation among the caregivers of young patients [16].

Engaging Young People in Their Healthcare

The term "patient activation" is often used interchangeably with "patient engagement." However, Hibbard and Greene (2013) clarify that patient engagement refers to a broader umbrella concept that includes activation [17]. An assessment of patient engagement in young people must take into account the individual's developmental state, knowledge base, and emerging abilities to advocate for their own needs [18].

Promoting patient engagement with their clinical care can be enabled through accessible, youth-friendly rheumatology services and supportive staff. Clinicians can encourage adolescents to gradually attend medical appointments independently and work with them to develop goals for their treatment based on their values. They can also use decision aids to help patients to make informed choices about their care (see Box 20.2). If feasible, clinics could also set up young person advisory councils to advise on other ways to support engagement based on the patient perspective.

Promoting Shared Decision-Making with AYAs and Providers

Some clinicians have been shown to deliver care that matches their own preferences rather than those of the patient [19]. This approach may lead to clinician-centered decisions and hinder patient engagement in following their disease management plan. "Shared decision-making" refers to an approach to care that enables patients and healthcare providers to make joint decisions that take into account the best available evidence of treatment options and the patient's individual values and preferences [20]. The use of decision support interventions can help to optimize this process [21, 22] (see Box 20.2).

Box 20.2 Resources to Support Clinicians in Promoting Shared Decision-Making

Pediatric Rheumatology Care and Outcomes Improvement Network (PR-COIN)

- Shared decision-making tools for youth with RMD and their caregivers
- Freely available for download on the Cincinnati Children's Hospital website: https://www.cincinnatichildrens.org/service/j/anderson-center/evidence-based-care/decision-aids

Dartmouth-Hitchcock Decision Support Toolkit

- Stepped framework for clinicians to implement patient decision-making into practice
- Freely available at the Dartmouth School of Medicine website: https://www.dartmouth-hitchcock.org/decision-making-help/professional-resources
- *SHARE Approach Curriculum Tools*
- Printable tools for clinicians to support shared decision making
- Freely available at: https://www.ahrq.gov/health-literacy/professional-training/shared-decision/tools/index.html

Supporting Self-Management in the Clinic Setting

Specific self-management strategies identified as important by adolescents with RMD included the process of "letting go" from their caregivers as essential to gaining control over their disease management [9]. Specific skills that were reported to facilitate this empowerment were:

(i) Listening to and challenging healthcare providers
(ii) Acquiring skills to communicate with doctors

(iii) Managing pain and discomfort
(iv) Managing emotions
(v) Acquiring knowledge and awareness about arthritis

Study results also emphasized the importance of providing adolescents with communication skills and assertiveness training to enhance their ability to be more active and decisive participants in their care [9].

Overall, it is recommended that all rheumatology clinics should implement strategies to support self-management of AYA. These strategies should particularly focus on supporting mastery of the specific self-management skills that AYA have identified as important. See Box 20.3 for clinical resources to measure and support self-management efforts as well as strategies for clinicians to use in daily practice.

Box 20.3 Resources to Support Clinicians in Promoting AYA Self-Management

Institute for Healthcare Improvement, Cambridge, Massachusetts

- Toolkits to aid busy clinical practices to support AYA and families in day-to-day self-management activities. For example, help AYA to understand their central role in managing their condition, collaboratively develop visit agenda and care plan, support patient goal generation, and organize follow-up support to help AYA to sustain positive behavior change.
- Link: http://www.ihi.org/resources/Pages/Tools/SelfManagementToolkitforClinicians.aspx

How Can I Measure Self-Management Skills in My Patients?

- The Self-Management Skills Assessment Guide is a 21-item tool designed to measure AYA's ability to make decisions relevant to their healthcare needs [23].

(continued)

Strategies for Clinicians to Support Self-Management in Daily Practice

- Work with AYAs to develop a plan of care based on their values.
- Discuss the pros and cons of different therapeutic strategies and listen to the AYA views.
- Encourage AYA to set personalized functional goals that are specific, measurable, achievable, realistic, and time bound (i.e., SMART). Discuss strategies for AYA to work toward their goals and support them to problem-solve solutions to potential barriers.

Digital Strategies to Address Self-Management

There are a growing number of self-management programs designed for AYA with RMD including a movement toward using digital technologies such as web-based interventions and mobile apps to reduce care disparities related to geographical, financial, and health literacy barriers [24–26]. An advantage of these digitally mediated programs is that they can enable nonspecialists and peers to be trained to provide self-management support, thereby improving accessibility for AYAs living in remote and rural areas [27, 28].

Teens Taking Charge: Managing Arthritis Online

Stinson et al. developed a web-based self-management program for adolescents with JIA using a phased approach including a scoping review and qualitative needs assessment [27]. A pilot randomized control trial was then completed with the intervention (Teens Taking Charge website and weekly health coach calls) and attention control (educational websites and weekly control calls) [27]. Participants in the intervention group demonstrated significant improvements in JIA knowledge and exercise adherence as well as a reduction in pain intensity compared to the control group. Both groups exhibited high compliance with weekly calls (91% and 90% for intervention and control groups, respectively).

A subsequent full-scale randomized controlled trial (N = 333) demonstrated overall reductions in pain intensity ($p = .02$) and pain interference ($p = .007$) for intervention group participants compared with those in the education-control group. Significant improvements were also observed for health-related quality of life related to problems with pain ($p = .02$) and problems with daily activities ($p = .01$) among intervention participants. Lastly, significant effects were observed over time ($P = .008$) with the intervention group demonstrating improved health-related quality of life by 12 months compared with education control.

The Teens Taking Charge Arthritis program is now freely available: https://teens.aboutkidshealth.ca/jiateenhub.

The website is divided into 12 interactive modules and covers topics such as managing symptoms and emotions, relaxation, physical therapies, communication with doctors and teachers, lifestyle issues such as nutrition and sexuality, and self-advocacy skills. Two parent modules are designed to help caregivers to encourage self-management skills in their children and learn how to "let go" control over disease management. Individual modules can be "prescribed" to young people and families based on identified clinical need.

iPeer2Peer: A Skype-Based Peer Mentoring Program for Youth with JIA

Peer support interventions have been reported to improve behavioral and emotional symptoms of young people [29]. iPeer2Peer is a peer-mentorship program for youth that provides modeling and reinforcement by older peers. Participants are matched with a trained peer mentor with the same condition, and together they complete ten Skype-based mentoring sessions over an 8-week period [30]. In a waitlist pilot randomized controlled trial, trained peer mentors with arthritis (aged 16–25 years) were matched to participants (12–18 years) and randomized to the intervention group to provide peer support and education for effective self-management of arthritis. Participants reported high program satisfaction, and all reported that they would recommend it to their peers. Participants who completed the iPeer2Peer program demonstrated improvements in their perceived ability to manage JIA ($p < 0.04$), compared to controls [30]. The iPeer2Peer program has been licensed to the Arthritis Foundation (http://blog.arthritis.org/juvenile-arthritis/arthritis-foundation-pilot-peer-mentorship-program-juvenile-arthritis/). Young people who wish to become mentees or mentors in the iPeer2Peer program can apply through the Arthritis Foundation.

Conclusion

In summary, the development and practice of self-management skills are integral to the successful management of RMD during adolescence and young adulthood. This developmental period represents a critical window of opportunity to introduce and establish positive self-management behaviors in order to promote continued practice of healthy self-management strategies as adults and minimize future disease-related disability. Clinicians have an important role to play in supporting AYA with RMD in health and disease self-management and should consider taking advantage of existing resources to support these efforts.

Key Management Points

1. Develop an early therapeutic alliance with AYA and their families in order to support them to develop into independent, functioning adults.
2. Emphasize the gradual shift in responsibility from you (the clinician) to the parent, and ultimately to the AYA.
3. As the AYA ages, encourage them to actively participate in different aspects of their disease management (e.g., setting up appointments, taking responsibility for pre-

(continued)

scription renewals, learning to self-administer injections, generating a list of questions for discussion at appointments).
4. Remember that the roles of AYA, families, and the healthcare team should change over time with the clinician eventually moving into a consultant role and the young person eventually becoming the primary supervisor for their own health.
5. Set clear expectations with AYAs regarding responsibility for specific disease management activities.

Acknowledgments Thank you to Cleo Davies Chalmers (Research Student, The Hospital for Sick Children, Toronto, Ontario) for assisting with the literature search for this chapter and drafting the abstract. Thank you to Fabiah Mahmood (Nursing Research Intern, The Hospital for Sick Children, Toronto, Ontario) for assisting with the updated literature search.

References

1. Modi AC, Pai AL, Hommel KA, Hood KK, Cortina S, Hilliard ME, et al. Pediatric self-management: a framework for research, practice, and policy. Pediatrics. 2012;129(2):e473–85.
2. Arnett JJ. Emerging adulthood: what is it, and what is it good for? Child Dev Perspect. 2007;1(2):68–73.
3. Jastrowski Mano KE, Beckmann EA, Fussner LM, Kashikar-Zuck S. Executive functioning in adolescents with chronic musculoskeletal pain. Children (Basel). 2020;7(12):273. https://doi.org/10.3390/children7120273.
4. Packham JC, Hall MA. Long-term follow-up of 246 adults with juvenile idiopathic arthritis: functional outcome. Rheumatology (Oxford). 2002;41(12):1428–35.
5. Lawson EF, Hersh AO, Applebaum MA, Yelin EH, Okumura MJ, von Scheven E. Self-management skills in adolescents with chronic rheumatic disease: a cross-sectional survey. Pediatr Rheumatol Online J. 2011;9(1):35.
6. McDonagh JE. Transition of care from paediatric to adult rheumatology. Arch Dis Child. 2007;92(9):802–7.

7. Hazel E, Zhang X, Duffy CM, Campillo S. High rates of unsuccessful transfer to adult care among young adults with juvenile idiopathic arthritis. Pediatr Rheumatol Online J. 2010;8:2.
8. de Oliveira RJ, Kishimoto ST, de Souza DP, Fernandes PT, Marini R, Appenzeller S. The importance of transition from pediatric to adult rheumatology care in juvenile idiopathic arthritis. Expert Rev Clin Immunol. 2021;17(2):155–61. https://doi.org/10.1080/1744666X.2020.1865157.
9. Stinson JN, Toomey PC, Stevens BJ, Kagan S, Duffy CM, Huber A, et al. Asking the experts: exploring the self-management needs of adolescents with arthritis. Arthritis Rheum. 2008;59(1):65–72.
10. Clemente D, Leon L, Foster H, Carmona L, Minden K. Transitional care for rheumatic conditions in Europe: current clinical practice and available resources. Pediatr Rheumatol Online J. 2017;15(1):49.
11. Reid GJ, Irvine MJ, McCrindle BW, Sananes R, Ritvo PG, Siu SC, et al. Prevalence and correlates of successful transfer from pediatric to adult health care among a cohort of young adults with complex congenital heart defects. Pediatrics. 2004;113(3 Pt 1):e197–205.
12. Hibbard JH, Mahoney E. Toward a theory of patient and consumer activation. Patient Educ Couns. 2010;78(3):377–81.
13. Hibbard JH, Stockard J, Mahoney ER, Tusler M. Development of the Patient Activation Measure (PAM): conceptualizing and measuring activation in patients and consumers. Health Serv Res. 2004;39(4 Pt 1):1005–26.
14. Greene J, Hibbard JH, Sacks R, Overton V, Parrotta CD. When patient activation levels change, health outcomes and costs change, too. Health Aff (Millwood). 2015;34(3):431–7.
15. Huang JS, Terrones L, Tompane T, Dillon L, Pian M, Gottschalk M, et al. Preparing adolescents with chronic disease for transition to adult care: a technology program. Pediatrics. 2014;133(6):e1639–46.
16. Pennarola BW, Rodday AM, Mayer DK, Ratichek SJ, Davies SM, Syrjala KL, et al. Factors associated with parental activation in pediatric hematopoietic stem cell transplant. Med Care Res Rev. 2012;69(2):194–214.
17. Hibbard JH, Greene J. What the evidence shows about patient activation: better health outcomes and care experiences; fewer data on costs. Health Aff (Millwood). 2013;32(2):207–14.
18. Howland S, Fisher K. Looking through the patient lens—improving best practice for young people with juvenile idiopathic arthritis transitioning into adult care. Springerplus. 2015;4:111.
19. Lipstein EA, Brinkman WB, Sage J, Lannon CM, Morgan DE. Understanding treatment decision making in juvenile idiopathic arthritis: a qualitative assessment. Pediatr Rheumatol Online J. 2013;11(1):34.
20. Makoul G, Clayman ML. An integrative model of shared decision making in medical encounters. Patient Educ Couns. 2006;60(3):301–12.

21. Stacey D, Légaré F, Lewis K, Barry MJ, Bennett CL, Eden KB, et al. Decision aids for people facing health treatment or screening decisions. Cochrane Database Syst Rev. 2017;12(4):CD001431.
22. Stacey D, Kryworuchko J, Bennett C, Murray MA, Mullan S, Légaré F. Decision coaching to prepare patients for making health decisions: a systematic review of decision coaching in trials of patient decision AIDS. Med Decis Mak. 2012;32(3):E22–33.
23. Williams T, Sherman E, Mah JK, Blackman M, Latter J, Mohammed I, et al. Measurement of medical self-management and transition readiness among Canadian adolescents with special health care needs. Int J Child Adolesc Health. 2010;3:1–9.
24. Macea DD, Gajos K, Daglia Calil YA, Fregni F. The efficacy of web-based cognitive behavioral interventions for chronic pain: a systematic review and meta-analysis. J Pain. 2010;11(10):917–29.
25. Lalloo C, Jibb LA, Rivera J, Agarwal A, Stinson JN. "There's a pain app for that": review of patient-targeted smartphone applications for pain management. Clin J Pain. 2015;31(6):557–63.
26. Armbrust W, Bos JJFJ, Cappon J, van Rossum MAJJ, Sauer PJJ, Wulffraat N, et al. Design and acceptance of Rheumates@Work, a combined internet-based and in person instruction model, an interactive, educational, and cognitive behavioral program for children with juvenile idiopathic arthritis. Pediatr Rheumatol Online J. 2015;13:31.
27. Stinson JN, McGrath PJ, Hodnett ED, Feldman BM, Duffy CM, Huber AM, et al. An internet-based self-management program with telephone support for adolescents with arthritis: a pilot randomized controlled trial. J Rheumatol. 2010;37(9):1944–52.
28. Connelly M, Lee RR. Technology to assess and treat pain in pediatric rheumatology. Rheum Dis Clin N Am. 2022;48(1):31–50. https://doi.org/10.1016/j.rdc.2021.09.004.
29. Ahola Kohut S, Stinson J, van Wyk M, Giosa L, Luca S. Systematic review of peer support interventions for adolescents with chronic illness. Int J Child Adolesc Health. 2014;7:183.
30. Stinson J, Ahola Kohut S, Forgeron P, Amaria K, Bell M, Kaufman M, et al. The iPeer2Peer program: a pilot randomized controlled trial in adolescents with juvenile idiopathic arthritis. Pediatr Rheumatol Online J. 2016;14(1):48.

21 Can't Do or Won't Do? Adherence in Adolescent and Young Adult Rheumatology

Lauren Huckerby, Janet E. McDonagh, and Nicola J. Gray

L. Huckerby (✉)
Department of Paediatric and Adolescent Rheumatology, Alder Hey Children's Hospital, Alder Hey Children's NHS Foundation Trust, Liverpool, UK

Department of Paediatric and Adolescent Rheumatology, Royal Manchester Children's Hospital, Manchester University NHS Foundation Trust, Manchester, UK
e-mail: l.huckerby@nhs.net

J. E. McDonagh
Arthritis Research UK Centre for Epidemiology, Centre for Musculoskeletal Research, University of Manchester, Manchester, UK

NIHR Manchester Biomedical Research Centre, Manchester University NHS Foundation Trust, Manchester, UK

Manchester Academic Health Science Centre, Manchester, UK
e-mail: janet.mcdonagh@manchester.ac.uk

N. J. Gray
Department of Pharmacy, University of Huddersfield, Huddersfield, UK
e-mail: N.J.Gray@hud.ac.uk

C. Ciurtin, J. Hackett (eds.), *Adolescent and Young Adult Rheumatology In Clinical Practice*, In Clinical Practice,
https://doi.org/10.1007/978-3-031-82102-8_21

Introduction

It is important to adolescents and young adults (AYA) with childhood onset RMD, that they learn to manage their own condition [1] (see Chap. 20). This is also fundamental to successful transitional care (see Chap. 23). Although the terminology in this area is continually debated, the term adherence will be used in this chapter as unlike concordance, it can be measured and lacks the implied passivity of the term compliance (Table 21.1). Adherence is not just relevant to medication, but to self-management activities like blood test monitoring, hospital appointments, therapy exercises and healthy lifestyle advice. Adherence may also vary according to the task, e.g. young people may take medicines but not do blood tests, or may attend clinics but not take their medicines. Adherence is linked to better health outcomes, but it can be a challenging area for young people, family and professionals alike.

Table 21.1 Terms and definitions [2]

Terms	Definitions
Compliance	The extent to which the patient's behaviour matches the prescriber's recommendations Implies lack of engagement, or passivity of the patient; therefore, other terms preferred
Concordance	*The active process* by which the patient and prescriber form a therapeutic contract. Cannot be measured, unlike adherence and compliance
Adherence	The extent to which the patient's behaviour matches agreed recommendations from the prescriber

Types of Nonadherence

Nonadherence can be divided into two types—unintentional and intentional. This division is somewhat simplistic as there is also likely to be overlap between the two types, e.g. forgetfulness can potentially be both intentional and unintentional. It is important to distinguish between these, however, as the strategies to address them will differ (Table 21.2).

When considering risk factors for nonadherence, it is important to consider what aspects can be changed and which aspects will be more challenging to change, but professionals still need to be aware of them (Table 21.3, acknowledging Professor Rachel Elliott, University of Manchester).

Table 21.2 Types of nonadherence

Unintentional nonadherence ("can't do") may occur because of practical or cognitive difficulties in taking medications, e.g.:
Forgetfulness
Problems with dexterity, e.g. getting tabs out of blister packs, administering injections
Difficulties carrying/taking medicines in certain settings, e.g. during school day, privacy
Complexity of regimes
Poor understanding of—and access to—the repeat prescription/refill system
Poor understanding of how to access an emergency supply
Ability to pay for prescriptions
Intentional nonadherence ("won't do") to medication may be the result of:
A lack of information about the advantages and disadvantages of the treatment
When the benefits of treatment are not obviously apparent
The psychological adaptation required to see oneself as in need of treatment
Fear of visible side effects
Unwilling to disclose to others

Table 21.3 Risk factors for nonadherence and ability to change

Things we can't change, but must be aware of:	Things that we might be able to change:
Milder illness Having the illness for a long time Having side effects Problems with relationship with caregivers No stable family structure One adult only in the house No family routine Problems with school access to medicines	Forgetting Caregivers worrying about side effects Not knowing about the illness and medicines Not sure whether the medicine works/is needed Not feeling in control or able to change things Not feeling "normal" or looking forward to the future Number of medicines/doses per day Not convenient or pleasant to use Inability to use medicines, e.g. size of asthma inhaler device Poor relationship with the doctor

Challenges to Adherence for Young People with Rheumatic Disease

The frequently reported barriers to adherence are not unique to specific diseases, with the top five in recent reviews being physical well-being, forgetting by coincidence, strive for normality, relationship with peers and relationship with caregivers [3, 4]. Examples of these challenges are detailed in Table 21.4.

As with all aspects of healthcare for young people, acknowledging the impact of adolescent and young adult development on adherence is imperative (see Chaps. 1, 2, and 3). Of particular relevance is the stage of cognitive development.

Formal operational thinking (or abstract thought) develops in early to mid-adolescence but can be delayed by chronic illness. Even in young adulthood, young people may have logical competencies similar to adults but will exhibit differences in decision and risk-taking due to the different social and emotional factors at this life stage (see Chap. 2). Moreover, even in those young people who have moved into abstract thought, a traumatic event—such as the diagnosis of a long-term condition in

Table 21.4 Challenges to adherence for young people with rheumatic disease

AYA development
Cognitive
Psychological
Social development
Medicine/therapy
Dose regimes, e.g. frequent daily doses or infrequent dosing e.g. weekly
Delay of therapeutic effect, e.g. methotrexate
Have to take when well and in remission, e.g. methotrexate and biologics
Reminder of ill health
Side effects—Nausea (including anticipatory)
Cosmetic issues, e.g. steroid side effects
Complexity of regimen
Need for planning, e.g. parenteral administration
Organisation
Taste
Pill size
Treatment perceptions—Understanding of risk benefit [if risk outweighs benefit, then there is risk of nonadherence]
Interference with normal activities—e.g. methotrexate and alcohol
Privacy issues for administration
System barriers including supply disruption, cost and complex repeat prescription systems
The condition
Chronic nature
Relapsing nature
Unpredictability of flares, symptoms
Relative visibility of condition
Acceptance of condition (risk if in denial)
Interference of activities particularly peer and leisure activities

adolescence—could make them revert to concrete thought (see Chap. 1). Cognitive developmental stage has therefore an impact on adherence due to a reduced ability to plan and prepare using abstract concepts. For example, using future motivators ("if you don't take your etanercept, you will end up with joint damage") with a concrete thinker is likely to prove less effective when trying to improve adherence than the preferable immediate motivators ("if you don't take your etanercept, you are unlikely to be able to play football this summer"). This is particularly pertinent when there is a delay before improvement is seen following commencement of medication, and/or when medication with significant side effects has to be continued, even when the actual disease is in remission, as is the case with methotrexate ("I forgot to take my methotrexate and my arthritis was fine so I'm not going to take it anymore").

Psychological development during adolescence encompasses the development of a sense of self, and during mid-adolescence, this is often expressed as a sense of being invulnerable or "bulletproof"—"I know all the risks Doctor, but it won't happen to me." During adolescence, young people will strive for normality, and young people with rheumatic disease are no different. If therapeutic regimens interfere with their normal activities, then there is a risk to adherence. The goal of medicine-taking in rheumatic disease should be to maximise both physical and emotional wellbeing; addressing the physical symptoms should reduce anxiety and low mood about their impact [5].

Social development may similarly be impacted if such regimens interfere with relationships with peers, siblings and/or caregivers. During adolescence there is a gradual increase in peer influence that may come into conflict with parental influence. Likewise, there is a shift in responsibility for health management as young people grow up and become more autonomous in looking after their own health and, in the case of young people with rheumatic disease, their treatment. This can prove a challenging time for all concerned—the young person and their caregivers, as well as the health professional—and needs to be negotiated carefully and sensitively (see Chap. 4). When considering the social context of young people with rheumatic disease, disclosure of their condition can be challenging, particularly to peers. Nondisclosure could be a marker of nonadherence as the young person may be unable or unwilling to create the private space needed during school, college or other work to manage their therapies.

In addition to taking the stage of adolescent-young adult development into consideration, coexisting learning difficulties/disability/cognitive impairment also need to be acknowledged. It is important to realise that although some of these young people may never be truly independent in self-managing their condition, they may be able to do certain components with appropriate supervision. This should be explored with both the young person and their caregivers if age and developmentally appropriate. Strategies to increase independence in medicine-taking, particularly when young people have learning challenges, require sufficient time in the consultation to elicit their medicine-related concerns and those of their carers. Young people with learning challenges may also be taking psychotropic medicines; joint working across medical teams may improve their holistic care.

In addition to AYA development, the actual medicine/therapy and the rheumatic condition can present particular challenges to young people, examples of which are listed in Table 21.4.

Assessment of Adherence

Assessment of adherence is a core component of reviews with young people, particularly once a management plan is in place after diagnosis. As with all encounters with young people, assessment of what stage of development (see Chaps. 1, 2, and 3) they are at is vital, whilst acknowledging the potential for delay and regression in chronic illnesses. An underlying learning disability and/or secondary cognitive impairment may also be present—the latter may occur in such conditions as SLE (see Chap. 8).

The most important task for the health professional is to normalise nonadherence. So rather than ask "Do you take your meds regularly?", it is preferable to ask, "When was the last time you forgot?" Questions to help understand the context of their lives are important: "How do you manage to fit taking your medicine into a typical day?" "What makes it difficult to take your meds?" Using the HEEADSSS approach [6] (see Chap. 4) is useful in this regard. As well as being a strategy to engage young people, it can help identify risk as well as resilient/protective factors and furthermore provide information which will assist the formulation of adherence-improving strategies.

Once nonadherence is identified, it is important to assess their motivation to change, if any. Motivational interviewing techniques (see Chap. 4) are extremely useful in the AYA rheumatology clinics [7–9], as well as addressing resistance and ambivalence to change; they also emphasise self-responsibility in changing or modifying one's behaviour. Trigger questions to assess motivation to change are detailed in Table 21.5. Once gathered, subsequent questioning can include *"what will it take to move you from a 5 to a 7 in confidence?"* and over time at subsequent reviews "*are you still at a 5/10 in confidence?"*

Table 21.5 Trigger questions to assess motivation to change

Trigger question	Exemplar responses with strategies	
"*On a scale of 0–10,*	Example A	Example B
How much of a **priority** is it that you *start to take your meds regularly?*	10	7
How **important** is it that you *start taking your meds regularly?*	10	4
How **confident** are you that you could succeed "*in taking your meds regularly*?"	5	10
Possible strategies	No need to address knowledge but rather address why lacking in confidence; use confidence building techniques	Assess their knowledge of the medication including risk and benefit and also what is of greater priority

Strategies for Optimising Adherence

As previously suggested, information collected during HEEADSSS screening [6] (see Chaps. 3 and 4) is useful in the development of AYA-centred strategies with the young person in question, taking into account the life and developmental context of the AYA. Examples of such strategies are detailed in Table 21.6.

Table 21.6 Strategies for optimising adherence

Education—Accurate and individualised
Knowledge includes:
Diagnosis and its acceptance
Honest explanations
Anticipation of common side effects, and provision of advice about what to do if these happen
Risk/benefit
Treatment goals
Future effects on fertility
What if I miss it?
What if I can't take it?
Clear instructions about dosing—Check understanding, including that of caregiver
Address impact on activities—Vocational, social, leisure, etc.
Address beliefs—This includes the priority that young people assign to both the positive and negative effects of their therapy
Address disclosure issues
Therapeutic relationship
Honesty
Attention to their lived experience
Enable venting of their thoughts, beliefs and feelings, regarding therapy, hospital attendance, blood monitoring, etc.
Encourage their own questions
Encourage problem-solving
Participatory
Support lone consulting, i.e. young person seen independently of caregiver for part/all of visit

(continued)

Table 21.6 (continued)

Behaviours
Positive reinforcement
Link with daily routines
Need to use immediate more than future motivators, particularly if at concrete stage of cognitive development
Cueing e.g. calendar to support monitoring, post-it notes
Aids e.g. mHealth interventions, mobile app, text reminders [4, 10–12], dosette boxes
Time out, e.g. drug holiday
Simplify regime
Any regimen should be built around the life context of the AYA [13], acknowledging that this is likely to change as the young person grows up—Particularly at the points of transition whether health, social or vocational
Ideally once or twice daily regimes
Try to avoid dosing during school/college/university/work hours when possible
Encourage development of problem-solving skills (e.g. they work out a way to get into a dosing routine and remember each dose)
Ensure uninterrupted supplies
Support from others
(i) Parent/ caregiver
Act as operational and long-term memory
Tend to collect prescriptions on the young person's behalf
Move from shared to self-management during adolescent development (see Chap. 20)
Likely to still be involved to some degree in young adulthood
(ii) school, e.g. teachers, school nurse, university disability support services, etc.
(iii) peers—Requires discussion with young person as this involvement will vary according to developmental stage and disclosure issues
(iv) health professionals
All members of the rheumatology multidisciplinary team
Pharmacists—Hospital and community pharmacists are an underused resource in the rheumatology multidisciplinary team. In particular, a youth-friendly community pharmacist should be identified during adolescence as a useful and easily accessible resource for the young person as they become more autonomous regarding their medicine management [14]

(continued)

Table 21.6 (continued)

General practitioner—Of increasing importance as the young person becomes more autonomous and particularly at the time of transfer to adult rheumatology care
(v) Health care system [15] (See Chap. 20)
System changes such as scheduling of appointments outside of school/college hours, improved continuity of care
(vi) Credible online resources

Key Management Points

1. Education and skills training in adherence to therapy and healthcare is core to AYA rheumatology service provision.
2. Adherence is not just about taking medication but also encompasses other therapies and attendance at appointments.
3. Nonadherence should not be perceived as always intentional on the part of the young person.
4. Some risk factors for nonadherence are more amenable to change than others.
5. During adolescence and young adulthood, young people with rheumatic disease face particular challenges in adhering to therapies and care provision.
6. Health professionals require developmentally appropriate communication skills and a range of strategies to engage and motivate young people to optimise adherence during adolescence and young adulthood.

References

1. Tong A, Jones J, Craig JC, Singh-Grewal D. Children's experiences of living with juvenile idiopathic arthritis: a thematic synthesis of qualitative studies. Arthritis Care Res (Hoboken). 2012;64(9):1392–404.
2. Horne R, Weinman J, Barber N, Elliott R, Morgan M, Cribb A. Concordance, adherence and compliance in medicine taking: report for the national co-ordinating centre for NHS service delivery and organisation R & D (NCCSDO). London: NCCSDO; 2005.

3. Hanghøj S, Boisen KA. Self-reported barriers to medication adherence among chronically ill adolescents: a systematic review. J Adolesc Health. 2014;54(2):121–38.
4. Rohan JM, Winter MA. Ethical considerations in pediatric chronic illness: the relationship between psychological factors, treatment adherence, and health outcomes. Paediatr Respir Rev. 2021;39:48–53. https://doi.org/10.1016/j.prrv.2021.05.008.
5. Gray NJ, Wood DM. The role of medication in supporting emotional wellbeing in young people with long-term needs. Healthcare (Basel). 2017;5(4) pii: E84 https://doi.org/10.3390/healthcare5040084.
6. Doukrou M, Segal TY. Fifteen-minute consultation: communicating with young people -how to use HEEADSSS, a psychosocial interview for adolescents. Arch Dis Child Educ Pract Ed. 2018;103(1):15–9.
7. Naar-King S, Suarez M. Motivational interviewing with adolescents and young adults. New York: Guildford Press; 2011.
8. Motivational interviewing network of trainers. http://www.motivationalinterviewing.org/. Last accessed 2 Feb 2018.
9. Schaefer MR, Kavookjian J. The impact of motivational interviewing on adherence and symptom severity in adolescents and young adults with chronic illness: a systematic review. Patient Educ Couns. 2017;100(12):2190–9. https://doi.org/10.1016/j.pec.2017.05.037.
10. Slater H, Campbell JM, Stinson JN, Burley MM, Briggs AM. End user and implementer experiences of mHealth technologies for noncommunicable chronic disease management in young adults: systematic review. J Med Internet Res. 2017;19(12):e406.
11. Stinson J, Ahola Kohut S, Forgeron P, Amaria K, Bell M, Kaufman M, Luca N, Luca S, Harris L, Victor C, Spiegel L. The iPeer2Peer program: a pilot randomized controlled trial in adolescents with juvenile idiopathic arthritis. Pediatr Rheumatol Online J. 2016;14(1):48.
12. Santo K, Richtering SS, Chalmers J, Thiagalingam A, Chow CK, Redfern J. Mobile phone apps to improve medication adherence: a systematic stepwise process to identify high-quality apps. JMIR Mhealth Uhealth. 2016;4(4):e132.
13. Gray NJ, Christie D, Coyne I, Fonseca H, Philippe CD, Sawyer SM, Tuchman LK, Versnel J. The use of medication by adolescents and young adults: a position paper of the society for adolescent health and medicine. J Adolesc Health. 2017;61:396–9.
14. Gray N, Shaw KL, Smith FJ, Burton J, Prescott J, Roberts R, Terry D, McDonagh JE. The role of the pharmacist in the care of young people with chronic illness. J Adolesc Health. 2017;60(2):219–25.
15. Rapley T, Farre A, Parr JR, Wood VJ, Reape D, Dovey-Pearce G, McDonagh J, Transition Collaborative Group. Can we normalise developmentally appropriate health care for young people in UK hospital settings? An ethnographic study. BMJ Open. 2019;9(9):e029107. https://doi.org/10.1136/bmjopen-2019-029107.

22 Developmentally Appropriate and Youth-Friendly Rheumatology Services

Albert Farre, Kerry Jobling, and Martin Lee

Introduction

Adolescence and young adulthood is a major developmental stage covering a wide age range (10–24 years) and several key developmental stages—early, mid- and late adolescence and emerging adulthood. Adolescence and young adulthood also encompasses major life transitions such as entering secondary education, puberty, finishing mandatory education, moving away from home, moving into higher education or the workplace, making friends beyond the family, engaging in romantic relationships, the development of greater autonomy and independence in

A. Farre (✉)
School of Health Sciences, University of Dundee, Dundee, UK
e-mail: a.farre@dundee.ac.uk

K. Jobling
Royal Victoria Infirmary, Newcastle upon Tyne, UK
e-mail: kerry.jobling@nuth.nhs.uk

M. Lee
Mediclinic Parkview, Dubai, United Arab Emirates

Mohammed Bin Rashid University, Dubai, United Arab Emirates
e-mail: martinlee@doctors.org.uk

C. Ciurtin, J. Hackett (eds.), *Adolescent and Young Adult Rheumatology In Clinical Practice*, In Clinical Practice,
https://doi.org/10.1007/978-3-031-82102-8_22

addition to moving from child- to adult-centred services including health (see Chaps. 1, 2, 3, 4, 5, and 23). These factors add complexity to the requirements that AYA with long-term conditions have of a health service and are a key reason why any AYA service, whether located in adult or paediatric services, should recognise AYA as a distinct patient group with unique healthcare and psychosocial needs. Furthermore, these needs change as the young people move through adolescence and young adulthood, thus requiring a health service which can be responsive to these changes.

Why Is It Important that Rheumatology Services Are Both Developmentally Appropriate and Youth-Friendly?

Developmentally appropriate and youth-friendly healthcare are two complementary approaches that play a pivotal role in ensuring that rheumatology services can address the unique needs of AYA living with rheumatic diseases. Tailoring healthcare services to meet the developmental, emotional, physical, and social needs of this demographic as well as their preferences is vital for fostering a positive healthcare experience for AYA and for achieving better health outcomes.

The concept of *youth-friendly healthcare* is associated with practical guidance and frameworks to assess and improve the quality and experiences of AYA services using standards, indicators and criteria informed by AYA perspectives [1]. Examples of this can be found in many countries as well as globally, e.g. the World Health Organization (WHO) proposed global standards for quality healthcare services for adolescents [2] and, in England, the Department of Health (DOH) published the recently revised 'You're Welcome' criteria for youth-friendly services [3].

The concept of *developmentally appropriate healthcare*, in contrast to the service-focussed nature of youth-friendly healthcare, addresses the clinical approach required to meet the changing developmental needs of AYA [4, 5]. AYA undergo distinct developmental stages, each with its unique challenges and milestones comprising biological, psychological, social, and educational/vocational aspects. However, chronological age is recognised to be a poor indicator of developmental status, particularly in the context of a long-term health condition [6], thus developmentally appropriate healthcare focuses on biopsychosocial development (rather than chronological age) as a defining characteristic of healthcare delivery. A developmentally appropriate approach recognises these stages and aspects of development and adapts healthcare interventions accordingly [7–9] based on a biopsychosocial approach to clinical interactions [10]. This should include a comprehensive (i.e. physical and psychosocial) evaluation in an atmosphere of trust and confidentiality, considering developmentally appropriate communication, education materials and involvement of parents and caregivers.

Therefore, the different emphases of youth-friendly and developmentally appropriate healthcare can be combined to provide health services that are meaningful and consistent from both the AYA and provider perspectives. This echoes the WHO call for policy makers to move from adolescent-friendly service delivery towards systems that can respond to the health and developmental needs of adolescents [11].

Characteristics of Developmentally Appropriate and Youth-Friendly Services

In 2013, Ambresin et al. [1] published a systematic review of youth-friendly healthcare based upon the literature from young people's perspectives. This review identified eight core indicators of a youth-friendly service:

1. Accessibility
2. Staff attitude
3. Communication
4. Medical competency
5. Guideline-driven care
6. Age-appropriate environment
7. Involvement in healthcare
8. Health outcomes

Table 22.1 Core indicators of a youth-friendly service from the AYA's perspective [1] and some examples of how to translate them into practice

Indicator	Example
Accessibility	Is the location of the healthcare service accessible and affordable for young people?
Staff attitude	Are staff respectful, supportive, honest, trustworthy, friendly and caring towards young people?
Communication	Do staff provide clear, age-appropriate information to young people? Do staff engage in active listening?
Medical competency	Are staff competent at medical procedures?
Guideline-driven care	Do staff provide comprehensive, guideline-driven care that respects the confidentiality and autonomy of young people?
Age-appropriate environment	Are appointment times flexible? Are waiting times reasonable? Do young people have access to separate physical space with age-appropriate health information?
Involvement in healthcare	Are young people actively involved in their healthcare?
Health outcomes	Is pain management and quality of life considered?

Table 22.1 provides some examples of how the eight indicators can be translated into practice.

Further work has progressed in this area to not just consider youth friendliness in service delivery but also the impact of biopsychosocial development. The focus then becomes how developmentally appropriate a service (and indeed the system it exists in) might be [5, 12]. Five conceptual dimensions of such care as perceived by practitioners have been identified [5] which potentially provide a framework for developmentally appropriate healthcare provision:

1. Holistic care addressing biological, psychological, and social development
2. Acknowledgement of AYA as distinct from children and older adults
3. Adjustment of care as the AYA develops
4. Empowering the AYA by integrating health education and health promotion into their care
5. Interdisciplinary and inter-organisational work

These in turn echo the core indicators of youth-friendly services as perceived by AYA themselves (Table 22.1) thus facilitating the adoption of a combined approach to ensure that health services are meaningful and consistent from both the AYA and practitioner perspectives.

Table 22.2 provides some examples of how the five conceptual dimensions of developmentally appropriate healthcare can be translated into practice.

Table 22.2 Examples of how the five conceptual dimensions of developmentally appropriate healthcare can be translated into practice [7]

Conceptual dimensions	Examples
1. Holistic care addressing biopsychosocial development	• Routine biopsychosocial developmental assessment and approach to the AYA adjusted accordingly. • Use of psychosocial screening tools such as the HEEADSSS psychosocial interview as a routine component of clinical consultations with AYA.
2. Acknowledgement of AYA as distinct from children and older adults	Acknowledgement of age and developmental stage-specific issues and how these may change during adolescence and young adulthood: • Confidentiality and rights • Privacy issues • Peer support • Accessible services (e.g., after school/ college) • Dedicated clinics/space • Longer appointment times to enable time to see young person independently of parents • Information and resources
3. Adjustment of care as the AYA develops	Flexibility in approach and acknowledgement of regression during active phases in relapsing conditions: • Change in communication style with respect to cognitive development • Impact of physical growth and pubertal stage on condition and therapy

(continued)

Table 22.2 (continued)

Conceptual dimensions	Examples
4. Empowering the AYA by integrating health education and health promotion into their care	• Support for the young person and parent as they move from shared to self-management of health (within their individual capacity). This includes knowledge and skill development in both health and disease management as well as health care utilisation skills • Information and resources
5. Interdisciplinary and inter-organisational work	• Effective team working • Staff training in adolescent health • AYA responsive staff and services • AYA-specific issues addressed in policies and guidelines; • Support of key interfaces with education and vocational agencies, social care, youth work reflecting holistic approach to care • Coordination/continuity/consistency across roles, professionals and shifts • Coordination/continuity/consistency throughout a patient's journey through the healthcare system

In addition to reports of AYA rheumatology services [13], several toolkits have been developed to assist practitioners in the promotion of the implementation of such developmentally appropriate and youth-friendly health services whether it be at the consultation level or at an organisational or institutional level [3, 14, 15].

Implementing Developmentally Appropriate and Youth-Friendly Services

Young people with rheumatic musculoskeletal disease (RMD) should have access to a high-quality developmentally appropriate healthcare service throughout adolescence and young adulthood (10–24 years of age). This is a key stage of life as many health-promoting and self-management behaviours are becoming established. This healthcare should be structured around the principles and indicators discussed above. The service should address not only management of the young person's RMD but also psychological, sexual, social and educational/vocational aspects of their care.

At the consultation level, many professionals involved in AYA care use psychosocial screening tools such as the HEEADSSS assessment tool [16] (see Chap. 4) to engage young people and identify both health-risk behaviours and resilience factors in AYA. This has been further adapted into a smartphone app for trainees [17] and a further iteration of the screening tool—THRxEADSSS—to cover transitional issues [18] (developmentally appropriate approaches to engaging with young people in clinical consultations, including the importance of assuring confidentiality, are detailed in Chap. 4).

At the wider organisational level, it is important that AYA learn to navigate the health system beyond the rheumatology clinic, and learning which service to access and when and how is core to the knowledge and skills framework underpinning a developmentally appropriate and youth-friendly rheumatology AYA service. Therefore, it is important to ensure that developmentally appropriate and youth-friendly care is supported at organisational level, and that key features of such care remain consistent across the multiple services that AYA often require for their care. Research has shown that putting in place an organisation-wide strategy or policy, together with an associated package of in-house training for clinicians and service leads, offers the greatest potential for developmentally appropriate and youth-friendly services to become embedded in routine practice [12].

The Importance of Training Healthcare Professionals in AYA Care

In order to run a successful developmentally appropriate and youth-friendly rheumatology service, it is vital that all members of the healthcare team involved in that service should be interested, engaged and adequately qualified [19].

Healthcare professionals should be aware of how RMD present in childhood and how they are managed, as well as the impact of adolescence and young adulthood development itself on RMD and vice versa. Increasing knowledge about AYA development offers significant opportunities for service improvement [12]. Services underpinned by developmentally appropriate healthcare have been reported internationally as a potential key mechanism to improve health outcomes for AYA [20, 21] and pave the way for adolescent-responsive healthcare systems [11].

Training in communication skills specific for AYA care is essential as the ability to discuss areas of health such as emotional well-being, social, sexuality and reproductive health issues with AYA is necessary (see Chap. 4). Healthcare professionals are required to be respectful, supporting and caring towards AYAs as well as be willing to actively involve AYA themselves in decisions about their healthcare. Training programmes and curricula are available in adolescent care that cover some of these specific issues [22, 23, 24].

Summary

As AYA grow up, they seek active involvement and decision-making opportunities in their healthcare and condition management [1, 9, 25, 26, 27]. They report a need to "strive for normality" and a desire for respect and involvement in their own healthcare [25]. Young people feel well looked after in a context that acknowledges their lived experience [26, 27] and provides them with guidance to make their own healthcare-related choices.

Developmentally appropriate and youth-friendly rheumatology services for AYA should recognise AYA as a unique patient group, treating them holistically within their wider psychosocial context, taking into account the life changes and transitions that shape this stage of development. Flexible, person-centred healthcare in this group of individuals will help to foster independence, promote engagement and empowerment and increase their confidence in self-management. The potential impact of AYA care may have significant benefits both in terms of the health of AYA with chronic RMDs and also health economics. Providing a good quality, well-resourced service for AYA is likely to reduce rates of non-attendance and the potential for AYA to become lost in the transition process, as well as improve patient adherence and outcomes [9, 25, 26, 27]. Through developmentally appropriate and youth-friendly effective communication, education and psychosocial support, the journey of AYA living with RMD can be transformed into one marked by resilience, knowledge and improved quality of life.

Key Management Points

1. Healthcare services should recognise AYA as a distinct patient group with unique and changing healthcare and psychosocial needs, and adapt healthcare interventions based on a biopsychosocial approach to clinical interactions.
2. AYA want a service that provides flexibility, the potential for peer support and developmentally appropriate information that acknowledges their lived experience and provides them with guidance to make their own healthcare-related choices.
3. Principles and criteria for developmentally appropriate and youth-friendly healthcare can be combined to provide health services that are meaningful and consistent from both the practitioner and AYA perspectives.

References

1. Ambresin AE, Bennett K, Patton GC, et al. Assessment of youth-friendly health care: a systematic review of indicators drawn from young people's perspective. J Adolesc Health. 2013;52(6):670–81.
2. World Health Organisation (WHO). Global standards for quality health care services for adolescents. 2015. http://www.who.int/maternal_child_adolescent/documents/global-standards-adolescent-care/en/. Accessed 22 Mar 2024.
3. Department of Health (DoH). 'You're Welcome': establishing youth-friendly health and care services. 2023. https://www.gov.uk/government/publications/quality-criteria-for-young-people-friendly-health-services. Accessed 22 Mar 2024.

4. Farre A, Wood V, Rapley T, et al. Developmentally appropriate healthcare for young people: a scoping study. Arch Dis Child. 2015;100(2):144–51.
5. Farre A, Wood V, McDonagh JE, et al. Health professionals' and managers' definitions of developmentally appropriate healthcare for young people: conceptual dimensions and embedded controversies. Arch Dis Child. 2016;101(7):628–33.
6. Wright EK, Williams J, Andrews JM, et al. Perspectives of paediatric and adult gastroenterologists on transfer and transition care of adolescents with inflammatory bowel disease. Intern Med J. 2014;44(5):490–6.
7. Farre A, McDonagh JE. Helping health services to meet the needs of young people with chronic conditions: towards a developmental model for transition. Healthcare. 2017;5(4):77–10.
8. McDonagh JE, Farre A. Are we there yet? An update on transitional care in rheumatology. Arthritis Res Ther. 2018;20(1):5.
9. Farre A, Lunt L, Lee R, et al. Addressing education and employment outcomes in the provision of healthcare for young people with physical long-term conditions: a systematic review and mixed methods synthesis. Patient Educ Couns. 2023;112:107765.
10. Farre A, Rapley T. The new old (and old new) medical model: four decades navigating the biomedical and psychosocial understandings of health and illness. Healthcare. 2017;5(4):88.
11. World Health Organisation (WHO). Towards adolescent-responsive health systems: steering the transition from adolescent-friendly projects to adolescent-responsive health systems. http://apps.who.int/adolescent/second-decade/section6/page8/adolescent-responsiveness.html. Accessed 22 Mar 2024.
12. Rapley T, Farre A, Parr JR, et al. Can we normalise developmentally appropriate health care for young people in UK hospital settings? An ethnographic study. BMJ Open. 2019;9(9):e029107.
13. Fay M, Lee MA. What young adults want from a young adult rheumatology service. Rheumatology. 2017;56(suppl_2):292.
14. McDonagh JE, Farre A, Gleeson H, et al. Making healthcare work for young people. Arch Dis Child. 2018;103(6):623.
15. Royal College of Physicians. Acute care toolkit 13: acute care for adolescents and young adults. https://www.rcplondon.ac.uk/guidelines-policy/acute-care-toolkit-13-acute-care-adolescents-and-young-adults. Accessed 22 Mar 2024.
16. Doukrou M, Segal TY. Fifteen-minute consultation: communicating with young people—how to use HEEADSSS a psychosocial interview for adolescents. Arch Dis Child Educ Pract Ed. 2018;103(1):15–9.
17. Young People's Health Special Interest Group (YPHSIG) of the Royal College of Paediatrics and Child Health. The YPHSIG App. https://www.yphsig.org.uk/resources-1/app. Accessed 22 Mar 2024.
18. Chadi N, Amaria K, Kaufman M. Expand your HEADS follow the THRxEADS! Paediatr Child Health. 2017;22(1):23–5.

19. Michaud PA, Schrier L, Ross-Russel R, et al. Paediatric departments need to improve residents' training in adolescent medicine and health: a position paper of the European Academy of Paediatrics. Eur J Pediatr. 2018;177(4):479–87.
20. Patton GC, Sawyer SM, Santelli JS, et al. Our future: a Lancet commission on adolescent health and wellbeing. Lancet. 2016;387(10036):2423–78.
21. National Institute for Health and Care Excellence (NICE). NICE guidelines [NG43] Transition from children's to adults' services for young people using health or social care services. 2016. https://www.nice.org.uk/guidance/ng43. Accessed 22 Mar 2024.
22. European Alliance of Associations for Rheumatology (EULAR) and Paediatric Rheumatology European Society (PRES). 11th EULAR/PRES online course in paediatric rheumatology. https://esor.eular.org/. Accessed 22 Mar 2024.
23. European Training in Effective Adolescent Care and Health (EuTEACH). https://www.unil.ch/euteach/en/home.html. Accessed 22 Mar 2024.
24. Health Education England (HEE) and eLearning for Healthcare (e-LFH). Adolescent health programme. https://www.e-lfh.org.uk/programmes/adolescent-health/. Accessed 22 Mar 2024.
25. Hart RI, McDonagh JE, Thompson B, et al. Being as normal as possible: how young people ages 16-25 years evaluate the risks and benefits of treatment for inflammatory arthritis. Arthritis Care Res (Hoboken). 2016;68(9):1288–94.
26. Tong A, Jones J, Craig JC, Singh-Grewal D. Children's experiences of living with juvenile idiopathic arthritis: a thematic synthesis of qualitative studies. Arthritis Care Res (Hoboken). 2012;64(9):1392–404.
27. Farre A, Ryan S, McNiven A, McDonagh J. The impact of arthritis on the educational and early work experiences of young people: a qualitative secondary analysis. Int J Adolesc Med Health. 2021;33(4):20180240.

Transitional Care 23

Lucy Gossens, Janine Hackett,
Hanaa Rajabally, and Judy Ammerlaan

Transitional Care for Young People

Living with a rheumatic disease is challenging at any age but particularly difficult for AYA with RMD since their chronic condition and treatment affects both physical and psychosocial development (see Chaps. 1, 2 and 3). Whilst treatment has improved in recent years, a cure for RMD remains elusive [1], and many AYA grow into adulthood with RMD. In the context of these challenges, a move from paediatric to adult healthcare becomes a significant and inevitable event.

L. Gossens (✉)
Amalia Childrens Hospital, Radboudumc, Nijmegen, The Netherlands
e-mail: lucy.gossens@radboudumc.nl

J. Hackett
Division of Occupational Therapy, Queen Margaret University, Edinburgh, Scotland, UK
e-mail: JHackett@qmu.ac.uk

H. Rajabally
University Hospital of North Durham, Durham, UK
e-mail: hanaa.rajabally@nhs.net

J. Ammerlaan
Department Rheumatology and Clinical Immunology, University Medical Centre Utrecht, Utrecht, The Netherlands
e-mail: J.Ammerlaan@umcutrecht.nl

C. Ciurtin, J. Hackett (eds.), *Adolescent and Young Adult Rheumatology In Clinical Practice*, In Clinical Practice,
https://doi.org/10.1007/978-3-031-82102-8_23

Transitional care is defined as 'the purposeful, planned process of transferring a young person's healthcare from a child-centred to an adult-orientated care setting that comprehensively addresses the medical, psychosocial, educational and vocational needs of that young person' [2].

Health transition, however, is just one facet of a wider set of educational, personal, family, and social transitions young people make during adolescence and young adulthood. Transitional care needs have been well described in the literature [3–6], alongside growing reports of how transition programmes can support a successful transition process for young people and their families [7, 8]. Barriers hindering the delivery of effective transitional care have been discussed for many years [9], however, remain an ongoing challenge. Barriers including lack of leadership and institutional support, narrow focus of care and inadequate support for young people to develop skills, insufficient parental involvement, and lack of training in adolescent health care, have all been highlighted in the recent UK National Confidential Enquiry into Patient Outcomes and Death [10].

Like all other adolescents growing up, young people with RMD need to develop their own identity and acquire skills for greater independence (see Chaps. 2 and 3), but in addition, have the added burden of becoming more responsible for the management of their health-related condition. From the perspective of AYA with RMD, there may also be daily challenges in relation to managing the consequences of having a chronic disease in the context of ongoing medical treatment and other issues such as pain and disability [11]. In this period of change, AYA also have to navigate the complexities of transferring from child-oriented services to adult care systems which can lead to a period of vulnerability.

A broad range of social and psychological factors have been found to impact on transfer readiness, [12], underscoring the need for holistic, person-centred assessment and developmentally appropriate interventions that are tailored to meet the diverse and unique needs of AYA [2, 13, 14]. To do this, effective AYA friendly communication is essential (see Chap. 4) as the perceptions and perspectives of healthcare providers and AYA can often reveal gaps between health care professional's goals and priorities, and those of young people. In Boxes 23.1 and 23.2, a health professional describes her own experience of this [13].

Box 23.1 Anne [1]: A Patient Story

The paediatrician introduced the next patient in the outpatient clinic as a "vulnerable young girl," with no friends and severe systemic juvenile arthritis. The door opened and there was Anne, a young girl of 17 years, sitting in a wheelchair. Her mother pushed the wheelchair into the consultation room. Her father came along too. He walked in with the coats and the bags of Anne and her mother, and in a second, the consultation room became filled: Anne, the paediatrician, the family, a wheelchair and me. The paediatrician started the consultation and asked: "How are you today, Anne?" Anne replied, quietly, as she looked at the ground, "good," whilst her father and mother looked worried. I looked at Anne's nose and lips displaying impressive piercings. I also noticed a bracelet on her arm with the name of a popular festival on it, a sign that Anne had been there. Mother took the floor and expressed her concerns. She had tried not to interfere with the medication regime and to leave it to Anne, as had been agreed in the last consultation, but it had not worked. Anne had not taken her medication and mother felt helpless. Father also took the floor: he was worried about Anne. She attended school but seemed to have no interest in her future. Discussions about this subject gave rise to a lot of stress, and for 2 weeks, father and daughter had not been on speaking terms, due to this situation. Anne gave her father the silent treatment. The paediatrician nodded understandably and tried to make eye contact with Anne. He cleared his throat and stressed the importance of taking the drugs and of focusing on the future. Anne nodded too and murmured that she understood what he was saying. The parents still looked worried. Anne looked at the ground.

(continued)

Box 23.2 Anne [2]: A Patient Story

Due to a technical problem with the computer, the paediatrician took Anne's parents to another room to discuss the X-rays of Anne's hands. Anne did not want to go. I asked her why she was not interested in her X-rays. From her point of view, she already knew the results: "ugly hands and painful hands." So, Anne and I stayed behind. It was suddenly strangely silent, and Anne sighed. I smiled at her; she smiled back. "You're a nurse, right?" she asked. I nodded, tears dripped from her eyes, and she squeezed her hands forcefully. "Can I ask you something?" she said. I gave her an encouraging nod and moved my chair closer to her wheelchair. "A few weeks ago, I had sex at a party and did not use condoms. I think I am pregnant." I nodded and swallowed. It became somewhat hotter in the consultation room.

Key Components of Transition

No model of transition has been proven to be more effective than others, nevertheless, there is growing consensus on the key components of the transitional care process [10, 15, 16]. The European League of Arthritis and Rheumatism (EULAR) provides standards and recommendations for transitional care of AYA with RMD, based on available evidence and opinions of both patients and multidisciplinary teams (MDTs) in paediatric and adult rheumatology [17]. Box 23.3 provides an overview of key components of transitional care [15–18].

Box 23.3 Key Components of Transitional Care [15–18]

(a) AYA with RMD should have access to high-quality, coordinated transitional care, based on individual need, delivered in partnership with healthcare professionals, young people, and their families.

(continued)

(b) The transition process should start as early as possible, in early adolescence (usually by age 12) or directly after diagnosis in adolescent-onset disease. The transition process begins within paediatric services, but continues into adult services and is therefore, by definition, a paediatric and adult concern.
(c) Transition should never be considered as the event of transfer between paediatrics and adult care, rather it must be considered as a developmentally appropriate process, addressing the psychosocial and educational/vocational aspects of care, in addition to the traditional medical areas. Transition services must be AYA focused and address the complexity of young adult development.
(d) There must be direct communication between all key stakeholders during the process of transition. Before and after transfer, there should be formalised contact between paediatric and adult rheumatology teams.
(e) Individual transitional plans should be developed with the AYA and his/her family/caregivers to optimise and facilitate each AYA towards self-management, and progress should be carefully documented in the medical records.
(f) Every rheumatology service and clinical network (paediatric and adult) must have a written, agreed and regularly updated transition policy. In the policy, there should be a clear written description of the multidisciplinary team (MDT) involvement in transitional care, locally and within the clinical network. The MDT should include a designated transition coordinator.
(g) Healthcare teams involved in transition and AYA care must have appropriate knowledge and skills to treat the individual, and holistically support the AYA, based on need. Healthcare teams therefore need continuing professional development in relation to adolescent health,

(continued)

developmentally appropriate care health, communication, and childhood-onset RMD.

(h) Secure funding for dedicated resources to provide uninterrupted clinical care and youth-friendly services for young people entering adult care, should be in place.

(i) Increased research is needed to improve evidence based knowledge and practice to improve outcomes for AYA with RMD.

Transitional Care in Practice

Transitional care is an integral part of developmentally appropriate care (see Chap. 22) and attends to the wider psychosocial aspects of the AYA's life [3]. It aims not only to equip young people with the skills, knowledge, and confidence to better manage their health condition, but to help young people thrive and promote participation in current and future life roles and activities. The process is similarly designed to support caregivers, as they too navigate this period, relinquishing some of their caregiving roles as the AYA gradually assumes more responsibility and increased levels of independence (see Chap. 5).

Transitional care is the responsibility of the whole team [17, 19] and must involve the AYA and their caregivers [10]. Crucially, it must reflect the individual's developmental level rather than chronological age. The transition process starts early, usually around the age of 11 or 12, which coincides with the transition to secondary school and is therefore perhaps easy to explain and initiate at this stage. The process remains ongoing until the age of approximately 25 years [17]. Transitional care is therefore a central pillar of practice for all those working with this age group. During this period, formal individualised transition plans are essential and are recommended by EULAR [17] and NCEPOD [10], as they provide a record of the identified needs of the AYA and caregiver and provide plans of how these will be met. They also chart progress and serve as a method of team communication and coordination of transitional care, which promotes consistency in follow up.

There are a number of transition plans available for use, all of which mirror the stages of adolescent development and reflect the multifaceted nature of the transition process. One example is the Ready, Steady, Go, (RSG) Hello, transition programme [20] which provides a suite of transition plan templates which are freely available and can be translated into a variety of languages. An early plan (Ready template) is initially used for those typically aged 11–14, with the practitioner introducing the concept of transition, outlining an overview of the differences between paediatric and adult care, and how over time the AYA will develop skills and assume greater responsibility for their health. During this period opportunities are also provided to slowly start increasing levels of independence and ensure participation in developmentally appropriate activities at home and at school. This plan is then replaced with a mid-transition plan (Steady template) around 14–16 years, which progressively builds on skills and is then followed by a late plan (Go template) typically around 16–18 years, where life post completion of compulsory education, becomes a key focus. Once the AYA moves to adult services, a 'Hello' template is initiated which welcomes them and addresses their ongoing transitional care needs until the age of 25. The transition plan templates outline several associated domains in relation to self-advocacy, skill and knowledge development, lifestyle and emotional wellbeing, self-care, leisure, and productive occupations, which include education and work, and finally, transfer to adult services. Largely based on previous iterations [9, 21], each plan reflects the ages and stages identified above, but notably the RSG templates omit self-management of pain, which is a significant feature of RMD for many, and thus an important skill to master. Importantly, the individual plans clearly outline actions required of team members to address issues, review progress, and intentionally create opportunities for the AYA to develop capabilities and practice skills.

Appropriate caregiver involvement is also important during this process as this can lead to better long-term outcomes for the AYA [2], therefore an individual transition plan for caregivers is also important to document their needs. Practitioners should spend time with caregivers, as they too require support and knowledge, particularly in relation to their specific role during this process [22], and how they can best support the AYA to gradually develop skills and assume new roles both at home and in the wider community.

During clinic visits AYA must be supported to develop skills and confidence to be seen alone, and once ready, an opportunity to practise these skills in communication and self-management. This also allows AYA to discuss any concerns they may have in a confidential environment, also affording the clinician the opportunity to assess adherence and risk-taking behaviours [23]. In addition, provision of teaching and learning opportunities which are developmentally appropriate and reflective of learning style including, information giving, workshops and skills-based sessions are also important and are key facilitators to a successful transition for AYA [6].

Attention must also be given to the AYA aspirations for the future and their own perceived participation and satisfaction in school/work and leisure activities. These are not only important components of transitional care but are also viewed as priority research areas by AYA and their caregivers [6]. Since education/work is central to the lives of AYA, addressing needs in the context of RMD is important within the healthcare setting [24]. Unfortunately, vocational readiness is often a neglected practice area and has been found to be addressed in only 50% of transition plans [23]. Recent evidence-based recommendations to address education and vocational needs in healthcare settings suggest that this can be done relatively easily with only minor adaptations to practice and includes signposting and liaison with teachers and employers [24].

Creating innovative opportunities for peer support can also be valuable [25] and might include group work, summer camps, signposting to third sector organisations or providing peer introductions in clinics.

Multidisciplinary Team

Team flexibility and creativity is key. Developmentally appropriate care for AYA, means acknowledging and responding to the challenges of living with a RMD at this important life stage, consequently, care should be responsive, convenient, and flexible enough to accommodate the busy academic priorities and work lives of AYA [24]. Similarly, to address the holistic and ever evolving needs throughout the transition process, different members of the rheumatology MDT will need to assume a variety of roles, however individual skills and preferences should be acknowledged. Coordination of the transition process is essential and an identified member of the MDT from any professional background should act as a Transition Coordinator. Their role is to be a link for the AYA and their family, ensure ongoing implementation of transitional care plans and help bridge the adult and paediatric divide to ensure a smooth and coordinated hand over of care and ultimate transfer [17, 23, 26]. Prior to transfer to adult services, joint clinics with paediatric and adult services are considered best practice [5, 10] and have been shown to improve outcomes and satisfaction at this potentially vulnerable time [2]. Meeting new adult care team members offers an opportunity for the AYA to gradually get to know their new care provider and orientate them to the new setting. This also allows adult colleagues an opportunity to meet the family, understand the AYA needs and address concerns, as well as offer continuity of care. Effective interaction with primary care practitioners and other professionals and institutions is also essential.

Figure 23.1 offers an overview and visual representation of the transitional care process. Although indicative ages are included, the plans must be developmentally appropriate and tailored to the AYA.

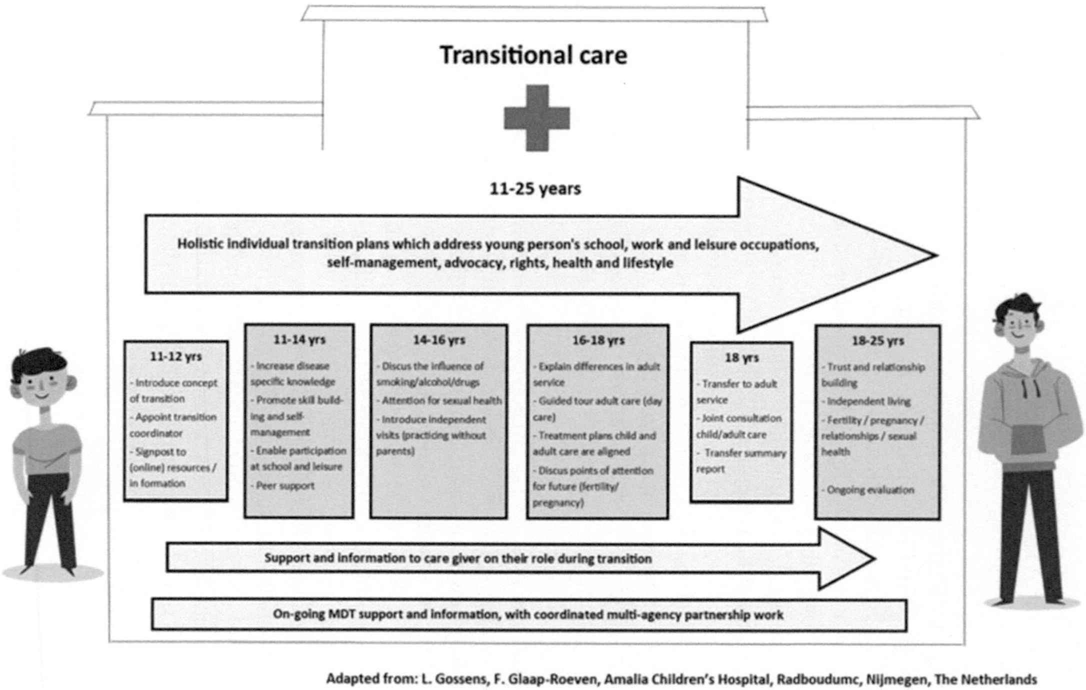

Fig. 23.1 Transitional care process in practice

Strategies for Implementing Transitional Care in Clinical Practice

Implementing new innovations and introducing new ways of working in practice seldom work immediately, particularly if they require complex changes in clinical practice, such as changes in organisation of care, interdisciplinary working, or changes in patient behaviour [27]. Since the introduction of transitional care requires complex changes in all these facets [17], an implementation strategy is key. In the absence of a universally accepted implementation strategy, the following steps are important, encouraging the active involvement of AYA in all steps [26].

- *Assessment and dissemination:* identify barriers and facilitators for implementation [8, 10]. Examples of these facilitators can be identifying key individuals, involving young people and families, agreed policy, written communication, training, and clarity of roles within teams [17]. All these interventions will require sufficient funding or reimbursement to implement transitional care as a standard part of healthcare practice [17].
- *Adoption:* all interested parties, including AYA, families, healthcare professionals and institutional managers, should develop and approve the transition policies, as equal partners [20, 23, 28] and they must be approved by hospital or institutional managers to facilitate appropriate resources to support the implementation within the clinical departments [17].
- *Implementation:* Multi-disciplinary adoption of a developmental practice framework [14], and a commitment to interdisciplinary and interagency working [19]. Motivation and flexibility within the healthcare team is also required to reorganise existing work practice and access available resources [23]. The multidisciplinary team also requires training in transitional and developmentally appropriate care [29] and capacity to fulfil the role of transition care coordinator [17].
- *Evaluation* of outcomes: Agreed indicators need to be established to evaluate the success of transitional care programmes.

An example of an implementation strategy of a transition outpatient clinic in the Netherlands [13] is outlined in Box 23.4.

Box 23.4 Implementation of a Transition Outpatient Clinic in the Netherlands

Health policy in the Netherlands directs young people to make the transition from child to adult care at the age of 18 years. In the University Medical Center Utrecht, up to 40 young people make this transition annually, moving from the children's department to the adult department, which are housed in different buildings. In the past, continuity of care was dependent on a summary of the disease history within the medical record of the AYA. Despite good intentions, communication between the children and adult team was poor, even though both teams were experiencing significant problems during the transition. These problems were mostly caused by mutual prejudices and high rates of treatment dropout and non-adherence to medical treatment Gradually, paediatricians and rheumatologists realised that their mutual mistrust and lack of communication and coordination interfered with optimal care. They concluded that sharing responsibility and working together on developing knowledge and supporting the AYA were needed.

To bridge the distance between the two departments and improve understanding and coordination between paediatricians and rheumatologist to better support parents and the young people towards adolescence, young people were invited to share their experiences on growing up with a rheumatic disease and to reflect on their experiences, needs and preferences for support from healthcare professionals. Two questions were posed: "What is the most important for you?" and "How would you like us to organise your treatment?"

The answers were honest, simple, and down to earth. *"Listen more and speak less," "I don't want to be an exception," "your recommendations should fit into my daily life,"*

(continued)

"information should meet my language" and *"I want to be prepared, and I want to be in charge."* The young people not only identified needs, but also shared solutions. These included; the use of the Internet as a contact point and to provide developmentally appropriate information, as well as the need for access to a professional whose main focus is "self-management and helping with the consequences of rheumatism in daily life." Based on the outcomes of the conversations with the young people, an outpatient transition clinic was developed where young people, and their parents/caregivers can meet their future rheumatologist at an early age and where a transition nurse guides and supports them during the transfer from child to adult care and self-management. To improve the AYA's knowledge and to meet the needs for information suitable for their language and preferences, an informative website with written and video information was developed [30]. To encourage active involvement and increased feelings of control, a web-based portal with access to the personal medical record, self-monitoring and eConsult functionalities was also developed. Young people who used these eHealth tools expressed their needs for a training programme, where they could practise self-management skills. To meet these needs, two versions of a self-management training programme were developed: a face-to-face and a web-based version both led by young people.

A UK Adult Rheumatologist shares her experience of implementing transition care in practice in Box 23.5.

Box 23.5 A UK Adult Rheumatologist Reflects on Her Experience of Transitional Care

Working with young people aged between 16 and 18 years gave me a fresh perspective on aspects of rheumatology

(continued)

care, which I had previously taken for granted. I had to develop my communication skills, find creative solutions when young people declined procedures or treatments and explore their reasons for doing so. I had to tailor management plans around their education to suit their specific needs to promote engagement in healthcare.

It is rewarding to be involved in the medical care of young people, and it helped me grow as a Rheumatology Consultant as I fine-tuned my skills to develop a person-centred approach to transitional care.

The adult Rheumatology Higher Specialist Training I received in the UK did not give me much experience in Transitional Care. Therefore, I had to seek out additional training opportunities by networking with colleagues who are already experts in the field. I would strongly encourage doctors who wish to work in this area to join local and national networks, like the Barbara Ansell National Network for Adolescent Rheumatology (BANNAR) in the UK, where they can access clinical resources, promote best practice, share advice, and gain support from more experienced colleagues. It is important to be mindful of one's training needs and show commitment in building skills and knowledge to be able to deliver evidence-based care.

I found attending Paediatric Rheumatology clinics helped me build relationships and trust with paediatric colleagues as well as the AYA and their family and learn about their journey. Receiving comprehensive MDT transfer summaries and having meetings with the Paediatric Rheumatology team is also helpful in identifying key issues that require ongoing attention as they transition into adult services.

The major challenge for transitional care remains lack of resources in adult services in terms of time allocated per patient in clinic, availability of AYA-friendly infrastructure, support of Specialist Nurses and ease of access to Allied Health Professionals. Age banded clinics might prove use-

(continued)

ful and provide a relatively easy way of offering young people opportunities for peer networking and informal support.

On a personal level, I found it difficult to promote independence for the AYA while still allowing caregiver involvement. To overcome these challenges, it is important to seek ongoing constructive feedback from AYA and their caregivers and show a positive attitude to promote change where needed. In terms of my vision for the future of Transition Care, acknowledging resource constraints, and the need to optimise outcomes, I am very enthusiastic about the use of technology in enhancing the standard of Transitional Care and hopeful that digital tools such as websites with built-in educational videos, smartphone apps and chatbots may be developed in collaboration with young people and their caregivers to achieve this. A number of resources and academic papers are available on this topic (see further reading).

Transitional care is an emerging area of Rheumatology, and it is an exciting and meaningful time for those interested in working in this field as there are lots of opportunities for professional growth, service development and creation of resources to make a lasting positive impact on young people.

In this chapter we have briefly outlined key components of transitional care within a practice setting, however, we acknowledge varied factors will influence local service delivery [23]. Importantly, implementation of transitional care needs commitment, leadership, flexibility, and teamwork.

Transitional care is an integral part of developmentally appropriate care which must include efforts to give voice and include young people in their own care, as well as involve them in service design, policy development and research if we are truly committed to improving outcomes for young people with RMD.

Key Management Points

1. Transitional care is an AYA-centred developmentally appropriate approach to care which attends not only to medical needs and eventual transfer to adult services, but addresses wider holistic needs to support young people's health, well-being and participation.
2. Transitional care is a key element of practice when working with young people aged between 12 and 25. It is responsive to the ever-changing needs of the AYA and begins in early adolescence and continues into young adulthood.
3. Transitional care is multi-dimensional and involves a team approach including members of the paediatric and adult rheumatology teams, caregivers and professionals in the wider community.

References

1. Bridges JM, Mellins ED, Cron RQ. Recent progress in the treatment of non-systemic juvenile idiopathic arthritis. Fac Rev. 2021;10:23. https://doi.org/10.12703/r/10-23. PMID: 33718940; PMCID: PMC7946384.
2. Colver A, Rapley T, Parr JR, McConachie H, Dovey-Pearce G, Couteur AL, McDonagh JE, Bennett C, Maniatopoulos G, Pearce MS, Reape D, Chater N, Gleeson H, Vale L. Facilitating transition of young people with long-term health conditions from children's to adults' healthcare services—implications of a 5-year research programme. Clin Med (Lond). 2020;20(1):74–80. https://doi.org/10.7861/clinmed.2019-0077. PMID: 31941736; PMCID: PMC6964170.
3. McDonagh JE, Farre A. Transitional care in rheumatology: a review of the literature from the past 5 years. Curr Rheumatol Rep. 2019;21(10):57.
4. Kelly A, Niddrie F, Tunnicliffe DJ, Matus Gonzalez A, Hanson C, Jiang I, Major G, Singh-Grewal D, Tymms K, Tong A. Patients' attitudes and experiences of transition from paediatric to adult healthcare in rheumatology: a qualitative systematic review. Rheumatology (Oxford). 2020;59(12):3737–50. https://doi.org/10.1093/rheumatology/keaa168. PMID: 32413124.

5. Jiang I, Major G, Singh-Grewal D, et al. Patient and parent perspectives on transition from paediatric to adult healthcare in rheumatic diseases: an interview study. BMJ Open. 2021;11:e039670.
6. Bitencourt N, Lawson E, Bridges J, Carandang K, Chintagunta E, Chiraseveenuprapund P, DeQuattro K, Goh YI, Lee TC, Moore KF, Peterson RG, Roberts JE, Ronis T, Sadun RE, Smitherman EA, Stringer E, White PH, Chang JC, Childhood Arthritis and Rheumatology Research Alliance (CARRA) Transition Workgroup. Pediatric to adult transition literature: scoping review and rheumatology research prioritization survey results. J Rheumatol. 2022;49(11):1201–13.
7. García-Rodríguez F, Raygoza-Cortez K, Moreno-Hernandez L, García-Pérez R, Garza Lopez LE, Arana-Guajardo AC, Jáquez-Quintana JO, Villarreal-Treviño AV, de la O-Cavazos ME, Rubio-Pérez N. Outcomes of transitional care programs on adolescent chronic inflammatory systemic diseases: systematic review and meta-analyses. Pediatr Rheumatol Online J. 2022;20(1):15. https://doi.org/10.1186/s12969-022-00670-1.
8. Şahin N, Sönmez HE, Aktay Ayaz N, Sözeri B. Addressing the unmet needs of transitional care in juvenile idiopathic arthritis. Rheumatology (Oxford). 2024;63(3):619–29.
9. McDonagh JE, Southwood TR, Shaw KL. Growing up and moving on in rheumatology: development and preliminary evaluation of a transitional care programme for a multicentre cohort of adolescents with juvenile idiopathic arthritis. J Child Health Care. 2006;10(1):22–42. https://doi.org/10.1177/1367493506060203.
10. The national confidential enquiry into patient outcome and death. 'The Inbetweeners' 2023. London. https://www.ncepod.org.uk/2023transition/The%20Inbetweeners_summary%20report.pdf.
11. Sattoe JNT, van Staa AL, Hilberink SR, editors. Self-management of young people with chronic conditions. A strength-based approach for empowerment and support. Cham: Springer Nature Switzerland AG; 2021.
12. Howsley P, Dunkley L, Calvert R, Hawley S, Tattersall R, McMahon A-M, Hawley D. Psychological/social factors associated with transfer readiness in young people with juvenile idiopathic arthritis. Clin Rheumatol. 2022;41(12):3777–82. https://doi.org/10.1007/s10067-022-06237-5.
13. Ammerlaan JW, van Os-Medendorp H, de Boer-Nijhof NC, Prakken B, Bijlsma JWJ, Kruize AA. The most important needs and preferences of patients for support from health care professionals: a reflective practice on (transitional) care for young adults with Juvenile Idiopathic Arthritis. Patient Educ Couns. 2017;100(10):1961–4.
14. Farre A, McDonagh JE. Helping health services to meet the needs of young people with chronic conditions: towards a developmental model for transition. Healthcare (Basel). 2017;5(4):77. pii: E77

15. Suris JC, Akre C. Key elements for, and indicators of, a successful transition: an international Delphi study. J Adolesc Health. 2015;56(6):612–8.
16. Sattoe JNT, Hilberink SR, van Staa A. How to define successful transition? An exploration of consensus indicators and outcomes in young adults with chronic conditions. Child Care Health Dev. 2017;43(5):768–73.
17. Foster HE, Minden K, Clemente D, Leon L, McDonagh JE, Kamphuis S, et al. EULAR/PReS standards and recommendations for the transitional care of young people with juvenile-onset rheumatic diseases. Ann Rheum Dis. 2017;76(4):639–46.
18. Nederlandse Vereniging Kindergeneeskunde. Kwaliteitsstandaard—Jongeren in transitie van kinderzorg naar volwassenenzorg. 2022. https://richtlijnendatabase.nl/richtlijn/kwaliteitsstandaard_-_jongeren_in_transitie_van_kinderzorg_naar_volwassenenzorg/startpagina_-_jongeren_in_transitie_van_kinderzorg_naar_volwassenenzorg.html.
19. Farre A, Wood V, McDonagh JE, Parr JR, Reape D, Rapley T, Transition Collaborative Group. Health professionals' and managers' definitions of developmentally appropriate healthcare for young people: conceptual dimensions and embedded controversies. Arch Dis Child. 2016;101(7):628–33. https://doi.org/10.1136/archdischild-2015-309473. Epub 2016 Mar 4.
20. Nagra A, McGinnity PM, Davis N, Salmon AP. Implementing transition: ready steady go. Arch Dis Child Educ Pract Ed. 2015;100(6):313–20. https://doi.org/10.1136/archdischild-2014-307423.
21. McDonagh JE, Hackett J, McGee M, Southwood T, Shaw KL. The evidence base for transition is bigger than you might think. Archiv Dis Childhood Educ Pract. 2015;100(6):321–2. https://doi.org/10.1136/archdischild-2015-309204.
22. Heath G, Farre A, Shaw K. Parenting a child with chronic illness as they transition into adulthood: a systematic review and thematic synthesis of parents' experiences. Patient Educ Couns. 2017;100(1):76–92. https://doi.org/10.1016/j.pec.2016.08.011. Epub 2016 Aug 16. PMID: 27693084.
23. Clemente D, Leon L, Foster H, et al. Transitional care for rheumatic conditions in Europe: current clinical practice and available resources. Pediatr Rheumatol. 2017;15:49. https://doi.org/10.1186/s12969-017-0179-8.
24. Farre A, Lunt L, Lee R, Verstappen S, McDonagh JE. Addressing education and employment outcomes in the provision of healthcare for young people with physical long-term conditions: a systematic review and mixed methods synthesis. Patient Educ Couns. 2023;112:107765. https://doi.org/10.1016/j.pec.2023.107765. Epub 2023 Apr 17.
25. Zimmerman C, Garland BH, Enzler CJ, Hergenroeder AC, Wiemann CM. The roles of quality of life and family and peer support in feelings about transition to adult care in adolescents with gastroenterology, renal, and rheumatology diseases. J Pediatr Nurs. 2022;62:193–9.

26. Ammerlaan JW, Scholtus LW, Bijlsma HJ, Prakken BJ, Kruize AA. An urge for change: transitional care for young adults with juvenile idiopathic arthritis. Patient Educ Couns. 2013;92(1):127–9.
27. Wenger M, Grol R, Grimshaw JM, editors. Improving patient care: the importance of change in health care. 3rd ed. Hoboken: Wiley Blackwell; 2020.
28. Jensen PT, Karnes J, Jones K, Lehman A, Rennebohm R, Higgins GC, et al. Quantitative evaluation of a pediatric rheumatology transition program. Pediatr Rheumatol Online J. 2015;13:17–015-0013-0.
29. Rapley T, Farre A, Parr JR, Wood VJ, Reape D, Dovey-Pearce G, McDonagh J, Transition Collaborative Group. Can we normalise developmentally appropriate health care for young people in UK hospital settings? An ethnographic study. BMJ Open. 2019;9(9):e029107. https://doi.org/10.1136/bmjopen-2019-029107.
30. Ammerlaan J, Os-Medendorp H, Scholtus L, Vos de A, Zwier M, Bijlsma H, et al. Feasibility of an online and a face-to-face version of a self-management program for young adults with a rheumatic disease; experiences of young adults and peer leaders. Pediatr Rheumatol Online. 2014;25(12):10. https://doi.org/10.1186/1546-0096-12-10.

Further Reading on Use of Technology

Butalia S, Crawford SG, McGuire KA, et al. Improved transition to adult care in youth with type 1 diabetes: a pragmatic clinical trial. Diabetologia. 2021;64(4):758–66. https://doi.org/10.1007/s00125-020-05368-1.

Husted GR, Weis J, Teilmann G, et al. Exploring the influence of a smartphone app (young with diabetes) on young people's self-management: qualitative study. JMIR Mhealth Uhealth. 2018;6(2):e43.

Lopez KN, O'Connor M, King J, et al. Improving transitions of care for young adults with congenital heart disease: mobile app development using formative research. JMIR Format Res. 2018;2(2):e16. https://doi.org/10.2196/formative.9963. Epub 2018 Jan 29. PMID: 30574573; PMCID: PMC6298756.

Xu L, Sanders L, Li K, Chow J. Chatbot for health care and oncology applications using artificial intelligence and machine learning: systematic review. JMIR Cancer. 2021;7(4):e27850. https://doi.org/10.2196/27850.

Resources

CanChild. My transition App. https://www.canchild.ca/en/research-in-practice/current-studies/apply-the-mytransition-app-in-transition-applyit-study/mytransition-app.

Royal college or paediatrics and child health. Health transition resources. https://www.rcpch.ac.uk/resources/health-transition-resources.

Transition and Patient Empowerment, Innovation Education and Research (TIER). Ready steady go programme. https://www.readysteadygo.net/home.html.

Index

C. Ciurtin, J. Hackett (eds.), *Adolescent and Young Adult Rheumatology In Clinical Practice*, In Clinical Practice,
https://doi.org/10.1007/978-3-031-82102-8

MIX
Papier aus verantwortungsvollen Quellen
Paper from responsible sources
FSC® C105338

If you have any concerns about our products,
you can contact us on
ProductSafety@springernature.com

In case Publisher is established outside the EU,
the EU authorized representative is:
Springer Nature Customer Service Center GmbH
Europaplatz 3, 69115 Heidelberg, Germany

Printed by Libri Plureos GmbH
in Hamburg, Germany